"Once again, Dianea provides us with a book that emanates incredible openness and liberating truth. Readers cannot help but be mesmerized by her life journey toward self- reclamation, personal experiences and perennial inquiry into the healing power of tears is commendable. Dianea's own quest will encourage others to dare to venture toward reclaiming that vulnerability rightfully theirs – inner peace of the heart, mind, body and soul.
   — *Jodi J. DeLuca, Phd, Psychologist, Neuroscientist*

"*Evolution of an Orgasm* invites us to re-examine the way in which we relate to our own orgasm. Brilliantly honest and forthright, Dianea once again challenges our awareness in places sacred, and rarely explored, yet often visited. It is truly an evolution."
   — *Kathleen P. Kelly Ciavolella, MA, Interdisciplinary Scholar*

"*EVOLution of an Orgasm* is one of the most important books currently available in the emerging Spirituality-Sexuality arena. Dianea weaves accounts of her own profound erotic experiences with her expansive knowledge of emotional release therapy and her deep spiritual insights into the power of orgasm. Having read *Evolution of an Orgasm*, I will never again experience my own sexual ecstasy – or that of my partner— as an explosion of pleasure resulting in carnal satisfaction, but as a channel to the Divine. Love.
   — *T. Morrow Fairchild, management consultant*

"Crying makes me happy"

— *Muhammad Arif, Computer specialist,*
Cornell University, former client

EVOLution
of an
Orgasm

Dianea Kohl

Chelan Publishing, Ithaca, New York

Special appreciation to George Foster,
for the awesome cover design,
And to my friend Adriana Rovers
for the colorful author photo.

For Gregory,
Once soulmate, and essential catalyst
For opening my heart to a profound Love
I had not known possible.

I, Dianea, have a dream,
that someday, tears will be as easy as laughter
then truly, they will be tears of joy.

"When the shell of my heart breaks open, tears shall pour forth
and they shall be called the **pearls of god**."
— Rumi, 13th century poet

"It's so simple, I remind myself: **Just sit down and have a good cry.**
Just stay with the feeling, including the fear;
including the aversion to the fear,
including the judgment that I'm a coward;
including the actual sensation in the chest, in the belly;
including the sadness.
By staying with the feeling, I'm actually, genuinely loving myself.
The feeling is naked.
It doesn't need to wear a story, though I have a closet full of stories.
The feeling wants to be naked, to feel its own skin.
The feeling is more alive than the stories.
The feeling is the healing.
When I stay with the feeling, **I feel god's presence** –
not as an abstraction, but here in this flesh,
in this shame that <u>tears</u> wash away."
—*Sy Safransky, editor of the SUN magazine*

"When you cry, your tears are always for yourself."
—*Elizabeth Kubler-Ross, M.D.*

"The soul would have no rainbow if the eyes had no tears."
—*Native American proverb*

"Grief is not a problem to be cured,
it is only a statement that you have loved someone."
— *author unknown*

Appreciations

So many appreciations, how do I count them all? Where do I begin?

With my parents, without whose sexual bodies I would not have been conceived. Yet, more importantly, is my non-biological dad, Michel Colbert, who got down on his knees to ask my mother to marry him, when she was in Tarrytown, New York considering putting me up for adoption. He not only wanted me, he loved me very much, as much as his two biological children, my younger brother and sister. He was a gift through many lifetimes for me.

Next are my daughters, Erin and Megan, who as children are my guiding light into what love is meant to be. As are my granddaughters, Denali and Riley Shea.

My best friend, Susanne Ottander, has been in my heart for twenty years, and by my side since 1998 when she joined me in weekly crying-therapy sessions, to support each other on this most remarkable healing by tears journey. Tanya Konefal, my other best friend, is also a constant source of shared love.

The men whom I have loved and been loved by are in the story of this book. I still give them love and find ongoing friendship because real love does not die. I must give special acknowledgement to Johnny, who is exposed most vulnerably and with whom I was most vulnerable with my tears at orgasm.

Also, many thanks and love to my clients with whom I learn while I support them on their healing paths. Thanks especially to Moe Arif for his computer support, whereby this book and others would not have been completed.

Those who have read parts of my manuscript and endorsed my book: Jodi DeLuca, Kathleen Kelly Ciavolella, and T. Morrow Fairchild, you are courageous souls. Thank you from the welcoming of my heart.

Then, my steady editors, George Mermagen, and Kristie Snyder. You have made my writing clearer than this novice writer could ever have known.

Finally, all the authors before me that have contributed to our Human Being awakening to Real Love, many mentioned in the recommended reading list. Arthur Janov being my primary mentor, author of the *Primal Scream*, and many other books thereafter.

Contents

Preface

Another book on Love? What can I say that is new? Can I direct people to LOVE better? Isn't Love what our spirit thrives on? Isn't love the greatest or highest reason for being sexual? God is Love, right?

I am the annoying child who is always asking questions until the exasperated parent ends up saying, "I don't know…guess you'll have to ask 'god'."

But where and who is god? The religions of the world seem to think they know. Yet, literally, they fight over which way to god. Witness the Crusades, "Holy War," and the tragedy of the World Trade Center on September 11. Religion doesn't seem to know how to manifest the loving spirit, which many are now referring to as "spirituality."

Matthew Fox, the well-known author and ex-Roman Catholic priest, aptly defines the difference between religion and spirituality: "Spirituality is about *experience*, while religion, unfortunately ends up being about the *organization* of the experience… Spirituality is connecting with the source of creativity, justice and compassion." I would add Love, which encompasses those three.

Because I was raised in a strict religious family and church - I know I can write about my spirit becoming free of the oppression of religion. I FEEL the difference between spiritual and religious. I have cried floods of tears about Sunday School robbing me of my innocence, bible teachers instructing me as a preschooler that I was a sinner, born in sin, and unworthy of god's love! And I am a more genuinely loving person (not obligated to love) <u>because</u> of the tears, and their healing power. This book will tell how this power transformed me.

It is my healing into real Love that my brother noticed when he said (in 2002) with amazement, "I have to give you a lot of credit for taking care of the mother who abused you." And I truly do not feel resentment toward her, like my religious sister does. Yes, in the past I resented my mother too. And no, I did not wish or think my resentment away. Instead, I raged and cried my pain away, like a storm that leaves a brilliant rainbow in its (a)wake.

"The soul would have no rainbow, if the eyes had no tears," - Native American saying.

My life as a psychotherapist has privileged me with a spiritual journey into my heart where my soul-spirit resides. During my marriage to Gregory, I found myself triggered into childhood pain, the depth of which this "self-aware professional" had not known. I sobbed and threw temper tantrums like a two-year old. Since 1993, I have learned to let myself cry deeply and to access the deepest emotions through my tears, and sexual climax. I have learned not to suppress or run

i

away from my tears, my agony, *or* my ecstasy. As a result, I have become more sensitive to my spirit, which has made me more loving and less judgmental. Now compassion comes easily to me – for the killer as well as for the victim. This book shows how this happened for me and how it can happen for others.

My compassion and passion is unleashed by true stories like Billy Crowley's. In 1997 Billy killed his grandfather who had beaten him and his sister and his wife all of Billy's 20 years. His grandfather had threatened to come after Billy if he tried to run away. He lived in great fear. The extended family and others living in their small Georgia town were aware of the abuse. No one stopped it. It was observed that the jury exercised compassion by convicting Billy of manslaughter instead of murder. They sentenced him to five years in prison. But, in addition, he received a *life sentence*, because after he killed his grandfather, he took the $400 dollars from his wallet to pay bills. The judge's decision was upheld even though the jury wrote to him, protesting that the sentence was unjust. Not enough Love to render justice. Outrageous!

Why did I digress to this example of injustice? It is my belief, building on Matthew Fox's "spirituality connects us with the source of justice," that injustice happens because most people are not wholly connected to their own spirits. Spirits, that are hiding in the emotional pain of their childhood. They are not free to cry, to grieve. They can't FEEL the experience of the people who commit crimes. All they can bring to bear is the structure and organization of the law, which leads them to revenge. I'm not condoning taking another's life. But I am protesting, for cases like those of Billy Crowley, the court's sin of omission by not taking into account the pain of Billy's experience that drove him to act violently. No one ever held the grandfather accountable for a lifetime of murder, murder of that child's spirit.

It is my objective in **Evolution of an Orgasm** to illuminate how injustice is done to our spirits when it carries shame of our sexuality.

We continue to be astounded by stories about "quiet" or "excelling" students who turn to killing either themselves or others. I know some clients like this through my psychotherapy practice. Just this week, Michael, a soft spoken thirty-three year old, recently married and expecting a baby, tells me that if someone would start a physical fight with him, he'd "kill him." In the same session he began to connect with the rage he has toward his father who beat him on several occasions when Michael was a child. The abuse was so obvious that a social worker from the school came to their home to investigate. Michael's father denied the allegations although bruises on Michael's back had been seen by his teachers. His mother was too afraid to tell the truth. After the social worker left, Michael's father told him, "*This* is abuse," and proceeded to hit Michael in the head where bruises could not be detected. Michael is a well-respected and admired teacher of high school physics, as well as a coach for several sports. And he is seething inside with unexpressed *and* therefore unresolved rage.

Stories like Michael's, characterized by physical, emotional and sexual abuse and their denial, abound. The same denial surrounds abusive religious indoctrination, which in reality is brainwashing of children, most apparent with the recent rule by the Muslim Taliban in Afghanistan. The brainwashing is subtle in examples like christian missionaries stripping Native Americans of their Great Spirit beliefs, which create a spirituality of respect of all of creation. Or in the fundamentalist christian religion where I, as a small, vulnerable child, was persuaded to believe in my own basic sinfulness and to deny my essential goodness. *Including* the essential goodness of my sexuality. And what choice did my parents give me but to believe these doctrines? None really. Because every child is afraid to be rejected, or unloved by their parents.

Victor Frankl, author of the international classic, *Man's Search for Meaning*, says it better than I. "**To be truly human is to be spiritual.**" In German, Frankl's native language, the words Geist (mind,spirit), Seele (soul), and geistig (intellectual, spiritual) do not mean anything religious…Longing for life to make sense, yearning after something really worth living for, is no sign of psychological disorder. Rather, it reveals the human spirit in its most authentic and honest hours, for when we have reason for peace or a good conscience, we no longer worry about them. It is not really happiness that we want, but something to be happy about," (*When Life Calls Out To Us*, by Klingberg, pg.8) **Like Love.** Every human thirsts for Love.

It is apparent that we are evolving to a greater consciousness of what it means to be truly human. Repression of our feelings has caused great pain to our **spirits**, and is many times visited onto the next generation of children until we find trust enough to expose what is happening behind closed doors. This repression includes the repression of our **sexual** feelings. Thus, the intimate connection between spirituality with sexuality. If we cannot freely express our "whole" selves - including our sexual selves - our spirits cannot be fully free. And if our spirits cannot be free, neither can we be free to be fully human and to Love. If we cannot Love, we cannot be at Peace - - individually or collectively. And stories like that of Billy, and Michael, and September 11, and Afghanistan, will continue to unfold.

But this is a book about love and sexuality and *orgasm*. In my first book, *TEARS ARE TRUTH…waiting to be spoken*, I showed how by giving ourselves permission to cry deeply, we provide ourselves access to a wellspring of healing and love. This book will show how sexual behavior acts out the repressed pain of the past, therefore limiting our spirit's ability to Love.

My purpose in writing *Evolution of an Orgasm…a coming to* **Love's*** call through the spirit of sexuality… is to help us improve our ability to integrate our spirit(uality) with our sex(uality.) Simply stated, to not just have sex, but to truly make Love. More fully. I demonstrate through graphic details of my sexual life how I have acted out my emotional pain through sex, (as I believe we all do) and therefore have limited my ability to have fuller more intense orgasms. More Love. Further, I show how orgasmic release, when fully and intensely experienced, can lead to deeper and more authentic Love – of one's Self and of others.

One interesting note that affirms the premise of this book: is the biological evolution of increasing numbers of animals to monogamy (or serial monogamy) as they progress in physiological complexity. (The California mouse is truly sexually faithful and 3-10% of mammals are socially monogamous.) My journey will demonstrate the function of monogamy as a facilitator in learning how to deeply love.

I hope my vulnerability will inspire others to take this rolling ride on the river of tears, (an ultimate experience is being able to cry at orgasm) to the rambunctious liberation of LOVE. To the ecstasy of an expanding orgasm of LOVE. Connecting the divine spirit within us all!

* Today, I'm musing with pleasure, that I just happened to be reading the page in Victor Frankl's biography which states, "Victor owed many pinnacles of insight to Scheler, and these 'aha' experiences of discovery he later called '**spiritual orgasms**,'" (*When Life Calls Out To Us*, pg.53). I'd never read this expression before now.

Introduction

"MAKING LOVE" – what an enthusiastic statement about evolution. Listen to the words we choose to express ourselves, which we so easily take for granted.

Like the first four letters of evolution – spell them backwards. EVOL = LOVE! So we are in a constant and certain evolving journey, learning to "make love."

As I stated in the Preface, I will describe in detail my own sexual journey that continues to integrate my body with soul-spirit.

In June of 2002, I met Johnny at a tango workshop. His deep brown eyes met my gray blue eyes in the dance studio's mirror. We began making love at that moment. I wasn't sure I'd fall in love with him, or even if he was available – although my heart intuited so. It was a month later that the clouds of life's activities lifted enough to present Johnny at my door.

We spent our first hours together hiking through forests, streams and waterfalls. Johnny told me that he wanted to walk our relationship in slow steps. He wanted to be able to be alone with himself, to be less dependent on commitments to women, having been married three times by age 48.

I was to be surprised by him over and over again. At the foot of Lucifer Falls, he wanted to undress so we could get closer, a better view. Of what? He called himself a nudist, an illustrator, drawer of human figures for years.

"Are you sure you want to do this?" I asked with trepidation. I say I am unashamed of my body, after forty years of being so – here was the test. I had emailed Johnny for four weeks; I trusted him. We were taking slow deliberate steps of spontaneity. The clouds laid low in the sky, and Johnny picked me up in his arms, carrying me through six steps of deeper spring-cold clear water.

It had been over a year since I had been with a man whose hand I wanted to take. It was as easy as birds flying through clouds to walk hand in hand with Johnny for the two miles leading us to this grand waterfall. We sat with a comfortable foot of black table rock between our nakedness.

We "made" long gazes reflecting blue and brown cloudy eyes between our words. Eye contact as steady as mountains, as new-found as the last decade's tears that have created openness of a new dimension.

I had always thought I had good eye contact with everyone, especially since 1985 when, while married to my second husband, I graduated with a Masters degree in Marriage and Family Therapy. But I had really just looked at others' faces, with fleeting eye connection. It wasn't until my fourth husband, Gregory, who became the catalyst to profound inner love only known to me through tears, that I would allow myself to cry at orgasm. That was eye -"I"- contact.

Back to Johnny, who gave me a greater surprise than any man had ever given me. (A greater surprise than non-sexual nudity on our first date.) It was like a gift my father might wrap for me. Dad would use extraordinary care to fold the corners of the wrapping paper, fitting them as tight as a rubber band. The bow would be tied and taped precisely in its place of design. Very special, like his love is for me.

As was my first date with Johnny, who readily offered to read some of his poems to me. Somewhere in our conversation about the subject of this book concerning the integration of sexuality with spirituality, and my previous book about the healing power of tears, Johnny said, "I'd like to cry at orgasm."

I had not mentioned to him how that is a special moment of healing for me. I felt excited and surprised by the first man to ever express that wish to me. Pure as the white of a sunshine cloud, tasting like wildflower honey.

My eyes widened in harmony with my smile. My heart beat louder. I began to "make love" with Johnny with my feelings. There is the possibility to have masculine meet feminine with a spiritual connection that goes beyond the body's sexual energy. Beyond what is known as "falling in love," although I believe that is an important part of "making love." The phrase "I love you" will take on deeper meaning, like a rainbow that is seen as double.

These concepts are demonstrated and explored throughout this book, with details describing my whole life's sexual journey, with the greatest emphasis being on the last decade of my life, when I began to cry at orgasm.

You will read how crying at orgasm essentially came after I was triggered to cry in daily interactions with Gregory, and then learned to connect those tears with repressed childhood pain. This deeply spiritual connection with my child-heart allowed me to trust my Self in a NEW DEEP way. I became open to my vulnerable f(t)ears. I could let go of control of my feelings more often, revealing my pure being – like innocent babies, who give love readily. Just look into their eyes! They are steady and ready to (make) love.

Most people who are in recovery, "making" themselves healthier, readily admit that they act out their past hurts: pain from growing up in a world inadequate to love fully or unconditionally. Our emotional pain is like a storm cloud waiting to let go of its tears.

Our pure loving spirits are crushed and hiding due to emotional, physical, and sexual abuses. The act outs resulting from these abuses range from overeating, alcoholism, smoking, and compulsive sex to shopaholism - and the list goes on and on. My act-out-isms were mainly religion, sex and running. (I talked too much too☺)

Dear reader, if you would like a more tender, fully present with feeling, expansive way of "making love" that connects your true spirit with another and simultaneously with your true Self and the Design of the Universe… come orgasm with me. *Spirituality* is finally connecting with what we were born with: an innocent and pure spirit full of love. *Sexuality* is the physical play where we can stop acting – fully let go - in orgasm. When they or we "come" together, we are fully spirit. LOVE.

I wish to conclude by saying that I hope the reader will be inspired by my true love story. That your fears will diminish as you let go of more tears. That your tears at orgasm will ignite the special light and love that burns when you unite with your Beloved within and without.

part one

◊

EVOLution of an Orgasm as Waking Up

The SEASON of WINTER...1969–1993

"Oh my God, you're in me!" rolls from my lips loud and clear, from a deep place in my chest, being by myself as I orgasm. It is an intensity that has climaxed after beginning its climb during lovemaking with Rosey the previous night. For a second, I thought about him being inside me, his muscular arms and lats embracing me. Simultaneously I thought, "God is in me." It's April 1999.

This was not the first time I've masturbated and connected with similar insights. How did this all begin?

I cannot remember my first orgasm with my first husband, Chuck, or even our wedding night's first intercourse. I was a virgin, 22, looking forward to being free of my religion's restraint: "thou shalt not have premarital sex." It was more than a restraint; it was a law, which when broken, brought you to the brink of hell. Or to the adoption of the "not nice girl" label.

I remember Chuck singing "Ich Liebe Dich" in his melodious first tenor voice that sprung tears from my eyes, while standing in my satiny wedding gown in front of the Tabernacle Baptist church's ugly gray pews. Our first married night together was spent at the Red Lion Inn, in Binghamton, New York. I am surprised that I did not, or we did not attack each other sexually like Siamese cats in heat. Where was the desire? Gone, because intercourse was no longer forbidden? It was May 1969.

We listened to the small tape recorder reiterate our wedding ceremony. Chuck's solo stood out: was I tearful? I do not remember. I am sad and disappointed now that these past feelings of our wedding night are so elusive. Not just the feelings about making love, but also about masturbating. I did not even know what masturbate meant at the not-so-innocent age of sixteen.

One sunny Saturday morning I awoke in my twin bed, the flowered, gauze-like bedspread rumpled to my side. Lying on my back, I was suspended in a very warm glow tingling between my thighs, naively excited like butterflies hovering near desired nectar-flowers. Probably that was my first orgasm, though I did not know how to name it. I did not know what a clitoris was either. Only as I wrote about this memory thirty years later, was I aware of my sadness, expressed by rapid breathing and tightened tummy, mixed with welled up anger and resentment that had piled up like unthrown spitballs all those many years.

As I began to write about "first love" in September of 1992: my first thoughts were of my first husband, Chuck, and my first daughter, Erin. My first loves. Then, my father, Michel: each love a different kind of soothing. I questioned whether I ever had a first love when it came to boyfriends. I didn't like my thought that **I had never known love that was not dependency**. I went with my thoughts of Chuck, whom I had met at the Tabernacle Baptist church, where my choices of whom I could love were constricted. God damn it – I never had the chance to have a first love of my choice! These thoughts were a bit scary – new to me.

What I did love of Chuck was so much of my father. I chose Chuck because he provided the safety for me to be myself as much as possible within those jailing religious rules, a prisoner of war within myself.

"Will I ever have a first love of my own?" I cried, reading my own words **out loud** in 1992, just before I met my fourth husband, Gregory, who became the catalyst that brought my defenses tumbling down. "I have never chosen my own love," was a startling revelation then. I didn't know what that revelation meant. Until now.

At that time, I continued to describe "good sex" as the eyes of a man staring steadily into the eyes of a woman without the need to get away, deep gazes of wanting me, not knowing where he stopped and she began. The overwhelming desire to have an orgasm rises between them, battling the conflict of not wanting to have the pleasuring come to an end, as if it might be the last time to climax. Or is the desire for more awareness? For more aliveness? Maybe "good sex" is a burgeoning exaltation to the loss of control, our vulnerability, our oneness. In 1992, I was still separating love from sex, unaware of how much I was still separate from my Self.

When Chuck left me, after coming out to his own homosexuality in 1975, I was given the opportunity to open up sexually ("*free* up my *spirit*") although I was still hindered by guilt from being a "born-again-fundamentalist-christian."

I had sex, or "made love," with a dozen or so men before marrying my second husband, Reid, whom I'd only known for three months. In between these two husbands, I had six years to explore new bodies, new penises, new beginnings with tongues. (My first husband reminded me 25 years later that I did not like oral sex while I was with him, having tried it only once.) Oral sex became one of my favorite ways to have an orgasm. I had always been a rebellious tiger in a cage - now the circus would begin!

Within the Big-Top circles of monogamy, of course, since I was still a married christian. But the divine spirit does not respect boundaries of humankind. This truth has been imprinted into my heart over and over again.

When I married Reid in 1982, I didn't know why I cried on our honeymoon when I told him I could not tolerate an extramarital affair. Yes, it would hurt, but why so much? While with Reid, I began graduate school classes part-time. I volunteered to be a teaching assistant for a Human Sexuality course at Cornell University. I allowed myself to question sexual practices, while I deeply doubted my christian beliefs during arguments with Reid. I began to break free of my religious chains, as I dared to test out an open marriage.

My apprehensions about losing Reid were outweighed by my fondness for freedom, catapulting me to leave Reid after only two years of marriage. During our time together, I allowed myself what I now see and know was a fuller picture of how separate I was from my Self. We enjoyed lovemaking in many positions and places, one of them being anal sex. Although Reid was gentle, the start of anal penetration always created discomfort, bordering on pain, until I could relax enough to let him enter me. Since I was on my stomach, and he was behind me, there was no chance for face-to-face contact, let alone eyes to peer into one another's souls. No connection at all, only pleasure we gave ourselves. I had to rub my clitoris in order to have an orgasm in this position. The only sense of connection was in our timing of simultaneous orgasms - only heard...not **seen**. The wholeness of my spirit was far from being seen.

After my amicable break from this marriage and religion, I had no desire to pursue anal sex with any of my future partners. I find this a pleasing evolve, to come *face-to-face* with my Self, as I more often *faced* my lovers during lovemaking, the reflection of which is love.

I completed my Masters Degree in Marriage and Family Therapy in 1985, along with my friendly divorce from Reid. Simultaneously, I had been released from nine months of individual therapy with a psychologist who said I didn't need any more therapy. I had been therapized as an expectation of the Master's program, having had no specific symptoms of anxiety or depression. Although I was aware of feeling some guilt and shame around the exposure of my body, I was "dealing with it."

Just like I had between marriages, I was being with new bodies, new penises, new muscles of men ten or more years younger than me. Yes, I was still looking for love - but wasn't it in all the wrong places?

One of those places was a place of power. He was 22; I was 38. He was a virgin, and my friend Bruce thought that I would be the right woman to deflower Steve. It was exciting to anticipate how we both would feel. I knew, consciously, that his orgasm would come quickly, and subconsciously, that my pleasure came from having this special moment of lost innocence be because of me: I would be special. Unconsciously, I would feel powerful, and thereby not have to feel the pain of the lack of (past or present) love.

I revolved from one boyfriend to another during variations of open relationships, with a couple of one-night stands thrown in, as casual as plain corn chips dipped in salsa. I thought I was so mature to challenge my society's expectations, like I had with Reid – sharing my husband sexually and being confident that I would be his primary love. I thought this would reinforce our 'love' for each other; I was not aware that I was acting out my pain of not being loved adequately by my parents, and especially not loved by my mother.

I became monogamous again when I married my third husband, Alain, five years after leaving Reid. Finally, having my freedom from religion, I felt I had to fly to find Me. For the first time, I lived with a man and prospective husband before our marriage in 1989, thinking I had cleaned up his smoking and drinking enough to trust that there were not obvious barriers to our intimacy. Within a few months, I was propelled back into therapy to search out my needs for closeness: connection on a deeper level than my workaholic husband was giving me. And he had returned to smoking.

Our sexual relationship bore out its own signs of distance. I had regular bombastic clitoral orgasms, making it easier for Alain to tolerate my inability to have intercourse orgasms, but it was all a ruse for the lack of true joining. Our eyes were usually closed during orgasms despite the desire to please one another. We could achieve close to simultaneous orgasms outside of intercourse, enjoy looking at each other's bodies, yet not connect through the eyes - the windows to our souls. I had not yet connected the tears from my eyes to the seat of my soul - my inner-hurt-child.

When Alain said he didn't need to change after six months of couple's therapy, I once again left another marriage in search of intimacy - the intimacy I was unaware that I did not have with my Self.

I wrote regular entries in my journal while with Alain, sometimes poetry, which helped create intimacy within my Self. I was not interested in writing on a formal basis until 1992, the year after my divorce from Alain. I began to write short essays about my sexual encounters as if they would open another door to my sheltered heart. How well the human spirit guides us...

...Even into a relationship with another Steve. He was not readily available to satisfy my "horniness." A queer word, to mean sexually aroused. It brings visions of horned toads, horned sheep, car horns, bull horns, sharpness and loudness of male reindeer racks crashing into one another in order to protect their harem for mating. Is their sexual drive so great that they need many females for themselves? I have learned that lions mate several times a day during their "in heat" season. I seem to be in heat after my menstrual period. I know I want orgasms more often if I have them more often. Not "once full, once satisfied." Maybe the physical fullness of orgasm does not satiate?

It is too separate. The sexual and the spiritual.

From my 1992 journal: "Without Steven, I must masturbate - with the wand of cream-colored-smooth-vibrator dripping with honeyed juices. No lips of his on mine, no eye-to-eye piercing through, no broad shoulders to envelope me. So many colors of orgasm. So much more brilliant when engaged and throttled to climax by a man.

I visualize Steven's mouth on my nipples, the sweetness of boyish face against my softness of nurturing breast. That giving of closeness is an innocent pleasure I remember with my two daughters suckling at my breast. What intimacy, what connection, what unity. I continue to vibrate my astoundingly sensitive clitoris, labia, lips of my vagina, all three, to an orgasm crying out for Steven's cock to enter me. The vibrator will not do! I want this soul to be with mine – a pleasure to *be shared."* Why not a <u>love</u> to *be shared*?

Why won't a laughing orgasm do? My next boyfriend, Carlo, and I are standing in the bathroom. He can no longer hold his position of swollen uncircumcised penis entering my labia, my soft, smooth, creamy untouched-by-the-sun derriere against his muscled abdomen. His thirty-five-year-old voice turns into a teenager's, gasping "I cannot hold it. I'm going to come." I brace myself against the sink, watching his grimaces of delight in the mirror, him gripping my waist like a rodeo cowboy on a bucking bronco. I am still; I am happy for him, so much so that I begin to laugh and laugh, and his laughs punctuate mine amidst his gasps for air. We laughed together- unified. I hear, "Te amo." I want to be more attracted to Carlo than I am; still, he's more than a really good friend. "I wish my seed could open more," are the words I wrote in 1992. And now I feel the tears of sadness of this truth. Frequent tears throughout the nineties enhanced my realization of their deeper meaning - truly I was but a seed of love in 1992.

The husks of that seed are cracking open on my forty-sixth birthday, when Steven tells me to close my eyes, as he sits astride my model-like thighs, looking down at me with his impish eyes. We are elevated in his loft-bed, where the ceiling meets his head, making it seem as if we are in a womb, just opening up to the sunshine of this, my birthday. I feel the lightness of electricity up and down my genitals, not quite able to distinguish its origins. It's not: blowing of air, fingers manipulating my labia as hummingbird's wings might, or marshmallow's softness rolling over my clitoris. I must peek. It's a gray and white feather, something I had mentioned to Steven as a pleasure I might enjoy. I was lightly disappointed because it did not arouse me as I had hoped. So different now, nine years later: the lighter the touch, the more excited I become: my increasing sensitivity to emotional feelings causes body/physical feelings to be enhanced.

An hour later, Steven surprises me again as I stand next to his bed. We are embracing, and suddenly I jump and let out a yelp! This does not deter Steven's pressured grip of an unknown vibrating force against my clitoris and perineum. I shiver with delight as I barely recognize the long gray handled probe with a circular end that reminds me of a miniature floor shampoo machine. Steven will not let up, and soon I am writhing with pleasure, the intensity approaching that of a Mack truck speeding down Mt. Washington, having lost its brakes. My legs are shaking; I must lie down. Steven pushes the vibrations around my buttocks and back again to my clitoris, which I believe is blossoming a head as big as that of a sunflower. The gray vibrator is now between both of our hardened genitals. Hard as a hammer and nail beating against each other. Suddenly, Steven is inside my juicy vestibule, but I cannot focus on that, nor do I want to, nor will I. I have burst into fireworks that are so loud, crashing at the hands of Steven's back massager.

I cringe, feeling regretful sadness seven years later as I rewrite this encounter, although I accept that it is part of my healing journey. The regret is to look at the separateness from my Self in this most mechanical of birthday orgasms. Little did I know that I was about to blossom like a Mo(u)rning Glory.

In October of 1992, I participated in a triathlon with my ex-third husband, Alain. We were still friends that continued to love each other in the best way we knew how -the physical. I have always been enthralled by his Herculean broad shoulders and hard-carved muscular legs. His wavy shoulder length hair added to his mythic romantic appeal.

On our way home in his red Mustang, Alain's well-practiced right hand traveled into my sweatpants, eliciting a trio of shivers from my clitoris. As I moaned, his penis rose to my hand's smooth firm strokes, higher and higher, until he was unearthed from his sweat pants, both of us panting like Bighorn sheep arriving at the peak of Mt. McKinley. My warm saliva dripped over his tip along my tongue, creating harmonious moans as we sped along the valleys of each other's legs, genitals, breasts, and eyes. We have nearly forgotten who is driving who or what.

It is an hour drive to my home. Could we stop and "make love" in the woods? It is too cool out, or is it that we want the comfort of our bed and the wonderfulness of anticipation to last, as if the warmth of amniotic fluid could bathe us nine months and longer?

Isn't it fascinating how similar infatuation with another is to the interaction we have with babies? This revelation came to me as I "came" less with sex and "came" more with love - Real Love. When there is a mutual attraction between two human beings, there is usually a speedy progression to hand holding, eye-to-eye gazing, and wanting to caress the other's body all over, thus the foot-touching under dining tables, and arms around shoulders in the movie theater. Just like how we automatically stare into baby's eyes, revel in them holding our pinkies, and snuggle into the softest skin folds of their necks. We make "goo goo" eyes with our new lovers, like we do with babies. It is the seed of unconditional love being planted.

Infatuation wanes, and like toddlers beginning to say "no" to their parents, lovers begin to say "no" to each other when their differences arise. How well we have been loved by our parents greatly determines how well we can say "no" honestly, or accept another's autonomy or independence, or, more basically, how afraid we are to express our true feelings. How often do couples play the game of who will say "I love you" first? Afraid that Love will not be returned. How often do we use sex to be close to someone as a substitute for love?

By November of 1992, I was beginning to become aware of the urgency of my body shifting down from fourth, to third, to second gear, in order to feel more than the outcome: the orgasm. Douglas and I were waiting for a table at a New York jazz restaurant, when he spontaneously nibbled my neck. I was so romantically moved that climax was not needed, orgasmically speaking.

Later, in his bed, it was not long before I wanted him inside me; yet, no, not yet, keep the changing intersecting of cock and genital area exploring, as if new patterns would make the excitement heighten. I wanted my body to feel in new ways, not just do what I routinely do, or know what feels good enough to bring me to climax. That tension of wanting to come and desire to learn anew was a whole new amusement ride for me; a ride that I wanted to last a lifetime. "The climax of life ever expanding into new frontiers of sexuality and spirituality mixing, like adding brown sugar, peanut oil, spices, and brown eggs into newer, tastier creations," I wrote in 1992.

Douglas' eyes closed, mine opened, during his orgasm. My eyes closed, his opened, as I screamed, "Oh my god, Douglas, it feels so good," so loud that Douglas could not help but laugh, "I won't be able to live here (apartment complex) anymore." Unbeknownst to me then, I was to move on, closer to the home of my heart. The real Me. To real Love derived from grieving my religiously repressed childhood pain, so that my spirit (love) could be integrated into my body (sex). "One's capacity to grieve is one's capacity to love," is expanded on throughout this book.

The mechanical electric waves felt from "asshole, cunt, clit, cock" were vocabulary I used back then symbolizing the harsh edge, like a knife, needed to feel alive, to cut through the unawareness of separation from my true Self. I also wrote, "I cannot hide my aloneness in their strong arms or daily kisses of hellos and good byes."

It is finally spring. 1993. Just a week ago, five of us were snowed in for the weekend by 28 inches of white fluff, unlike the purer substantial love between my two daughters, my granddaughter, Gregory, (my fourth husband) and me. It is completely sunny today. My heart sings as the chickadees play in the shrubs next to the woodpile, topped with a hat of snow which I am removing with my red shovel. Red as blood, the life force that allows me to love with pulses stronger, color fuller, the spectrum fully seen because I have no doubt that I love Gregory. We know many difficulties, yet I have never felt such surety with a man before.

We feel this even though we are just beginning our fourth month together. Melting snow over green needles is like his soul searching into me with soft penis, after many tender textures of kisses, blended with eyes staring as steadfastly as dolphins do. I cannot remember ever being kissed so completely in tenderness; even now tears dance in my eyes when I think of it. My lips and eyes have never been known so well.

Gregory's penis is recovering from a surgery and an unloving marriage, it stands up only partially, as if to say, "I'm hurting," and he must pay attention to that. We slide back and forth over each other's nakedness, for more than minutes, into hours, me enjoying the subtle crevices of a half-erect penis inside my labial folds. His head's rim is firmly rubbing my chasms into shivers I have never felt before from hard intercourse, from 50 or so men. His penis feels like fingering the frost's designs on a window pane or soft folds of a baby's thighs; he moves into my crevices where only birthing of two daughters has been known, where discovery of new souls is slowly born through labor and pain. His sorrow I see as his deep blues become reddened, ready to tear, but hold fast as I approach ecstasy while he pushes his hardened-jello in and out of me, over and over again. Our legs are intertwined like mating starfish, melting into the softness of jellyfish, where no form can describe our oneness.

His face portrays disbelief that I could be feeling so good from a soft penis, yet his penis is stiffening. We are forced to have patience and in so doing can feel the delicate designs within our bodies like winter frost's intricate patterns, only seen when trees are without leaves. Fog is frozen into sparkling tiny icicle gems lighting up pine trees' intertwining twigs and branches like our arms and legs intertwined into waves of intense passion.

Must the passion blossom last only seconds, like a hummingbird flitting from flower to flower? Or can the one hanging pot of blooms grow to fuller and bigger beauty throughout the summer? Yes, it can! As I walk up the deck stairs daily, my nose inhales the summer's sweetness, eyes stop to behold new open buds, fingers touch the bells, dropping to the wooden deck, ushering my footsteps to my beloved's homecoming - a rush of passion before arms squeeze our chests together after a day's work. I feel everyday intensity, fresh as morning brushed teeth, forever desired, routinely present, bright as laundered sheets on the drying line. Pin me and unpin me the rest of our lives!

Little did I know how sharp the pins of passion would become during the six years I was with Gregory as his spiritual and legal wife. There was a mystery being uncovered every moment we were together, not the obvious mechanistic hormone-run erection that has no particular meaning other than sexual tension, like a leap out of bed when the alarm goes off.

Due to our society's repression of expression of sexual feelings, it is not surprising that my daughter Megan, then eighteen, did not like to hear her mother being sexual, as if Old Faithful's eruption might overwhelm her with its explosion of power. Sometimes Gregory's kisses lingered into sounds like sugar smacks, and I heard Megan's annoyance when she said, "Must you kiss so loud?"

I told her sister Erin, then twenty-one, about needing to be at Gregory's home, two hours away, partly because I want to be free to be exuberant with my love-making, to not hold back as I did in order to respect Megan's feelings. I wanted the filter off the camera of love, and I felt the apprehension of talking with Erin about my sexual life, even though I did not want to feel that way. Erin told me that she used to hear me making love with my boyfriends, although I tried very hard not to be noisy. Erin showed surprise on her still-baby-pink cheeks in learning that I scream with orgasm because she doesn't. I told her that I had observed that, the one time I heard her and Kevin making love as I sat reading near the wood stove just outside her bedroom door. We exchanged a few more details about our orgasms and I felt the warmth and bubbles arising within myself toward Erin as we came to a climax of intimacy, to a degree of which we had never shared before. May "old Faithful" (spirit) continue to erupt in all its power.

"Even the hundreds of orgasms within three marriages and several boyfriends pale in the light of the five weeks I've known you, Gregory," I told him with a fervent heart. But, still, for months Gregory could not believe that I was satisfied with his half-erect penis, just like he couldn't believe that I didn't want to be with other men. Just like he couldn't trust me. Yet, it was so true - his large soft penis could find its way into crevices that a hard penis could not. Even into my heart! Even into my soul! (Mate) That fifth week knowing Gregory was the last week of January 1993, when, **for the first time** in my life, I was unable to shut my eyes during orgasm, and I careened into the longest orgasmic waterfall, crashing out the scream, "I love you, Gregory," with tears from newborn eyes.

The meaning of sex is so much more important than the act. Like snow clumped into the forks of tree limbs in no hurry to fall to the ground, which does suddenly when the moisture is so heavy and the temperature so warm that there is a spontaneous swoop to the earth below. The snow travels from limb to earth with unknown turns, undulations, sensations, never experienced before –like Gregory giving me more verbal expression of feelings than any man, or person for that matter, I had ever known. Colorful sunrises and sunsets were added to our lovemaking, not just daylight.

As a teenager, Gregory had been sexually betrayed by his girlfriend, who hid her sexual relationship with a college boy, then abandoned Gregory by not talking to him; he became suicidal. He had been the one keeping them from having intercourse, wanting to save that union for marriage. He didn't go home for two days, worrying his parents greatly. After this teenage betrayal, layered over an emotionally and physically abusive relationship with his mother, Gregory made a dramatic change in his sexual behavior. This monogamous fifteen-year-old became a promiscuous sixteen-year-old. He knew screwing 500 women during his high school years was his way of hating women, hating how they had hurt him!

As a forty-four year old, I believe Gregory had returned to distrusting women, holding onto his semen as a form of control; to protect him self from being hurt by them. A few months into our relationship, Gregory allowed more trust to literally erupt: ejaculating his semen into my mouth. Giving up his semen was a reflection of entrusting himself to me.

Like after 1984, the year I was liberated from religion's control, I began to enjoy forget-me-nots, buttercups, and wild violets splashing their colors throughout my lawn. I did not have to weed out the dandelions in order to make a perfectly green carpet. The periwinkle blues infringing over the borders of my lawn were welcomed. The freedom of this mixture of plants reflects the trustfulness of the universe in its diversity. Like the forget-me-nots, Spirit does not forget the goodness of itself, like Gregory continued to allow him self to plummet inside of me. Even though he was not totally erect like a tent with all its poles, the flap flew open, and he ejaculated inside of me for **the first** time, four months after the first time we made love. He said he ejaculated with those he loves and feels love from in return. He was beginning to trust me with his love, and my love gave sacredness to this union of our souls like the soft light-blueness of the forget-me-nots that stand out amidst the varied greens and still brings them all together, when uncut. As we let go of our defenses we are growing in awareness of connection to self, each other, and nature. Our spiritual-sexual oneness.

After being "in love" with Gregory for eight months, despite his ongoing mistrust that I was having sex with other men, and me becoming fed up with it; I added to the mistrust by kissing another man at a workshop. I am in need of loving that is not marred by the scars of mistrust. I did not know then how much I needed to uproot my pain of helplessness, pain caused by how little my mother and the church trusted me. I needed to believe and trust in *my* feelings, in my ideas of what *my* truth is!

As I healed emotionally through the process of connecting with my primal childhood pain, I had to release rage and sobs. This seemed to draw me closer to having vaginal orgasms through intercourse. The letting go of emotional pain allowed the obstacle of my defenses to fall further (less control needed to hold in my pain), relaxing me. I had never had an intercourse orgasm in my forty-seven years. In that same August of 1993, Gregory not only gave away his semen more often, but also added loud vocalizations to his orgasms, which I had not heard since our meeting, December 13th 1992. I felt like a very ripe watermelon splitting open in that hot sun of LOVE'S trust, eight months in the making, from black seed to red sweet water running down my chin, hands, even knees. We were beginning to be all there in the moment: all eyes, all ears, all beginner's love. I wondered if I enjoyed his orgasm as much as he did. I remember one of the positions we had been in was especially gratifying because of the physical hotness brought on by Gregory's rear entry. With my small back against his softer muscled pectorals, somehow he rubbed my G-spot so deliciously that I turned my head around, easily meeting his lips that felt like diamonds wrapped in satin. "No one has ever kissed me as tenderly as you, Gregory!" This position was so comfortable, maybe how a figure eight must feel to an accomplished ice skater?

After I come, **come**? Why come? It is more like letting go ...then, I wanted you to come inside of me, so I pulled you over me as I pushed your manliness once more inside my vagina, the hall of flame! I wanted you as close as possible: my lips caressed your shoulders, your lean biceps, your breath with wispy moans, especially when I sucked on your finger closely placed to your lips. I looked into your big eyes of blue, before me, above me. You rocked into a surprise explosion of orgasm with vocals unlassoed - we were **coming** home again. And a long road it is.

As we journeyed through our first year together simultaneous orgasms began to be our bill of fare. Like the day we were painting the dark brown paneling in our kitchen, the color of blue reflected off ponds on a sunshiny day. Everything seemed light as we shared this task together: the sweat on our upper lips and chins, the red T-shirt you had on showing a broad-branched tree with its deep, wide root system. I gave you this shirt because of the star placed over the tree, symbolizing the light that shines throughout our relationship because we are willing to grow. I could see you pleasuring me as our eyes locked into appreciation of one another's love and shamelessness. You told me you liked to look at my vulva and vagina; it's like a Morning Glory. I had never known it could be so beautiful to someone or feel so magnificent to be tongue-tickled or sucked in an upside-down position. You brought me to the heights of ecstasy over and over until I begged to be able to fly like an eagle in King's Canyon. My screams and your yelps were orgasmic music simultaneously played. Sometimes it was grand.

part two

◊

EVOLution of an

Orgasm as

Evolution of Love

The SEASON of SPRING...1993–1999

The dark side, like 3pm in the afternoon and it looks like twilight, almost like night. Gregory and I are in our bed; I'm on top of him looking down at his lips that kiss me better than anyone: tenderness, lingerness, spaciousness, both of us noticing the changes in pressure, angle, speed and feeling. This lovingness is broken apart by an intruder – you want me to tell a story, about my bachelorette party before our spiritual marriage celebration on September 18, 1993. Actually, I did not have this traditional ritual party; you want me to fantasize.

By now, we both know this is a replay of how your mother emotionally and physically abused you: she hit and yelled, worked up into a frenzy, then fainted, and you were left to pick her up. Then, she was sensually grateful, running her fingers through your hair as she said something like, "you know I love you." I say that I don't want to bring other men into our lovemaking so your erection can be harder, filled with anger and hate for what suffering you have experienced. Your eyes are almost begging me to "love" you this way, and my eyes are watering with sadness and fear that I will only reinforce this act out of your pain. And, I won't be seen or cared about. I want your erection to "come" from loving me, not from the story which culminates in you being loved the best by me, more than all of the other men, like a hot-air balloon with the brightest colors, flying the longest distance through the sky. The balloon has to land somewhere, fold up, let go of its hot air, so we can see the real colors of the sky: the rainbow, the moon, and the stars that twinkle and sparkle from their own substance, not from being spotlighted or compared with another.

We talk back and forth, as my vulvas do the same, I ride your swelling dick (a distancing word used in 1993) which is becoming stiffer as I tell you about fictitious naked men surrounding me. They are letting me have my way in patting their young rounded buns, holding their erections, as they undress me slowly, yet eagerly like brown sugar melting into hot cream of wheat.

My blue eyes are now gray with the ambivalence of enjoying your hardness inside my birth canal, and misty with the absence of lovingness. "I love a whore, my wife's a whore," my husband blurts out with an excited powerful voice, as he pulls my hips over his raised organ. I have to force my tears back as I tell him that I love him because he is who he is, he is special, not because he is the best man sexually in the world. Gregory's eyes glisten now with the tears that have rolled down my flushed cheeks, dropping into his iris blue-circled pupils.

In October of 1993, I write of Impatiens, the light-lavender-flowers hanging by a bungee cord in the corner of our Aster-laden deck. Impatient with the process of change, or is it our inability to surmount the fear of change? After a couple of months of rehashing my kissing a man twenty years my junior, Riyaz, we seem to be unstuck for a week, like gum pried off the bottom of a school desk after ten months stuck. Gregory calls me "starshine," and I do my best to bring that light into our room, an attempt to make love. He looks into my streaming blue eyes with the steadfastness of a blue anchor, connecting our lips with a tenderness I have never felt with any other man. This time there is no talk of other men, or "fucked cunt," which is his usual rise to a fuller erection - we don't want the past! We alternate "my darling, my soul mate, my husband, my wife, my best friend, my beloved, my love, my partner for life, I love you, I love you." Tears come, smiles stay.

Being "starshine," I do look to the stars for reassurance and validation of my journey as I learn more and more that everything in the universe is connected, that we are all ONE. Feeling the deep hurt of not being trusted by Gregory, I went to an astrologer, four months into our relationship, questioning if I could be patient with Gregory's mistrust of me. The astrologer said that Gregory's unconscious was "on fire" and may be cleaned up by the following year. It helped me hang on to the possibility of knowing Love that I had not yet fully experienced with Gregory. Or for my Self. The astrologer also said that I was "born knowing more about relationships than anyone ever figures out." WOW, I thought. "You are the fist in the velvet glove," he said.

In-no-sense can we fathom the acceptance of pain in our lives, although we easily throw around the cliché, "no pain, no gain." By October 1993, I had thought much about that saying, feeling more and more of my childhood pain of not being trusted by my mother, or my church's dogma. How that pain took away the **innocence** that I was born with – that we all are born with. We are as uncomfortable with the vulnerability of tears as a kitty is with a hairball in its throat, even though we love the vulnerability and honesty of children's feelings. How unusual it is to explore why a two-year-old swats us, the usual response being, "Don't do that, that's not nice." The child then sucks in his hurt, and anger, like the warm milk from a "left out" bottle, beginning to curdle.

Then, the tantrums begin, building into an adolescent rage of fist-fights, door slamming, violent sports, rape or anorexia. If only we could listen to our children's voices, like we view their first gaze long and hard into our eyes, before they learn to be afraid of daddy's temper or mommy's scowl or raised voice. Children, feeling unheard like the background hum of summer's crickets, learn to withdraw, defend, blame, until now, as a grown up, I am crying over a spontaneous question I ask of Gregory, "When did you get that message?" (on the message machine). "When do you think I got it?" he replies with annoyance. "Just think about it."

A simple question rebuffed, and I melt into tears. I cannot stop crying when I hear my twenty-two-year old daughter, Erin, coming through the door with her boyfriend, Kevin, father of precious granddaughter, Denali. After a few minutes in the bathroom, I appear with reddened, water-drowned eyes, part of me wanting to go unnoticed, the other part desiring to be "seen" in my sadness like dew sparkling on a spider's web, while an ant caught in the web struggles to get loose. Erin immediately asks, "What's wrong?" sending my eyeballs into a tub of swirling droplets, soaking into Gregory's turtleneck as he gently corrals me with his strong shoulders, recounting to Erin this most recent interaction.

We are somewhat aware of the layers of pain on which this incident focuses, if we are allowed to look at it with tenderness and kindness as Gregory's voice spoke it to Erin, whose eyes are blushing blue, open wide. **Openness** like that of a child, who is without fear of retribution, punishment, or its feelings being invalidated or ridiculed. At that moment, I felt like the innocent child, so dependent on my mother's understanding and acceptance of my questions, my feelings, still not received, until this moment in Gregory's arms, and Erin's eyes.

Like Gregory's (inner child's) innocence trying to be seen as an adult when he says, with angry eyes, "What about my hurt? You beat me (when you flirt with other men), then tell me you love me." Like his mother. His statement exemplifies that most inward essential feeling of mother's love not having been given. The past and the present are so clearly one! That is why we were committed to our healing journey to find real love. I am downstairs in the bathroom as I hear Gregory shouting, "I will not be used, fucked over, shit or pissed on, I am special, I am a good man." Even though it is difficult to see and hear his hurt, the reverberations of his childhood and first girlfriend's betrayal as a teenager, these most personal feelings bring *US* to deeper levels of vulnerability, and thus intimacy, if we can embrace grieving those hurts.

Until I began crying so freely, and deeply, because Gregory's distrust and acting out triggered my childhood pain, I hadn't been aware of the depth of my fear of losing Gregory, as well as the depth of my shame of exposing my body. Nor the need to define more precisely what a word means, such as the difference between lying and deception. Before Gregory, I would not have noticed the coolness of my calf muscle, because of the overwhelming sensation of my shin's hotness, when sitting in front of the wood stove. I am paying attention to subtleties that I was not concerned with in the past. I could now enjoy details of nature, whereas, before I could not hike slowly enough to <u>notice</u>. Not-ice☺

It's October 1993, and I am ten years freed intellectually from the fundamentalist chains of perfectionism, puritanism, and the denial of my own truth. But, am I really free? I am with a soulmate who is still smoking, having deceived me from the beginning, not admitting that he smoked. With a man who distrusts me. Yet, as we drive along, I am able to recount mornings where I am never bored with tender kisses, eyes pouring into eyes so frequently that one would think we were combination locks trying every sequence of gazes that unlock love's communication.

Then, the switch, so startling, "Are you going husband hunting today?" Gregory asks with sarcasm. Such hate is spoken out of nowhere except a past of sexual, physical, and emotional abuse that I remind him of when he sees flirtations on a dance floor twirling into an opera of betrayal. The melodrama speaks of deep pain, cutting my heart like a butcher's knife. He is intentionally cruel; I have never been.

I successfully let the darts of mistrust deflect off of me as we talk about getting over Riyaz, an infatuation of mine never acted on beyond the kiss, and told to Gregory 24 hours too late. He can only see my rare moment of deceitfulness. There is no room for understanding my fear – I should have known and been stronger. Just like the church and my mother would have expected from me. Now, I feel helpless, and that feeling is so hard to bear because I am that vulnerable hurt child again.

Still, I find myself kneeling between Gregory's legs, licking his very hard cock, as we again and again look into one another's jaded once innocent eyes, lowering me down onto his organ so full of blood desire. We move slowly, enjoying every moan, every crevice of delight, like Carlsbad Caverns stalagtites, stalagmites, rings of colors; my cave dripping drops of intense magnificent beauty through my vagina. As he pushes into my walls, I cannot believe where I am going. Moving toward a place I have never been in forty-seven years. I can barely keep my eyes open, yet I do. I am with you my beloved, as I careen into a new oneness, specialness, of my <u>first</u> intercourse orgasm, past thousands of orgasms I will never remember.

In late 1993, I write of my beginning consciousness toward a sacred sexuality and orgasm. I am surprised how unified I am with all of the universe's orgasm of beauty – not just the one of snowflakes swirling through the sunshine – of universal love. My journal's description: "Knights in shining armor, prince charming," Doctor Zhivago, and Rachmaninoff's piano concerto in C, all conjure up feelings of excitement, adventure intertwined with love, idealized like a dolphin carrying a drowning human to safety. Yes, it is true that this has happened, but it is rare. Rare as the ability for persons who love us not to disappoint us, or to love us unconditionally, as if we are babies getting all our needs met without even asking.

I wish I could be an otter, so genuinely playful, rolling over and under his or her buddies. Is work involved to find food? Or, I imagine being kept warm in the thick white coziness of polar bear fur, never feeling the coldness of the Arctic blowing against me. "You're not going to hurt me, too?" Gregory asks as he lays down beside me in his terrycloth bathrobe, smooth and navy. He's just taken a shower and his shoulder-length hair is slicked back wet, looking as sexy as Patrick Swayzy in "Dirty Dancing."

I am in the mood to make love, but he says, "I don't feel sexual, I'm too angry at all my losses." His abusive ten-year marriage, daughter Sara taken away by his wife for 11 days without any knowledge of her whereabouts, false charges of being physically abusive to his wife, losing the barn and house he dreamed of loving. Those romantic idealizations that things (or people) can replace our wish (need) for real love are like stones skipping across the water, thrown by a strong arm, hoping to reach the other side without sinking. I try to empathize by feeling the three losses of marriage I have experienced. The first (marriage) stone skip splashed me with a kind, accepting, non-controlling man, a lot like my father, except that Chuck's homosexual coming out allowed for this virgin to explore her sexuality. Six years later, I skipped into a marriage three months after I met Reid, still dominated by the fundamentalist belief that sex is only right within marriage. Guilt and fear were left behind by that divorce which toppled the Bible's "one way" of doing or believing. The next five years, I skipped through major controlling and caretaking issues while married to Alain, who wanted to stay where he was emotionally. It is now 1993, twenty-four years after my first legal (as compared to spiritual) marriage, and I am a psychotherapist in private practice – privately sinking deeper into mySelf and Gregory. I am no longer drowning in the overwhelming largeness of the ocean where there is no trace of land, or bird; now the stone is falling through the cattails, lily pads and tadpoles of a pond surrounded by conifers, maples, oaks, birch, beech, poplar, and huge-leafed sycamore.

The wildflowers on the pond's edge are leaning toward the light, like Me, as Gregory presses me to find, through painful intimate interaction and self-examination, distance, and love, the unromantic connection with all these living things. And, tears are pushing paths down my cheeks as I read this paragraph out loud, affirming its organic, exciting (orgasmic) TRUTH.

The previous writing shows the paradox of unconsciousness-consciousness of evolution toward an integration of spirituality and sexuality, but I did not have a grasp on its deep significance until the late 1990s. As the reader is aware from the beginning of the book, I ultimately had to leave Gregory because he refused to open his heart to his pain, and wanted me to act out sexually with other men. When I refused, he would become angry and sometimes extremely verbally abusive. Although I am still sad that I had to let go of our marriage, I know that I am happier and farther along into what real love can be.

After I separated officially from Gregory in November 1998, I was celibate until March 1999, as per our agreement, to see if there was any room for change toward more vulnerability on Gregory's part. To say the least, I was not readily giving up on this soulmate of mine.

Loss has radiantly shown me what is precious and also brought me to richer and higher relationships of love. I am finding that Vulnerability creates Happiness (not just pain). That Intimacy creates Intensity (not just closeness). Near the end of February 1999, I found myself in the shower screaming, because I felt a building of anger and it was mostly about being sick of emotional pain, especially the pain of not being taken care of – needing to be loved without giving away extraordinary energy. I began to spend time with a man named Fred, who is unusual in his interest and ability to explore deeper intimacy.

Fred was sorting out a separation from his wife, while being attracted to me. We would have long conversations about such things like the word "fully," being fully present, fully whole, fully intimate - what these all mean. How much can we be there for another if we are not fully desirous – like making love when the other may not really wish it – yet wanting to be there for the other. We want both at once, maybe that is truly loving, wanting/respecting oneself and the partner all at once. Fred said that the connection between us emotionally made the physical attraction secondary to him, although it was primary when he first met me. Later, when he held me, it was better than he had expected.

I could have done with less holding, but wanted to give us a chance. I liked his broad shoulders, but not his hairy back. (Not childlike enough, I wonder now?) Fred says I have a strong, youthful body, and something *new*. That when I dance, especially in wide skirts, like a girl, I'm more alluring – whereas I'd think being the woman in the long sensuous dress would be more so. Again, it is the innocence, playfulness that seems to motivate many to want to feel healthy and whole. That child! LOVED.

Fred kissed me after asking if he could, passionately, and it was fine, but a little more tongue than I like, especially on a first kiss. I've always felt that "French" kissing right away feels invasive when you don't know someone very well. It's like digging up tulip (two lips) bulbs before they've flowered. Green kisses are tender like young buds, lingering in the sun for warmth so they can bloom in the knowledge of love's gentleness.

I told Fred that he would have to tell his wife about me in order for me to feel respected about what I could take from him. I cried when he said that he didn't want to take from me, that he's happy to give to such an extent that he doesn't have to have sex, orgasms, kissing! I replied that I hadn't ever had a relationship where I was not the <u>heavy</u> giver. In a deep way we both want intimacy, which many others are scared of. Laughingly he says, "I'm such a <u>heavy</u> dude." And, "you have a light-joyful expression when you dance."

I laughed, and stopped for a moment to figure out why I was laughing - Fred's simple directness is childlike. It's delightful because of its honesty, its awareness, its simplicity. And sensitivity. The next time he was with me he kissed me without his tongue, without me having to tell him how I'd felt when we kissed the first time. He sensed from the way we kissed before that I didn't like it very much. He says he likes the way I kiss and enjoyed kissing me more the second time. He also tells me that if things were the way he wanted with his separated wife that he would not be interested in having sex with me or anybody else. Just how I felt and couldn't convey to Gregory, no matter how hard I tried. It feels great that a man understands. I shared that I feel very alone in my journey of deep emotional exposure, then, Fred honors how courageous I am. He says, "It's rare." I cry as I read this two years later. I am lucky to have him as a friend.

As spring approached in March of 1999, I found myself picking up the phone to call my third ex-husband, Alain. I wanted to be taken care of by someone I love, at least with some measure of love. He took me out for a yummy salmon dinner, soon after we watched the video "Parent Trap," and then we made love. For the first time in nine years! He asked if he could tell me, "I love you," and I replied calmly, "Of course, whatever feelings you have are okay."

I did not reply in kind even though I felt loving. I had told him at dinner that this encounter did not mean we were getting together again. He replied that he appreciated my honesty and that was one of the things he loved about me. I was ambivalent about Alain because of his lack of depth of feelings shared; that's why we divorced in the first place. Also, I was still thinking of Gregory, and his long softly firm Plenty between my legs – there was no orgasm as wonderful in my experience up 'til then. I was happy that I did not feel guilty making love with Alain. Orgasming. I was officially separated, and allowing life to give me some of its delightful gifts.

My crying session (what others call a "therapy" session) that week went again to a core, core, core, pain of my life…and what I believe is everyone's. Many many tears over why I can't be WHO I AM! It is my whole growing up, not allowing my true feelings – not letting myself have things without feeling guilty. I will continue to scream against that tasteless, "dull, lifeless" voice. Feelings are my meditation and medication.

One of those things I don't let myself have: accepting physical beauty as integral to the WHOLE as the emotional and spiritual. I was taught that the physical does not matter. Yet, it is what we awaken to everyday – the wildflowers, the sun, the trees, the sun, that makes us say, "What a beautiful day this is…to be alive!"

"I think one of the most romantic and loving things you can say to another person is 'LOOK.' There is a kind of love in which two people look at each other, but I don't think it's as interesting as the love between two people standing side by side and looking at something else that moves them both," says Kathleen Dean Moore, philosopher, and author of *Hold Fast: At Home in the Natural World.* It's all about being WHOLE. Now, I <u>feel</u> that the physical is part of the whole to be

true, and I'm learning to trust and honor what I want by listening to that innocent child, and not relying on the conditioned fear learned from what others
teach me. No more shame of beauty! Like when others tell me I have an expressive face. When I asked Rosey "How?" He said that when I smile, I have such clarity of eyes that it reaches inside of him. The childlikeness – again.

Rosey is an inch shorter than my five-foot-nine-inch frame, which is not what
I'd really desire physically. I like men to be taller and huskily muscular; he is only
the latter. As I talked with him about it, I realized that when a man is on top of
me I feel protected and sheltered which feels really good. It is an image of me
being taken care of, held to the fullest, soothing any fear I might feel. Those childhood feelings of fear to say my need to be held: "Please hold me mommy, daddy,"
unexpressed, unmet. Taught to be a "big girl" too soon.

When I looked into Rosey's eyes, while making love, tears would well up and
I would have to look away – I couldn't sob with him yet. "Oh god, is there ever a
bottom to the pit of not being SEEN for WHO I AM?" The feeling from intense
eye contact can no longer be avoided and for that I am glad! I am more and more
present with the REAL ME.

This same week of spring 1999, I find myself sobbing in my weekly therapy
session as I say, "to be a writer." Sobbing about being, I'm on the edge of being
born, it is so amazing, surprised to be crying so hard, like a faucet on full blast.
It's the glorious paradox of being: to be crying in pain, yet feeling wonderfully
alive inside that I can cry in order to BE. It's taken much crying out of my pain
to get here. *TEARS ARE TRUTH…waiting to be spoken!* NAKED AND CRYING
– like a newborn!!

How wonderful TO BE BORN **OUT** OF PAIN! The ONENESS of it all.

But of course, there is more pain to "come," as in orgasm. I had tears once
after kissing and looking into Rosey's eyes for several moments. But I didn't trust
enough for him to see my sadness, to "come" home to mySelf. I tell him he is a
wonderful lover, and he replies, "No, you are the wonderful lover," and that's
when the tears came. Because I am becoming one! Inside! With my lost "wonderful lover" the Child.

I'm aroused. I masturbate. I have a very intense orgasm. I'm saying, "Oh my
god, you're in me!" At first I was thinking of Rosey, but readily I connected with
meaning that god is in me! WOW! The sexual and spiritual connection is becoming clearer and clearer as the fog of emotional pain is cried away, like rain.

The more the eye contact, the more I feel my tears well up, the more the connection to the soul/spirit is made - because it is through the eyes that tears flow.
Truth flows. Grief flows, for keeping sexuality separate from spirituality for so
long. This is why I am no longer with Gregory. He wants sexuality separated
from love. To have me act out sexually with other men. To reenact his own mother's betrayal of him. It is because of connecting-to-repressed-childhood tears

that I am with more of mySelf. My true Spirit.

How clear it is that repression has betrayed me. (See my first book, *TEARS ARE TRUTH* for the process of connection to childhood tears, instead of "unaware" crying) As I wrote earlier, I cannot remember my first wedding night sexually, yet I remember playing the tape of our ceremony, and eating dinner at The Red Lion before we made love. So I call him in May 1999. He didn't remember our first sexual intercourse either. How sad. As I told Chuck over the phone, "I love you," tears spilled like a prayer from a child's lips. Sadness for being separate from my memory of my first sexual union because I was so separate from loving mySelf. Chuck said he understood how this was due to our repressive upbringing.

I talked a lot with Rosey about sex in relation to repression of the Self, and how we separate sex from love when we do not love ourselves. Then I realized that anal sex is a reflection of that separateness, when lovers are not face-to-face.

This resonated with experiences with a previous therapist and even the Primal Center, both wanting me to say "good bye" to daddy. Yes, I needed to become less dependent on my father emotionally, but that does not mean I need to say goodbye. A complete separation is not necessary. It is not black and white. I found mySelf sobbing while saying I shouldn't have to say goodbye to Daddy because it is like saying goodbye to mySelf. Your essence, Daddy, is part of me – the part that I always want to have with me – LOVE'S beginning. "You are the one part of me that lets me be alive." I sobbed again when I said, "I feel I'm betraying myself if I allow Rosey to not portray me as I am – the truth about me." He lied to his previous girlfriend telling her he did not have sex with me when she asked. If I'm not important enough or good enough to be told the truth about, it rings of the past message that the church dogma gave me. I am unworthy of Love. My personhood or feelings do not count! LOVE can only be a reality when the truth is being said!

THE MOST LOVING THING I CAN DO FOR MYSELF IS TO OWN THE TRUTH.

"Rather than love, than money, than fame, give me truth." Thoreau said. For Real Love can only be based on truth says I☺ There's nothing like the honest truth! I was kicking my legs in a session as I cried, "I can't remember ever loving myself! (In my head, I'd always thought I had.) Oh god, help me; to be so separated from yourself is just unbelievable." Instead, I go back to my father, the one string that (god, or the Design of the Universe as I call that supernatural force) gave me to find my lost Self. This is all so amazing – tears always connect us (my father and me). I'll be a warrior against religion; it has deeply hurt me and so many others. It is truly a form of slavery. It is not "Amazing Grace" when I'm seen as a "wretch like me."

Amazing grace is that I have found my own divine truth similar to that of

Mother Teresa's "**I have found the paradox: that if I love until it hurts, then there is no hurt, only more love.**"

Since leaving the controls of the church, I've followed my feelings into knowing that the universe is connected in as many ways as imaginable. Psychics allow for the spirits of other lifetimes to connect with us. Astrologers speak for the forces of the interplay of the planets and the well-known pull of the moon on the tides. These all affect us even if we do not slow down enough to notice. I gravitate toward seeing an astrologer every 2-3 years, and their specifics are 98 per cent correct in predicting my future. In May of 1999, I cried with Rick, an astrologer who said, "You're out of the woods on a new path." And I was crying while telling of my separation from mySelf, by separating sex from love. 1999 was the year I let go of Gregory entirely, knowing I was helpless to help him and that I was growing to trust my own way. The astrologer said I would change many aspects of my life, and that "others advice would be of little value." It is difficult for me to write that because I risk others thinking I'm narcissistic and writing me off. But that's what all great contributors have had to risk, like: Galileo's scientific discovery about the earth's rotation considered heresy by the church, or Henry David Thoreau living like a hermit in the woods. Being married to Gregory created an awakening to my own repressed pain, so now I can be"come" more sane - more whole.

I begin to believe what the astrologer told me in 1996: "You are a virtuoso on the keyboard of love." I still feel a small bit of embarrassment writing that.

I make another connection on Mother's Day, 1999. I've noticed that my fibro-cystic (benign breast lumps) disease hasn't been noticeable for a couple of months. That has continued to be true to the present. I wondered then if that is due to the sex/love/spirituality grieving I've been feeling. Those three, no longer separated from each other – more connected – like the seven colors of the rainbow bleeding into one another after a soaking-sobbing rain. That same May is the the month I stopped having my crying sessions written on a separate sheet of paper, then transferring them into my journal. Why not have Susanne write the notes directly into my journal? She has ever since. More connection, more integration☺

It is clear to me that we all use sex to feel "alive," even if for only a few minutes. The greater the intensity of the orgasms, the more "Oh my gods." We are searching for the divine within us. We will find it somehow, someday, through our tears. And outward beauty can be a reflection of the heart beauty. My nightly bowl of ice cream reminds me of my father's presence: the sweetness, the creaminess, the nuttiness, the "Death By Chocolate" flavor. Daddy's dead, but not his flavor.

A flavorful encounter of lovemaking with Alain, my third husband, that I will never forget happened on his birthday, May 22, 1999. It was like a trillium breaking free from a choking leaf before its spring explosion of new leaves. Alain's not a dancer, but he showed up for a Saturday night swing dance as I had requested. I went home with him, and found myself belly laughing as I struggled to put clean pillowcases on his king-size pillows. I hadn't laughed so hard in a long while, and it felt good to fully let go of control, as I do in orgasm. But I had no idea that I was preparing myself for a very special orgasm.

That night I was tired and not so sure I wanted to make love, but knew I wanted the closeness. Yet, I found myself enjoying our lovemaking, and "came" with his penis between my legs, one of my favorite ways to orgasm. He said that I had not done it that way ever before with him. I found that hard to believe, but could not remember how I usually climaxed with him. This night, he woke me up in the middle of the night and took himself to orgasm, while calling me "baby," an anonymous name which I told him I didn't like. He also said, "Oh my god," as he approached orgasm, and I commented how we invoke 'god' when **we are feeling so good**. So good. So free. So me. So **divine**. (Isn't it interesting to see that the word 'good' only needs an extra 'o' added to the word, "god?")

The next morning, over bagels and café au lait, while sharing more of my retrieved memories of my mother holding me down as a baby, nearly strangling me, I began to feel warmer than usual between my legs. I told Alain about my decision not to be sexual with Rosey any more because he won't tell another woman about being sexual with me. Alain told me he really likes how honestly I communicate all these things to him, and I felt a **deep respect** flowing over me like a slow-moving lover's hand. As I felt closer to Alain, and the overwhelming flow of self-respect in my body's cells, I had to respond to the hot juiciness between my labia, and the heightening of my clitoris into a monument of love. I had an undeniable desire to be gently licked. "A good lickin,'" as Alain put it. Sad, to think of his words in the context of punishing children, connected by the bridge of making love, the positive with the negative, the evolving out of abuse into desire for healthy love.

We began with intercourse, and sucking my nipples: a double connection that doubles my pleasure. Then, him licking my clitoris was like a tidal wave moving over us, taking its time, yet surely was going to crash over me. It took time that I wanted to take – no urgency, just prolonged enjoyment – no frustration – a wave of ecstasy that lasted probably ten minutes.

And, when I burst into orgasm, I screamed an all-out glass-shattering scream that sounded no fear, just joy! So primal. I did not feel like saying "I love you, Alain," but I did say before the scream, "Oh my god!" several times. I did tell Alain how perfectly beautiful he was helping (not making) me feel. He said that he enjoyed doing it for me. And, my clitoris had become noticeably larger, so the build toward orgasm was easy and intense because he had no trouble sucking it. I felt no holding back, a new freedom, my whole body shuddered. And my brains certainly felt like they became mush. It was a cloudlike expanded feeling of ultimate rest and fullness, like a child falling to the ground, exhausted from play, so happy.

After I became calm in Alain's arms, we talked more. He added, "I love you, Diane" and I responded, "I love you too," in a less determined tone. There will always be a basic love for each other. How special this day became for me when my third ex-husband admitted that he missed more than anything, "the touching, holding, more than the sex." The man who had had an ongoing affair during his first marriage. A man who finds it difficult to be vulnerable. Still, the inner child could come out, who always wants to be present! The child is the leader to the divine in all of us. That is, the FEELINGS of the newborn child. Innocence.

"Let the little children come unto me, for of such is the kingdom of heaven (and earth)." – Jesus (my parentheses)

The next week I find myself showing more respect for Denali, my five-year old granddaughter, when at the dinner table with other family members, she cries to have a chair instead of sitting on her mother's lap. Tone, Denali's mother's partner, did not want me to give in to her request, her tears, yet Denali deserves to have her needs or wishes met as much as adults do. As Denali said, "It's not fair." And it's not, that adults get more respect than children do. This incident demonstrates how my growing self-respect spills over to respecting children as equals, as important! As noticing on June 12, 1999 when I masturbated, saying something like 'love god, or loves me,' as I orgasmed. I had the unusual occurrence of an easy second orgasm, not needing it, just wanting it. Just loving mySelf.

On June 23rd, I masturbated just because I felt like having a beautiful feeling, and that's what I said when I orgasmed, "your're beautiful." But then, I could not go to sleep from 3:30 to 4:30am, which was unusual while not having interactions with Gregory, which have so often triggered me into my past pain. Yet, I was still grieving him, and his Plenty, but not his act out of wanting infidelity, where true intimacy is avoided. Infidelities are a way of using sex to avoid being close to one's pain. The pain cannot be let go of because it is not connected to its childhood source. (*Getting the Love You Want* is an excellent book by Harville Hendrix that can show you the way)

In August, I am aware that I have the possibility and desire for sexual liasons with Rosey and Alain, but I do not want long-term relationships with them because of their lack of desire to be more deeply connected to themselves, to their vulnerable feelings. I feel less need to be with them sexually, then ask myself, why not be able to have the harmonious balance of being connected and held? It is about me being able to be alone with my vulnerable feelings and not avoid them by acting out sexually. Not only do I have the chance to let go of more of my childhood pain while being alone – I must be alone to feel my aloneness – and immediately, after crying, I feel more compassionate for those around me that are lonely and alone. I need sex less and less outside the experience of a loving connection, with a man, or with mySelf. It's a beautiful circle of LOVE.

Simultaneously, I'm noticing myself creating more frequent direct eye contact. I've always looked at people in the face with sporadic eye contact but it is not steady, except with lovers, or little children – isn't that interesting? The true lover is the child! Another noticeable change is that I am wearing dresses more frequently not just while dancing. It's the softer, vulnerable side of me coming out in other areas of my life. Not just as the uninhibited child on the dance floor. Dresses are more exposing than pants. More skin. KIN☺ (remove the 's') Until my recent exposure through tears, connected to my inner child, my process could be analgous to meditation quieting the mind, but not necessarialy opening the heart.

At a waterfall in Vermont, I'm struck by the power and gentleness of water. It is the essence of life, more than blood, for without water blood cannot exist. It is easy to make the connection with the power of tears, which are water. We cannot fully love without them.

Surprisingly, in Victorian times, they made a tiny sterling-silver-over-glass vessel about the size of a foxglove blossom, called a "lachrymatory." A tiny jar of teardrops. In olden days it was one of the greatest gifts you could give someone. It meant you loved them, that you shared a grief that brought you together. It is what I would like to give to my daughters. I wish my thirty-year-old daughter, Erin, who has not told me she loves me for 12 years, would share her tears of hurt with me. Then, the gift giver and receiver, she and I, could mix our tears in the lachrymatory vial. I wish the same with Megan, my twenty-seven-year old daughter, who tells me, "I love you," on a weekly basis over the phone. I know our tears seal our love like a lock on a strongbox.

On my 1999 birthday I received the most unique gift! I was on vacation in Boulder, Colorado and had left more than one message on Gregory Ruth's message machine, a boyfriend from the 1970s. We had met while walking up Buffalo Street, in Ithaca, NY, after he said, "what beautiful legs," as he walked up behind me.

I had called Gregory's number and found it busy. I wanted to catch him before he went to work. Over the weekend, I had left a couple messages on his answering machine. It was just before 9am, when I called again, and after a few rings, Gregory's voice rang through to me like an echo traveling through the grand canyon of time. I hadn't heard his voice in over 25 years but easily recognized it. He readily took the morning off work and we met fifteen minutes later. I lit up like a sparkler.

He drove me to Boulder's city park where we walked for most of four hours, stopping for a lemonade while continuing our non-stop conversation.

Two things surprised me during our time together: within fifteen minutes of our walk, Gregory took my hand without hesitation. Firmly as a parent holds their child's hand, with love. Although Gregory wears his shiny fifteen-year wedding ring, reflecting his obvious pride of wife and two children, he shares his connection with me with his hands and heart. I'm crying as I write, remembering the lack of fear he showed, as well as his love and respect for his family. My sadness is for all the time I felt disconnected from Love due to fear I grew up with: to express my feelings with my voice, and subsequently with my hands. I could not show affection to the father I loved dearly from early on, due to stringent religious oppression opposing the body's need for touch, to express love fully! That may give rise to some sexual feelings. (I remember my mother telling my father not to walk around in his pajamas, to wear a bathrobe, although his pajamas were loose and revealed none of his body's shape.) Not even a close hug is innocent.

But not true for the last hug Gregory Ruth gave me as we said goodbye. Then, the second surprise. He took a few steps toward his car, then turned around and said clearly as a bell, "I love you," and of course I cried, as I am this very minute. I replied with ease, "I love you, too," tears underlining the truth: over and over I cry for the lost love for the child inside of me. Over and over I cry for the loss of being too afraid to say out loud, "I love you, daddy." Tears validate so intensely, like many exclamation points at the end of a sentence, how inadequately we love!! (I want to remind the reader that the tears do lessen over time, as the well of pain is drained off.)

I love you, Gregory Ruth, for taking that chance to <u>say</u> your feelings to me, and understanding how important (tears again) that is after we had talked about not saying it to our parents. That writing is NOT ENOUGH – it is too disconnected – it reflects the distance, the fear to say it – face-to-face, eye-to-eye. And real love casts out fear.

The next day, when waking up in my tent at Bear Lake in Rocky Mountain National Park, an hour from Boulder, I felt like masturbating with thoughts of Gregory Ruth, and his previous day's description of his daughter's birth, afterwards in intensive care for a short time. How she gripped his pinky finger, and opened her cloudy-blue eyes to him, where he saw "the galaxies, the wisdom, the serenity" of all time. And I added, "the innocence." Isn't this pure spirituality as seen in the unconditional love of a child given through their eyes? It reminded me of my husband Gregory Race's statement of how looking into his daughter's eyes at her birth was the greatest day of his life. Why is it that childbirth is the "greatest" day of our lives?

In April of 2001, after making love with Jack, I said, "It's hard to think of anything being more wonderful than making love," and paused, thinking to my self 'childbirth,' when Jack piped in, "Childbirth." And I added, "Just what I was thinking, and maybe playing with babies because they look directly into your eyes and give you unconditional love!"

Until we scare it out of them. Which is what is done to most of us while growing up. And when I masturbated thinking of Gregory Ruth, feeling our love for each other, after I climaxed, I cried while saying, "I'm sorry I haven't loved you more freely." Of course, that is about not freely loving mySelf first and then the resultant inability to give love freely. Gregory Ruth remembered how frustrated he was when we tried to make love in the 1970s and I was resisting having intercourse. We never did, and I loved him! I felt too guilty, due to my religious beliefs. Damn it!

I also remember how excited my speech became in telling Gregory Ruth how wonderful it is to make love when the physical, emotional, and spiritual connections are all there. "And I will have that someday!" Gregory agreed with me and has been faithful to his wife, not interested in other women other than to make eyes at college girls sunbathing in the park. He says he totally understands how one can be attracted to the beauty of others without wanting or feeling the need to be sexual with them. What a great counterpoint to Gregory. Yes, it is healthier to love freely, not to have sex freely. The spiritual "comes" when Love and sex become one and the same. Like crying as I said, "I'm more real now, more WHOLE, than in the 1970s and 80s. My feelings and thoughts are becoming more connected. Maybe more ONE and the saME."

In the early fall of 1999, I am aware that I have less need to masturbate even when I am awake for a half hour in the mornings before I rise out of bed. I still masturbate once or twice a week; it seems more to keep my body in tune – like a piano needing to be kept in tune. Like staying in shape with yoga stretches every morning, and running or walking three times a week. What is in use remains better functioning.

Now that I can be in my spiritual journey, having given up religious repression in 1984, I can and do inquire about my present relationships as to whether I have connections with them from past lives. I have done several regressions where I find my father has been with me in different lifetimes. I was curious as to my strong connection to Gregory Ruth, so I regressed myself to a time where I am a native American woman, not wanting to marry a man that I have been arranged to marry. I find myself sad, because my feelings are not being taken into consideration. Gregory Ruth, in this previous life, says he's sorry that he forced me into marriage, that he loves me still and wishes I loved him. Then, I sob. I couldn't love mySelf because of the church religion. I couldn't love mySelf so I could love him. And it showed in my present life's behavior, pushing him away from having intercourse, although in my heart I wanted it. I felt love for him! "I haven't learned to love mySelf yet" stimulated heavy tears, like a train engine building up a head of steam as it travels faster and faster. Religion had prevented my spirituality – to feel worthy of love – and my expresion of sexuality. My thoughts connected immediately to why I never give up looking for Real Love because my spirit is so strong it needs to find itSelf, as a WHOLE.

Love is connected with my need to dance, as well. Religion wouldn't permit me to dance. (Still, moderate muslims don't permit dancing.) I was told it is too "worldly" and leads to physical closeness and sexual temptation with men. Where, I now know, my spirit can be expressed more freely.

It wasn't until my fourth marriage that I could dance at my wedding. And now I cry in saying that I wanted to dance with my father. When I dance, I am closest to the little girl in me; that is where and why I want daddy to see me for who I really AM! "That's what dancing is all about for me – a possibility for being yourself." I cried in this September 1999 session while saying the church crushed me; and sobbed "god has forsaken me! And that's the god's honest truth, or I wouldn't be crying so much!" as I say those four words.

Before, I felt good and loved because a man loved me. Now, the foundation of love comes from me loving me, so I can give love more fully to a man, or any other person, animal or tree.

One October day in 1999, a radio-TV marketer asks me to advertise, "expert claims that crying will save your life." I write in my journal that that would be too hard to prove, and I guess I'm a bit mistrusting and afraid I will "lose my life" by having others demand too much of me. Isn't that a CORE feeling, I ask myself. The little girl's spirit was crushed by the demand to believe in a certain dogmatic way – my spirit's own truth could hardly be heard through the fear that I might not be loved. I spontaneously underlined the word "spirit" as I wrote, "The spirit within me is found through feeling! Crying! So automatic is the underlining, without thought! Spontaneous! That is the voice of my spirit that I could not hear as a child because I needed my parent's "love" for survival – the spirit's voice that I could not follow as a teenager into my sexuality."

I did not even know what masturbation was as a teenager. And now in the fall of my life as I orgasm more easily and freely, I'm saying as I climax "love me," and "in me." The emphasis is mySelf loving me, and mySelf in me! It is a different kind of feeling than having to get the love from someone else. It is like being the bulb of a tulip, and not the fertilizer or the soil. It's like the daisy that can reseed itself, and does not need the sower, just the gentle loving moist soil of Mother Earth in which to grow safely, being nurtured into my Self. It's that same Spirit that helps us remember if we take time to listen.

For a week, I had searched for my lost camera. Finally, on Friday night, before sleeping, I asked for the memory to find my camera. Being relaxed and focused, within a minute the answer came to me – in the little pack on the back of my bicycle. Wow! If you give room for the spirit's voice to speak, you can listen – and soon have your intuitive truth!

By thanksgiving 1999, I am aware that I am no longer running to a man to soothe my loneliness. Instead I am crying. I could be in Alain's arms, but I choose not to. I choose to take the time to listen to my feelings. FEEL them. Just like when I take the time to look at a photo of me as a toddler, a long look! I connect to that child inside of me, and I cry. I let go of more pain. Then, my spirit can fly higher. "THE PEOPLE WHO SEE YOU FOR WHO YOU REALLY ARE – ARE THE ONES WHO <u>REAL</u>LY LOVE YOU! WISDOM FROM TEARS!" I cry with my sister, Constance. "**In liberating our tears, we liberate our fears!**"

The sweet pain of sadness is ever more evident as I cry at orgasm. It is as if I am be"com"ing more whole. And interestingly, we look for that "hole" during intercourse. A man's penis fills the hole called a vagina. Connecting physically with another person so that we can feel the ecstasy of orgasm, many times substitutes for the ecstasy of LOVE our hearts (spirits) are searching for. How many times do we hear of couples having great sex after they fight? Somehow they have expressed important feelings, whereby they feel closer and want to become one. This isn't necessarily healthy if the fight is repeated over and over again and it becomes the usual way they connect. But it is a demonstration of the spirit's drive to learn how to love. Through <u>expressing</u> feelings. As most of us have experienced, shut-down feelings produce distance and depression.

There is the complementary reaction as well, where couples refuse to connect sexually because they fight. The anger and rage separates them, because they are not able to resolve their hurt that the anger covers up. At this point in my journey, I am not quite ready to give up "making love" with Alain, even though my dear friend Susanne is beginning to be sexual with Alain as well. After a dance, we made love satisfactorily, but I'm not satisfied emotionally, or physically. I asked Alain how he felt about "sleeping" with both of us. He replied nonchalantly, "Fine." I didn't pursue it; I'm tired of pursuing his feelings. I let a long silence elapse on the phone after telling Alain I am sad about my official divorce. No response from Alain. Static.

He does notice that I am wet when we make love, and is surprised because I have not had a period for over a year due to menopause. And even now in 2001, another year and a half later, I am still juicy when aroused. I give credit to my tears, which keep my fluids flowing, not backed up by the dam of pain. (I take no hormone replacement or supplements of any kind.)

I believe Alain's difficulty in achieving orgasm portrays his lack of connection with himself. I was slightly irritated that after we went to sleep around 1:30am, he woke me up around 3am, with intercourse again, and still he didn't climax. I was too tired to give, and if he can't ask more clearly how he wants me to help, that's sad. I am not responsible for his orgasm, although it would make me feel good to give that to him. Evidences of the disconnection between partners trying to learn to LOVE. If one is growing into the soil of feelings and the other is in the rocks of defendedness (or defensiveness)…one flowers and the other wilts.

As winter finds spring, my orgasms are less and less frozen in the past. I find my self "CRYIN' OUT LOUD." As I orgasm I am cryin' out, "loving me, loving me." Near this same time, I find myself crying in my session most intensely when I say the word, "exposed." Exposing my foibles, vulnerabilities, my true feelings! And that is the same as the exposure of orgasm. The total letting go of control…the moment of exposure to the divine within! Your heart and soul, even if only for a few seconds. "I am actually happy that I have a broken heart…I am broken open!" I say and cry simultaneously.

Exposed

That I hate being like my mother
With many 200 pounds of padding, fat,
Insulating you from yourself,
And that, I could have sat
On your lap,
Feeling your belly softness,
Suckling your breasts,
This silence never rests.
I've never seen you nude
I could intrude,
Once seen you run from the bathroom,
Towel around you; quick get the broom –
Sweep up armpits, buttock's cracks,
Pubic hair, even navel pregnancy tracks –
Never had to raise your arms to fix long hair,
Always short hair exposing pained face,
Large lips protruding,
Eyes closed
No feelings for me, not even a trace.
"I can't love myself," you say.
"If only I could help you," I pray.
So now I shy away from fat people
They bring back the pain –
kept away from your body and heart

> And now I cannot feign
> How I need you, to
> Remove the towel-
> <u>I'll</u> hang around you, awhile.
> —*July 1996*

Now, I readily connect with my 'dead' Daddy, thinking of how grand his love is for me. Love, large as a sunflower seed, not small as a mustard seed. As I cry I feel greater gratefulness…greater love for him. "Now, I can't tell you enough how much I love you, and wish I had told you face to face."

By New Year's 2000, I have completely let go of Alain. I can bear the aloneness. As I cry, "I want more for you, Susanne" (than a relationship with Alain who still smokes); I know I am crying for mySelf, as Elizabeth Kubler-Ross says, "**When we cry, it is always for ourselves.**" As I express the more difficult confrontations to Susanne, I confront my own fears of her rejecting me. While doing this same emotional work, she breaks through her irritation as well, and says, "I have oceans of love for you." Spontaneously, the tears flow like fingers over silk. I know deep within my sternum that oceans of tears become oceans of love. Letting go of money and material thing's importance has been a parallel process with the letting go of tears. Truly, tears replace more than fears!

And more light comes into my home, literally. I have lived in a home surrounded by trees since 1988. My first year there, I chain-sawed down one tree blocking my view from the living room deck. It wasn't until 1997, after I returned from the Primal Center in California, that the other hemlock at the corner of the deck had to go! Along with a couple of cherry trees too close to the house. Then, the following year, I had six more trees taken down that were leaning toward the house, one shading the opposite deck off of my bedroom. Weekly, I cried out past pain, allowing more room for light to enter my heart. I no longer needed the close protection of trees. I needed a greater expansive view, and sunlight shining into my windows amidst my forest of trees. In the spring of 2001, I sold my house, and now live in an apartment with a big view overlooking a wide green valley. Great light! Open view of tree tops, inclusive of the sky and the greater universe! Even a clothes(close)line on which to expose my laundry☺ And I live next door to my favorite park where there are many trees and waterfalls that I love and which love me.

Loving my increased eye contact as well. Steady. As I am more and more in contact with my deep feelings of sadness, (<u>bawl</u>ing) I am increasingly present with my Self, and therefore other's eye<u>ball</u>s☺

And do you notice my wish to mix humor in as I heal my emotional pain? I write in my journal near Christmas 1999, that a "few lighthearted flakes of fluff are falling, jumping, skipping to the ground as if having a party, maybe joyful.

And although I cannot say I am always joyful, I am content; sorta like my message machine saying, "white snowflakes make the nights lighter." In a December crying session, I find myself returning to a retrieved memory of myself as a little girl. Maybe I'm two, sitting at my bedroom window waiting for my father to come home because I do not feel safe with my mother. Although I had repressed it, I now know I was afraid of her. I felt like I had spent a lot of time alone in my crib. I'm sobbing as I say that last sentence. And, "How could you mom?" More sobs. "How could you let me cry and cry and cry?" I see mySelf in the crib, and she doesn't come and she ignores me. How could you be so cruel? (Refer to Aletha Solter's book where you let children cry while you HOLD them, *TEARS AND TANTRUMS*) While crying I connect my pain with why I've been sexual with Alain when really my heart does not want to. I am just soothing my childhood pain. Unwanted by my mother. Left alone by my mother. And luckily for me, I felt daddy wanted to be with me (like Alain.) I miss daddy greatly, and my present tears tell me so in loud sobbing truth!

I feel the sobs roll up my chest through my solar plexus like pressure that needs to be released from a pressure cooker. Held inside me all these years – like in all of us, unconscious, yet acted out in our everyday search for love. No wonder I react with anger when I hear the word "fuck." It is hostile, and demeaning, I hate the word; it is close to being assaultive. It is another way people cover up their hurt, their vulnerable hearts that "come" close to being unhardened when they have sex, and let go with an orgasm. No wonder there are many sex addicts in our society – that Hollywood and marketing make sex the center of our attention. Wake up, World, to the primary avenue to the divine within us all. I wish everybody could wake up to the tears that take us to true love!

"CRYING MAKES ME HAPPY!" my male Bangladesh, former muslim client said one day. As my daughter, Megan, told me at Christmas, "You want people to be vulnerable so there is more compassion for one another." She told me that this is how she said it to her dad. WhoopeeJ

It is now the first day of the new Millennium! I am reminded of the awesome feeling I had the other day as Canada geese flew over my A-frame, directly over. I watched one or two geese come out of formation from the rear to the front as if to say, "It's my turn to lead." I felt that need to lead within mySelf. Also, I was amazed that there was so much honking while flying – do they ever fly in silence? Do their throats get sore, maybe only when their wings get tired? They are quiet when grounded.

Like I am usually silent when I dance. Talking distracts me from feeling my body and how it is sensing itself. I notice I smile a lot while I dance, which others don't seem to do as much. I like that I connect readily with childlikeness, that I am free to express much spirit, whether in creative patterns or spontaneous moves. Like the Canada geese, or the water that flows beneath the ice! I don't believe a waterfall like Yosemite Falls ever stops. Is that why we are drawn to powerful waterfalls? There is always a flow underneath, like the spirit in my heart no matter how icy the defense becomes. My spirit flies more like the Canada goose as long as my tears continue to flow. My tears have helped me to go more "with the flow," be less controlling, as they do away with more and more fears – that is why I love them so. I just spontaneously smiled☺

Even in orgasm…my healing tears make my orgasm reach new heights, orgasm vocalizations honking as loudly as the Canada geese. Heart work – heard in my expanding orgasms. Tears gain more respect for mySelf, wanting more for mySelf, therefore not needing to have sex with Alain anymore, when my spirit is saying down deep, "I don't really want to." I no longer have to act out the pain of my mother not wanting me. As I cry at the beginning of the new millennium, choosing not to spend New Year's Eve with Alain, an idea "comes" to me. I will light a candle daily as a metaphor for the greater light in my life, begun with the small enduring flame of love from my father. All the ice around my heart is breaking up because of you, Daddy. Because of the tears I began to shed with Gregory. The sobs I wish I could have cried with you daddy!

There was something wrong with our hearts because we did not listen to them – the wee small voice of our spirit! You had a fatal heart attack. No wonder I had frequent earaches as a child, throughout growing up and the pregnancy of my second daughter, Megan. No wonder I had laryngitis every year until 1996. No wonder I was stuffed up with colds 3-4 times a year until 1994. No wonder the Mourning Glory is my favorite flower.

Hold on now – I even notice how there is more light in my life "coming" from my silverware! Sure, go ahead and laugh, I am☺ Three of my spoons had to be replaced because a housemate lost them, therefore they are shinier because they are newer. I prefer to use them because of the light they reflect. Also, I find myself selecting a different knife to use each morning as I spread butter on my bagel. There are eight knives piled on top of each other in the silver ware tray. I use a different knife each day, pulled from the bottom of the pile. I'm giving each knife a chance to be useful, a chance to be recognized☺ I usually use the same two or three bowls for ice cream: the blue which stands for the color of truth, the green one for the color of love and growth. I am smiling with the reader, to think of these connections being so silly. So what? I am the "silly goose" that I used to call my children, and now my grandchild, when we are having fun! This is the "light"- heartedness we all enjoy about life. Everything is connected – all ONE.

And I know this to be true because when I sobbed in my weekly crying session about the shiny spoons and silverware, I connected those tears with the feeling of being less important than the people around me, and the song, "This Little Light of Mine," I'm going to let it shine. Only, I could not let my light shine because I felt so unworthy of love, the message from birth, carried throughout growing up from the church's dogma, even the church song, "I am Not Worthy." The CORE pain of my life.

Shame (of Self) keeps all of our true hearts hidden, most blantantly, our sexual beings, which then causes us to act out sexually, as I did most pointedly with Gregory. I am pushing through my fear in this moment to write about my most embarrassing act out. As I have written previously, Gregory, out of his childhood pain, wanted me to not only be sexual with other men, but also come home and tell him about it, which would turn him on, and then he could call me a whore. Also, he thought the pornographic industry had its place in helping us free ourselves up sexually as a society although he did not think it was totally healthy. Still, in need of money, he thought it would be okay for me to be an "escort" or model for "soft porn" magazines. Being as naïve as I was, I decided I could model nude for magazines that were in good taste.

Gregory drove me to two interviews, and at the second, I knew I was in the wrong place! The second interview was especially **demean**ing. It was in a darkly lit office, a room that reeked of cigarettes smoked by poorly-cared-for youths. Attractive, while lonely. My heart was gripped with sadness as I signed in and gave them my driver's license to copy as a sign of their legally operated business.

After my nude photos were taken, a woman showed me some magazines that my picture would be displayed in: one was of small-breasted women that smacked only of objectifying sex. I was disgusted and left with shame covering me like the thick cloud of smoke suffocating that office. Once in the car with Gregory, he said, "I'm proud of you." I'll never forget those words. I replied with something like "I'm not proud of myself at all and I won't be a part of pornograpghy no matter in what light you see it." I had to endure his disapproval and anger but I was already becoming stronger in my own truth and knew I had to trust mySelf and feel the pain of his emotional abandonment.

Pain can be an avenue of enlightenment: transformed by tears. I noticed how the word "sob" is the abbreviation for "short of breath" and also "son of a bitch." Shortness of breath is the physical reaction to FEAR. Son of a bitch is the physical (vocal) expression of RAGE. Or anger – notice that when anger's letters are rearranged, they spell rage'n☺ See all the connections? Even in our language! It excites me to integrate all these aspects of life, and the way I have been able to do this is by weeping – tears that connect to our core pain. Not being adequately loved. Not just crying in the daily present situations.

How I have strayed from my theme of the 'sexual spirit joining with the spiritual orgasm'? (I love that phrase) I really haven't because the sexual and spiritual are the two foundational rungs of the ladder that climbs (and claims) all the combinations that make up the universe. In my crying session on January 13, 2000, I went to a memory of my mother holding a paint stick in her hand. I began sobbing as I saw her spank me so I wouldn't cry. She warned me, "If you cry, I'll hit you." In May 2001, I found mySelf crying as I read this journal entry. I wanted to go outside and pick the "Bleeding Hearts" waving their bright pink flower-hearts at me. Like the pink-heart of my clitoral masturbation that comes to an all-body exhilaration of love. It is like all of my body cells are alive with a low-volt level of electricity – a time-lapse photography of beauty flowering throughout my cells, as I say "Inside Me," at orgasm. Tears connected that form "Inside Me" not as a penis, but as "love" inside Me.

"Tears may be dried up, but the heart never," said Marguerite De Valois (1553-1615), French princess and scholar. But love is dried up and limited without tears which want to flow readily.

Like the tears that flowed as I spoke on the phone to Alain, in January 2000. He was telling me how difficult it was for him to draw up a will, and divide his assets between his two daughters. Mostly, I listened, except to say that these difficulties are here to teach us – to learn about what is truly important in life. He tells me how his dishonest clients make it hard for him to trust as he would like to. I cited the three months that Gregory told me lies about being sexual with several women, admitting later that he was trying to manipulate me into feeling free to be sexual with other men. That experience taught me to be more realistically trusting but still, I am basically trusting (more in mySelf), and I like that because trust is necesssary in order to REALly Love. I began to cry as I said that last sentence, and more tears ran free as Alain said he was glad I came into his life because he has learned so much from me. I **really** cried as I said how much I appreciated him saying that because when I tally up what he has given me materially, I cannot compete; but I feel I've given a lot to him emotionally and that can't be measured with money. He agreed. His acknowledgement was a surprise gift to me. I knew in part, that I was crying out old pain, not being appreciated by my mother and somewhat by my father, for the real Me. Partly I was crying in the present because I had rarely heard Alain appreciate me with his words. Those words of love, love I had tried to get by being sexual with him.

part three

◊

EVOLution of an Orgasm as

Peace of the Divine

The SEASON of SUMMER...2000–2001

LOVE, that I am still longing for from my mother. January 2000, I was being interviewed on public radio, about my first book, *TEARS ARE TRUTH...waiting to be spoken*. I was surprised to hear myself say, "I love you, mom," on the air. I was pleased and proud of my spontaneity, revealing how my tears have healed the deep wound of my mother not wanting or loving me. Inside of me, those three special words were held in silence for fifty years, in contrast to me saying them often to my children and friends. Those three special words, that I long to hear from my mother before she dies. She's actually admitted that I probably will not hear them. Yet, she says, "I love you," to my children and siblings. She's a born again christian whose heart is still filled with guilt and shame to have given her illegitimate child my name. It is her 'god' that says I am "unworthy of his love," heard my whole life growing up, my CORE, CORE pain, for which millions of tears have been shed, tears which healed me like much needed rain after a long drought. How can a child not be devastated in his or her spirit, hearing that message at least three times a week while attending church services?

In a crying session that same January, I am sobbing as I say that I hope that my mother tells me that she loves me before she dies. "I want you to tell me that so much; it would be wonderful if you could." I also talk about having lunch with my mother and Erin, my oldest daughter, when I asked my mother what I was like as a baby. She said that I didn't cry; now I am kicking and sobbing as I say those words devastating to my spirit. "Oh god! Oh god...where are you?" I learned early on not to cry and remember whispering to Erin, "I was probably depressed, because mom didn't want me." In contrast to Erin, who was very wanted and planned, and slept quietly for a positive reason. I slept quietly for a negative one. I'd given up.

"Oh Susanne, that hurts so much that I couldn't cry. My heart hurts; I had a broken heart in the womb." Physically, I could feel a huge hurt right over my heart, creeping up into my throat, like a steamroller bearing down on a tarbaby. My tears streamed as I said, "I love my father, 'cause he pulled me out from being a baby who couldn't cry...amazing with how much of this pain is inside me...crying all these tears that I couldn't cry before." My connected-to-childhood-pain tears have "saved" me, beginning with the seed of my father's love. So now I can love my mother, genuinely, while not feeling or hearing it in return.

And I can love more of my Self, like I did on a snowy morning, when I masturbated into a yummy orgasm, saying, "Oh my god," then, "I love you, Dianea." It's truly an evolving through the river of tears to loving oneself - the god within us all – the divine. Wouldn't "Divine" be a beautiful child's name?

Early 2000, I am aware that I masturbate once or twice a week not because I need to, but because I want to. It is no longer done to alleviate anxiety (fear) or as a sedative before sleep. It's a beautiful way to feel me loving my spirit, a present wrapped with the bows of sex and spirit.

I am not the whole package yet, as my meeting with Cipriam, my first lover of the new millennium, would teach me. I want to scream for joy – it's really happening. I am wearing a gray long-sleeved jumpsuit that flatters my small breasts and well-rounded butt in a 5'9" slender frame as I dance at a birthday party - a party I almost pooped out on due to the snowy night and it being 10PM on a Monday.

After a few swing dances I notice a tall, dark-brown-eyed man dancing by himself and I'm instantly attracted like a squirrel to a walnut. He handsomely showed off his husky broad shoulders, gracefully outlined in a loosely fitted white sweater. So rarely do I feel this magnetism. I join his gyrations, our eyes now connected in a dance of their own. Gigantic mutual attraction! But, he is too young.

That does not deter Cipriam from taking my hand and dancing with our bodies together. I can feel his delicious muscular back and shoulders with my dancing fingers. The electricity is crackling as he dips me into a loving oblivion. Our conversation reveals that he is a friend of the birthday boy's Romanian wife.

Maybe I can trust that he means what he says: "You're the most beautiful woman I've met in the USA, it's true," he repeats again later. He's a Romanian Cornell graduate student, here only four months.

As I sit, exchanging my dancing shoes for boots, Cipriam squats down and asks, "Can I tie those up for you?" So caring, so attentive, making it all feel more like love than a sexual attraction. "Can I walk you to your car?" makes my heart pound even harder, knowing kisses will mix with snowflakes. As I sit in my Jeep, the door open as I search for my keys, Cipriam French kisses me, which feels invasive, an intimacy that we have not yet entered. I stand up and take courage to say something I would not have dared to before this year. Maybe I feel like a green leaf turning red.

"May I show you how I like to be kissed?" I venture as a snowflake lands on my eyelash. My heart stops as our lips join passionately, tenderly. Writing this in my journal, I caressed tears of missing my mother's holding and tender kisses. Then, these two events became connected like the universe then having an orgasm of snowflakes hanging onto our hair and jackets. Tears now paint the picture of nature, love, pain, - all being connected.

As I drove away, I knew Cipriam wanted to "come" home with me. Without drinking, I was high as a rainbow when I arrived home, I could not sleep. I touched myself, unfolding a beautiful orgasm, imagining Cipriam's body all over me. That was not enough. Fifteen minutes later I orgasmed another smooth wave throughout my body. An hour later, another full-bodied orgasm. The next day when I told Cipriam about my orgasms while talking on the phone, he said I should have called him. But, I want to know him better before we make love, and not have just sex. I'm happy with myself, having not needed him so much that I acted out a one-night stand. Sex – not love. Unconnected, like I have been from mySelf, to my true feelings, all-my-growing-up. Unconnected to my true heart, where the divine IS!

It felt good not to be so needy of Cipriam's attention and still know that he wanted me, unlike (trying to make up for) my mother not wanting me. On Tuesday we talked for over an hour on the phone, Cipriam saying he wanted to see me that night. I said "No." To know, know, know you, is to make love with you. I want that loving-spiritual connection. I want to make spiritually sexy love, or is it that I want to connect with my sexually loving spirit? I suggested that we have dinner the next evening, before I left on a trip to Hawaii.

As I was stepping out of the car in front of Danos Restaurant, Cipriam picked me up like a bride (I wrote 'bridge' first☺) and carried me over the snow to the sidewalk. I was in lalaland to say the most. Could I be falling in love? It'd been so long ago. He's twenty-six and I'm fifty-three. His friend had told him that I was a grandmother before he met me! What are the bridges, here? "Maybe we are soul mates," said Cipriam, the first night we laid eyes on each other.

We shared about our families while eating our elegant dinner. Me eating; he watching me. I dribbled tears as I related how dad loved me and wanted me as much as his biological children. Cipriam asked several times how I felt about him, our dancing. I liked how he knew what he wanted and yet asked respectfully about what I wanted.

I wanted to touch and kiss and sleep together without intercourse and he said he could do that. It happened that way for maybe an hour but I knew I was giving in to the moment. Cipriam was too irresistible naked.

While his muscles were making some kind of love over me, he said, "Talk to me. Tell me what you are feeling." Like wow, I'm usually the one to say that! I felt very charged, up and down my spine, a force that overpowered at times, grazing that pleasure-pain edge. Like tears that relieve pain, I am happy.

When Cipriam orgasmed, it was without me really **knowing** it. Like I didn't know him. Or enough of Me. He said that he screams inside, and that he hasn't cried since he was fourteen, and that he wonders about it. So do I.

In flight to Hawaii, I had a stop over in San Francisco where I stayed in a Ramada Inn. Asleep by 10 PM, I awoke near 6 AM, thinking about Cipriam, and although I did not awaken feeling aroused, I desired to make love with him and when I climaxed, I was saying, "I want *it* just for you." 'It' meant LOVE.

Even though I was thinking only of wanting love and making love with Cipriam, I began to cry, sobs punctuating connected-feelings of needing love for the little girl inside me, not adequately loved as a child. I knew I was crying for my Self – not just missing Cipriam – it was about missing Love. He'd given me the best love that I had experienced, as beginnings go. I was a green leaf beginning to turn red. With maturing Love.

I guess I was a bit afraid to say 'love', knowing I'd want 'it' even more from Cipriam, but then again, that is the reflection of our lifetime, wanting and creating more and more love for ourselves, so we can give it more fully to others. A beautiful circle that a wedding ring symbolizes. The oneness of us all bound in Love.

During lovemaking Cipriam told me, "You're a giver." I cried when I wrote that in my journal because I have given too much, given up mySelf (feelings and beliefs) all my life in order to get Love. It has always fallen short of the real thing, now I realize it is our human journey to **evol**ve toward Real **Love.** I want to feel Love into infinity, that length and depth that makes love intensely beautiful. The spectrum, the prism of ever changing sparkling colors that become refracted and reflected by the water of tears, like the rainbow I saw fall into the ocean's depths off New Zealand. Love that deep.

Cipriam said he was jealous of Ken, a friend I would visit for a week in Hawaii, that I might be sexual with him. If Cipriam had not come into my life, I might have succumbed to Ken's big blue eyes, his attentions, or his erections. But my heart was taken by a Romanian prince, sculpted like a Greek statute, symbolizing the beauty of body and soul, an "Oh, god." Desiring monogamy drives us to pursue a deeper, purer Love. It's about learning to be true to one's Self – to feel love for that one person – to love in the most meaningful rich way. It makes sense that the evolution of our soul would parallel our biological evolution. There are increasing numbers of monogamous animal pairs, as they become more complex beings up the evolutionary ladder. (swans, mallards, penguins, gorillas, etc.)

While swimming in the Pacific Ocean with Ken, I noticed how my body continues to heal as I cry out oceans of pain, the obstacle to creating optimum body health. Ken went swimming in a wet suit; me in a bikini. As I waded in, my body acclimated to the cold as usual, but what was different was my ability to stay in longer and then not need a towel when I came out into the windy sunshine. I have little body fat, to keep me warm, so my blood must be circulating better, as my body and hands stay warmer longer. No longer cold hands, warm heart. But, warmer hands, warmer heart☺

The heart that has been pained most by being taught by my religious mother and the church that "I am unworthy of (god's) love." It is what I cry most deeply about and why I cried when I was appreciated at the emotional release workshop that I attended my first week in Hawaii. During this meditation circle, I heard new things other than the usual appreciation of my openness and vulnerability. That I have a lightness about me, "as if I was ready to fly like an angel." It is great to know I spread this lightness and not just the heaviness of tears. That others see my happiness because of my tears. As my male Bangladesh muslim client says, "Crying makes me (us) happy."

Joyce and Barry Vissell, married 35 years, leaders of this "Opening of the Heart" workshop, drove us to Hawaii's Volcanic National park. It is an amazing natural phenomenom of fire meeting water! Like rage meeting tears. Feeling my rage has released any barriers to experiencing tears of grief after beginning emotional release work in 1993. Tears that easily came when Barry cupped my face in his hands, looking directly into my eyes (tears now), telling me how precious I am. Just what I look for when making love – to see the love in my partner's eyes – as I orgasm WITH love. Not just sex.

In another group setting with the Vissells I stood up and pushed through my fear and embarrassment to expose shamed parts of my body. Telling about my sagging butt and my breast implants made me cry for little Dianea not accepting her body as it is. Joyce and Barry suggested that I take off my clothes in front of the group so I could more fully let go of my shame. Though scared, I was willing to do that, when a group member spoke up saying that she had noticed my "seductiveness" with her husband. Tears arose spontaneously as I felt the hurt of her statement. I felt my innocence was being questioned, and I said so. I did not want to be sexual with any men there even though I felt attracted to them. My feelings were with Cipriam alone.

There were mixed feelings about me becoming naked in front of the whole group so Joyce suggested that those who wished to support me would go into a separate room. Four or five of the ten who joined me were men. As my clothes fell to the floor, I felt shame go with them. Several said what a beautiful body I have with sincerity that seeped under my skin and into my heart. Several women said it helped them break through to their feelings of shame. And a male member of the group also released his clothes, claiming more acceptance of his body.

Joyce voluntarily said that she had not seen any seductive behavior, which she is very aware of picking up, between me and her husband Barry or any other man at their workshops. I needed and appreciated that validation. The innocent tenderness of holding and kisses on the cheek is what my tears wanted - what I had needed from my mother and wanted mostly from the father I loved and mostly trusted my whole growing up. But even our love was a beginning love, due to the distance created by guarding our vulnerable, hurt feelings. Humans are far from experiencing the best ingredients for making love.

The Glass Door

Through it all –
I lived with you eighteen years,
All too short,
Like the eighteen-year-old threadbare jean shorts
I wear, ready to fall apart –
As I do now with tears, never safe between us.
The heat of Death Valley's Desert
Exchanged for winter's down jacket
Feeling snowflakes melting on my cheeks,
mixed with salty sorrow of death's distance.
A distance felt long before your death,
Unreachable as full moon shining over Germany and the USA.
No pictures of you holding me as a
Child, to memorialize my first love.
Not yours; you wanted me,
Like picking a neighbor's flower.
I returned your love, unable to reach you –
I'm elated to see you standing next to me
Throughout my wedding reception line, in 1969.
I stare at the photo, me kissing your cheek,
Holding your hand, your other large hand touching
My arm with gentle strength.
I cry seeing the large ray of sunlight
Flowing between our bodies; a glass door
I could never pass through.
—*January 1998*

"Making Love" is a phrase that we take for granted. It is that innocent child in all of us, who knows how to (make) love, wriggling for hugs and kisses, cuddling and holding, wanting to hold off intercourse so the child-spirit can FEEL love and not just sex.

The last day at the Vissell's workshop, I woke up near 5:30AM and wondered about masturbating, although I did not wake up sexually aroused. I thought about Cipriam's body and being and when I orgasmed, I said outloud, "I do know that I love you," as if speaking to Cipriam - but I knew that I was talking to little girl Dianea, who cried as I said that sentence: "I do know that I love you." Truly I am "coming" closer to loving my Self.

The poem I wrote that morning is:

Sunrise of Love

Drinking my own tears
Is dissolving all my fears
Of "you" not loving me.
As I stand at the edge of the sea,
My heart pounding with the breakers
I know I am no longer a faker
For "you" to love me.
Now accepting fully my body
Sagging buttocks, breasts not big,
The ocean's pure white foam is bubbling
"you" to embrace me.
As I walk closer, over lava sharp,
Spiked with blackened pain –
Red-hot coral rays leap across the sky
For "you" to lighten me.
Even the gray-white clouds have fingertips of pink
Outlining the possibility of love
For "you" to believe me –
When the orange-gold globe of the sun
Bursts over my ocean of hope,
To open my lips and say,
"THERE YOU ARE" -
Emptying another tear of love for me to drink in –
For "me" to love me. And you.

As the reader may have figured out already, Cipriam soon exited my life, sadly, on Valentine's Day, the week after I returned from Hawaii. Oh yes, he was excited to see me and after a dinner of pizza, we made sweet and bombastic love of the infatuation-sort. He was more forceful than I was used to or like, although I felt electric-sensations all through my body. We did touch each other all over, I gave him a foot massage, and sucked his toes. But I could not let go and have a full orgasm, my body could only feel waves, not the breaker. I needed more time, to be more of mySelf.

During our lovemaking, Cipriam asked, "When did you have the best sex?"
I had to think. I just wondered why he asked that, then.
I answered, finally, "the best is when I am in love with the man." No reply. We

talked a day later about telling our family members, "I love you." Although he says he is close to his parents, he does not tell them "I love you."

"You just know it, because you feel it," Cipriam adds.

"But, you've said you like to hear me scream when I orgasm, although you scream inside," I counter.

"I've told two different women, 'I love you,' when I was 18, then 23. I was betrayed by them, finding out they loved another."

He says that he has never told this to anyone before; he's never been so honest. We've only known each other three weeks. Barely. More nakedly than inwardly. He tells me not to fall in love with him because he does not want to feel the hurt or suffer by seeing me hurt. I tell him he is not responsible for my hurt as long as he is honest with me. It is a GOOD hurt – to be able to love…go on to greater and greater love.

So when Cipriam said we were to be just friends, because he is open to his old girlfriend from Romania being his girlfriend again when she comes to Cornell, I cry, knowing I want to be with him. I'm glad I've had this short intense time with Cipriam – to be so wanted. Feeling unwanted since birth is the real pain I am letting go of as I sob. I'm letting go of tears in order to heal, like a parent who allows their toddler to fall and pick themselves back up again.

It prepared me for Valentine's Day with my mother. This time, it is she that brings up the painful subject…usually it is me. She must be adjusting to the vulnerability that I expose on a regular basis when we talk. She is worried that I am "twisting" Connie's (my sister) mind so that she will no longer be a "born again" christian like my mother is. She says that I am "powerful." I'm stunned but ask how I got that power. She repeats, "You're a powerful person." And I reply, "from telling the vulnerable truth." She is crying at this point, and I'm surprised that I am not when she says that I am cruel and that she doesn't feel love for me. Nor am I angry. I'm calm as pepper on mashed potatoes, not wanting to hug her like soft butter would. I cannot feel close to her when she says I'm going to hell. Someday, I'll hug her despite her negative beliefs about me. I feel that from the enlivened spirit within me…the little voice that is becoming louder and louder, and I trust more and more.

The "little voice" that yelled and sobbed as I related this incident in my weekly crying session. While saying, "Mom said I was more loving when I was a "born again christian." Well, you're right, Mom; I was a phony then, and now I feel so hurt having had to pretend much of the time. It just about kills me, it hurts so much!" I banged my fist on the mattress and cried without words for several minutes, then said, "I feel so sad for that little girl who was brainwashed and **heartwashed**. I now can **feel** that pain." As I spoke, I was spontaneously rubbing my hand up and down my breast(heart)bone, massaging it like one would a sore muscle. "How they (rigid religious beliefs) pained and nearly crushed my heart-spirit!"

My spirit has tried to break free through my passion for dance. While attending a dance weekend in February 2000 I was walking with a woman, Amy, whom I met there. Amy and I quickly moved into a conversation about feelings, because I shared what I do and she is active in co-counseling, an international group that focuses on emotional discharge of feelings between lay-persons. She said that when she cries deeply it is as good as sex. I had not felt exactly that way but certainly I could relate to the release crying gives, like orgasm does in that total loss of control, being utterly vulnerable to oneself and another.

When I go dancing, I usually have various partners to dance with, having been a part of the Ithaca Swing Dance Network for a few years. But sometimes there are not enough leaders so I find myself dancing by myself, many times in a rather sexy outfit. In the spring of 2000, I am solo dancing to the rhythm and blues of the Purple Valley Band, a local swing dance favorite. The lead guitar player said I was driving the band crazy while dancing in a form fitting sparkling black dress. My sexual energy is imaging my spiritual energy – my spirit signing up for flying lessons –to be free like child's love. One of my favorite parts of dancing is being dipped by my partner because I am entrusted into the arms that can hold me out in full exposure of myself – my heart is OPEN. Arms stretched outward, head back, held, like in orgasm. Dance (especially waltzing) is like love flowing at its best. Many tears splashed as I spoke to Susanne, underlining the words "My heart is open." It is the greatest truth of all – my sadness over my heart having not been truly open due to the religious oppression of my vulnerable feelings. I had to feel and believe as my religion dictated. I love my tears for giving me my own 'spiritual' truth.

And new laughter. The mix of pain and joy, like buying a gallon of my favorite ice cream, "Death By Chocolate," and receiving the second gallon free. "Oh god, the more I cry, the more I laugh," I write in my journal. As Jack Kornfield writes in *The Path With Heart*, "Somehow, in feeling our pain and sorrow, our own ocean of tears, we come to know that ours is a shared pain and that the mystery and beauty of life cannot be separated." And the daffodils are up…and I'm daffy☺

Like in orgasm, awake at 4am and after an hour of twilight, floating between wakefulness and sleep, relaxed, I masturbated into a full body orgasm, skin raised in praise, my voice saying, "It is so beautiful." 'It' is ME.

At this point in 2000, I am still having hot flashes six to ten times per day, mainly while sleeping. No menstral flow for two years. Still, I am wet vaginally when I masturbate, and while making love. My lovers are surprised. I sense that I am more wet due to the outward flow of my pain through tears. That I do not need estrogen replacement therapy. My grandmother lived well without it. My mother tried it and it made her ankles swell, so she went without it. I have no inclination to try it. I trust my body to heal itself, unclog its pain through the flow of tears, so that I do not have to dry up vaginally. Dry up my voice, dry up my ability to love fully.

"True feeling justifies whatever it may cost." - May Sarton, American writer

This same spring I meet George on Match.com. We connect on many levels: parent, writer, craftsman, outdoorsman, and he has no problem admitting to his tears. He's light in coloring, not my preference, with broad shoulders, definitely my preference. I try him out and he falls in love with me. I love him, but cannot find the "in love" feeling. He talks to me of his worry that he cannot maintain an erection with me, although he wakes up with one like that of a fifteen year old. I make love with him with reticence, not caring if I have an orgasm, until after he talks to me about this vulnerable topic, and then I do orgasm. Some connection with intimacy is so obvious. The spirit in me is awakened to connect, to love. Like I connect to my tears each week and this week it was sobs with legs kicking: "I had to shut my heart off." As a child, I did not feel safe enough to cry when I needed to: to be aware that GOD in me is **crying** out to be recognized. It is the greatest pain of all!

Let me tell you the story of Sachi:

"Soon after her brother was born, little Sachi began to ask her parents to leave her alone with the new baby. They worried that like most four-year-olds, she might feel jealous and want to hit or shake him, so they said no. But she showed no signs of jealousy. She treated the baby with kindness and her pleas to be left alone with him became more urgent. They decided to allow it.

Elated, she went into the baby's room and shut the door, but it opened a crack – enough for her curious parents to peek in and listen. They saw little Sachi walk quietly up to her baby brother, put her face close to his and say quietly, "Baby, tell me what God feels like. I'm starting to forget."

—Dan Millman, *Chicken Soup for the Soul*

And now, Susanne, my weekly cryin' partner says that I am "the most joyful person she knows!" It is now seven years into my deeply felt letting go of pain. It is painfully clear that certain core themes are cried about over and over again. Also, I see the <u>intensity</u> of the tears is lessening from sobs to streams. Also, I notice in my journals, how I leave out words that are key to the core pain repressed inside me. Like, "I'm having to pay even closer ( ) to myself from this cold." I left out the word "attention" - a word that is used instead of love when we say an acting out child (trouble maker) is "doing it for attention." Ah yes, attention-getting is his or her need for LOVE.

Another sentence from my journal, " 'I'm sorry Larry (client),'" which pro-moted more tears from him. It was hard to contain my own – but he didn't realize, being into his own tears – it just emphasizes again – the trauma and pain my little ( ) has had to bear, and contain for way too long!" Can you fill in the missing word? Yes, it is 'girl.' **Attention** for the **girl** was not permitted in an emotional way, a feeling way, due to the need to feel and think what my mother and her religion said I should feel and believe. It's really out<u>rage</u>ously sad to recognize how the spirit of the child is repressed in all of us…yet it is the baby's and child's spirit that we all love, in our unenlightened way. Tears will bring that child's spirit back to us all…so much so that my mother now called me a "sweet lady" this past (2001) Thanksgiving although she still cannot say "I love you," to me.

But I can make love to mySelf as I did in April 2000, masturbating to orgasm on my back, my heart open to the universe, saying outloud, "Oh goodness gracious Me – Oh god" all rolled into One! And, why did I say that at orgasm?

My seven-year-old granddaughter, Denali, whose spirit has not been dampened like mine or her mother's, can answer that from her free-child wisdom which once came to me while we were playing a game of Parkology. She asked me how to spell "why." I replied, "That's the best question in the world! Why?" She replied, "To always ask why!" YES! A cute inter**play** of words, I think to myself. Later that day I told Denali that I was feeling better, as I was getting over a cold. She asked, "Does that mean I can kiss you anywhere?" Is that spirit, or what?

"Why?"

Toddlers constant cheer
Curiosity always near
So appealing
Yet exasperating

…is the search for Truth.

Why do I do what I do, why do I say what I say? Like I asked George when he used the word, "obscene" to describe the sounds that women's vaginas make at times while having intercourse.

Why obscene? I liken these sounds to the smacking of one's lips during or after a superb dinner.

This is a picture of how our perceptions of the world changes when we can truly connect the heart (feeling) with the head (thoughts.)

George and I had an interaction that clearly brought this home to me. I was discussing how oppressive religion is to the human spirit, and that it took me 38 years to get out. He said that he couldn't understand why it took me so long to get out when "you're a smart, bright woman." I cried as I said something like: "it's about the HEART – who couldn't feel truly, deeply for so long. You don't get that I was brain and therefore heartwashed as a child, unworthy of love, besides not being wanted by my mother. And, my father believed it as well. I couldn't risk losing my father – the only bit of love I knew."

"They broke my heart, you don't get it; I don't expect you to understand." I ran downstairs with tears running down my cheeks and a trace of anger on my lips. George followed me downstairs, and I said, "Don't touch me." Who wants to be comforted by someone who does not understand? When he said, "I'm sorry I hurt you," I could let him hold me. I tell you this, my reader, because it illustrates the division of head and heart so easily split when the tears have not washed away the barrier of pain between thoughts and feelings. This is the root cause for so many misunderstandings, so much of the hate in the world. And George adds, "You are amazingly non-judgmental." The cleansing pool of tears brings a new vision of Love. A new communication of feelings, which is why I sometimes talk to him while we make love…which he says no woman before me has done with him.

George sees our relationship as "one of the most spiritually moving times of my life." He is "in love" with me, and I can't find that feeling for him. My mother says that "in love" feeling is not important; just that we get along. How sad! I have found the most growth in me has been by following my heart to the "in love" relationships, and the more deeply I have felt that way, the more willing I am to stay and work through the difficulties and my pain. I was most "in love" with Gregory, my fourth husband. Of all the love relationships I have had…it was the most painful and it was the relationship I learned the most about mySelf and real Love.

That "in love" feeling reaches down to the spirit and can capture that repressed spirit-child <u>only</u> if we <u>feel</u> our <u>past pain</u> in a <u>connected-to-the-source</u> way. Letting our tears (and rage) lead the way. Our vulnerability is our pathway to the stars of real love.

Past the "Illusion" of love, the word "Illusion" creating gushers of tears because the church would not let the real Me be known, or be understanding of my feelings, My Truth. In 2000 there are fewer screams about that "one way" illusion that prevented me from being understood so I couldn't feel loved. The façade I had to create while growing up is dissolving in my tears☺ And enhancing my enthusiasm to find more truth.

Enthusiasm means "god-filled" or as Webster's dictionary states, "a belief in special revelations of the holy spirit, a strong excitement of feeling." The way a child feels as they open their eyes to a new day when their parent picks them up from their crib, or the way adults feel when they desire to make love. Not out of obligation, or duty. It's REAL.

Although the physical pain over my heart while sobbing (not present in daily life) is lessening over the past seven years of connected-crying, it is still present occasionally when I'm sobbing about never being really loved, the religious love being a falsehood, except for daddy's love which was not enough. Too much fear loomed like an ever constant mist.(missed)

When Susanne put her hand on my heart, I cried more, and felt my nose stuff up, which rarely happens these days, unlike when I began my grieving process. The stuffiness cleared out quickly after this session, another sign of lessening pain, and more healing of the heart broken open, not having to have a heart attack to break it open, like how my father died. Mine is a positive broken heart☺creating new tear-oxygenated blood flow.

"When the shell of my heart breaks open, tears shall pour forth and they shall be called the pearls of god." —Rumi

Tears cause me to own what others accuse me of: self-absorption. We are all self-absorbed if we are really honest with ourselves. Even when we do things for others it is out of a need to feel good about ourselves by helping others. The difference, I believe, is that I am being self-centered…we become centered if we let go of the self-pain that keeps us off-center. The center IS a growing love that brings us to a self-trust in what is right for us, not what others think is best for us, and results in no need for disconnecting judgments, prejudices, revenge, or hate.

The "in-love" feeling is the strongest pull our spirit has to lead us into healing, that small voice of the child that "comes" out loud as adults when we fall "in love." It is the glue of possibility of REAL LOVE, where each person has the opportunity to become conscious of his or her own childhood (and possibly pastlife) pain that is carried into adulthood, grieve it, and thereby become a more trusting whole human being. It is why I hung in with Gregory and healed more of ME than ever before, because I was totally there with him. So many tears are shed because of our parents not being "totally there for us" as children. The spiritual journey of love.

Religion is no longer needed or matters. "I love my tears because they tell the truth that no one can dismiss or invalidate!"

Like my orgasms in 2000, more and more evolving to: "Oh god," less specific images, more inclusive images of nature and the many loves of my life, or even to just "ahhhh" or "ooooh" – the sounds of the universe? Like a tightrope of excitement balanced throughout my whole body. Where balancing becomes easier and easier, being able to have an orgasm on my back becoming as easy as on my stomach. An upward opening to the universe versus a downward hiding of my face while self-loving (masturbating).

Like the universe has no boundaries, neither does LOVE. And that is why "only" sex does not satisfy. Sex by itself is limited. And now I know why I have never been satisfied by one night stands…and have usually tried very hard to develop relationships with the men after the sex the first night that I met them. We all want love and act out our need for it by having sex, the frame of love, without the picture☺ (Or act out our need by refraining from sex, or eating too much, and all the other too muchs☺ or too littles)

It is why I cried when my stepdaughter's mother called me to ask me not to come to Sara's high school graduation. She said something like, "You have two daughters and a granddaughter, why are you still after Sara?" Tears came as I said, "I may be divorced from Gregory, but that doesn't stop me from loving Sara – LOVE has no boundaries."

Mid-year 2000, I'm noticing that I masturbate once or twice a week and more often it is in the morning, no longer at night, when used as a way to fall asleep. And I don't usually awaken aroused but develop a feeling of desire to love myself. Like one morning, after some foreplay with myself, I decide to become focused. On my back and within two or three strokes around my clitoris there is an unflinching buildup. I come with the force of a locomotive, like a rocket launching. I treasure the whole physical feeling and there was no one there but ME! No images of men, nature, no words, just "oooohhs" and "aaahhhs," the universal sounds that connect me with mySelf and all living beings. Like my lilac "bush" so tall, I see all its pinks through my dining room window. And it "arches" over the walkway into my "home" – my birth canal to me! I even smell its sweetness as I put my nose into its petals. No wonder men say women's genitals are like flowers. I self-love to keep the nectar flowing, to continue flowering, not out of need to soothe my anxieties. I am a perennial flower, not an annual. I want to open to as full a blossom as possible.

Thereby, I find myself asking more of my partners to open their eyes with me. Not just while making love but also when I said goodbye to Danny, a man I met through the personal ads. He later told me "how powerful" a feeling that was for him to experience. Appreciative of a deeper connection, of being seen, and not hearing criticism of the manner in which he kissed me.

That powerful experience is what I know to be a strong connection with the innocence with which we ARE all born. George was not the first man to say that he was attracted to my innocence. But he was the first I asked what he meant by "innocence." He said, "that you don't believe in evil…your openness, honesty, sweetness." It was what Gregory had said he was attracted to, "your naivete," which means "childlike, lack of worldly wisdom." "A genuine, innocent simplicity." Both dictionary definitions. I'm glad for this, that I can still believe in the basic goodness of humankind…that I can basically trust. George believes in evil, and that revs me up, because I know in the deepest crevice of my heart that it is not true – how could anyone look into a baby's eyes and see evil?

Child development research supports the experience that children born physically healthy develop emotionally (spiritually) according to how well they are loved…and yes, we have a long way to evolve in the ways of LOVE, but that does not mean that there is an evil force battling a force of love, or perfection. There is convincing evidence that we bring in some past pain from past lives. But still, just as there is no (human) perfection on this planet, there is no (human) evil. Such a belief traps us in fear…like of hell. Fear keeps us from being more conscious, aware of the small voice within us all that wills us to **evolve**…to **love** better. The same drive that makes sex so appealing…to experience the perfection of Love's orgasm.

I wish everyone could view the documentary "Child of Rage," which portrays a very abused child adopted by two loving parents. Their love and kindness was not enough. They took the child to a clinic where they used "holding therapy" for approximately six months. This seven-year-old girl, who could not cry, could stick needles in their pet dog's eyes, full of hate because she had been severely abused. She would kick and scream, until one day she broke through to tears. As she cried out her hurt in loving arms, her behaviors became kind and loving! Some of this child's innocence returned with Love. Tears of Love.

While I was reading to my friend Sue, I cried as I spoke the words, "I love you because of your innocence." My innocence had been taken away, mostly through being taught that I was born in sin and thereby not worthy of god's love in Sunday School, and at home from my mother. It is not just the fundamentalist religions that teach that we are born in sin. <u>God's love cannot</u> <u>incorporate sin</u> <u>with innocence</u>. **Innocence means to be "free from guilt and SIN."** How babies are born. When my daughter Megan read my essay, "Almost Innocent," she emailed me: "you are innocent in a way, just like you always say that children are. That is the child in you. The way you view the world and the people in it, so much hope and optimism for all."

Even Batman falls in love with a psychotherapist, saying "emotions have always been the mind of true justices!" And my tears are what have washed away the pain that shut away my innocence and ability to have "just" compassion. LOVE.

"ComePassion" that can be heard in my orgasms, which sometimes can be heard for miles into Ithaca, according to George. Isn't it interesting that "coming" is a word we use for estastic feelings of "passion." One time mid-2000, when I masturbated, nurturing myself, I said as I climaxed, "How sweet it is!" Sweet as children who have such unabashed passion, such freedom to feel and express…they "come" to life with LOVE. Why we respond to them so gushingly! The "Oh, Yes" of orgasm.

These concepts may seem profound…meaning I know something because I feel it deeply. With a client, tears came to my eyes as I said the word, PROFOUND, as we both identified with this deep "knowing feeling." Pro means forward, and found means bottom or deep…to truth and healing evolving from tears, if we allow them to connect us to our soft hearts of love. It reminds me of when I was sixteen, walking up the basement stairs into our kitchen, sitting on a stool while telling my father about this feeling inside me that lets me know that I am a separate entity unto mySelf…a **real**ization that had just **come** to me. I felt and spoke **passion**ately about it as I tried to express this to my father, whom I knew would understand. It was probably my first glimpse that I could be something other than what my religion told me to be. I'm glad I remember sharing this with him.

It is all so A-maze-ing - a maze which I am finding my way through, to my true spirit - the wonder of tears - that push me along, out of half-hearted love or lovemaking with men with whom I am not truly in love. The "force of love" that spouted out of my mouth after Susanne said "thank you" for bringing her to further awareness, adding, "you are a good force." Tears rushed out with my response, "The force of love." Tears that show and grieve the sadness of that birthright spirit-force being squashed out of me, now being revived like CPR. (Child Passesby Religion☺)

For more than five years I've had this fascination with simple small white churches, usually situated in rural areas. My attention is always drawn to them as I drive by. I notice their simplicity, purity of white, no facades, just bare truth, like a new fallen snow. They are old and sturdy, no puritanical airs like those of Queen Victoria and religion where one acts one way Sunday morning and unkind and angry much of the week. Where money and gold domes are not the priorites, but the "poor in spirit." Like me. A 66 year-old man I met at one of my book signings underlined this point by saying how deeply his christian religion hurt him, that he "knew no love, just hated himself."

It is still difficult for me to fully embrace what an astrologer told me in 1996: "You are a virtuoso on the keyboard of love." When I told that sentence to a woman at an Omega workshop in 2000, tears pierced through underlining how sad it is that I have not known enough love in my life, yet thankful my tears are bringing me and others home to REAL LOVE. Being sensitive enough to feel tears like I did with a client when he said, "I almost killed you," meaning the spirit of his son by not allowing expression of his son's true feelings. I noticed as I wrote this in my journal that if you remove the "k" of kill, then you have ill. We are an ill people because we do kill our spirits everyday that we deny and do not express our tender feelings. Like the word "said," if you remove the "i," then you have sad. Therefore, when "I" do not say what I feel I become sad! Amazing how so many words in our language convey these inner truths! Everything is wonderfully connected in this universe.

Therefore the **whole meaning of love** is found in being able to express how you feel, like children do until we tell them they shouldn't feel a certain way or to feel a certain way. No freedom to BE oneself. Again, that freedom that is found in orgasm: letting go of control, feeling "Oh god" in me.

By letting go of control of our tears, which lets go of fears, we can find the *Three Magic Words* written about by U.S. Andersen in 1954. He states these words to be "YOU Are God." I agree, and like many others, this author tells us, "Love makes the world go. It will make you go too. Just let it!" Like Nike says, "Just do it!" All the words in the world cannot help us "Just let go" or "Just let it." The process of letting our defenses down in order to feel our vulnerable hurt spots is not easy. I know how it has been easy for me to resist "going there," (to the emotional pain) as my clients say. That's why it is not just retraining the mind to think differently, because the feelings still creep in to destroy the thoughts we so wish to believe. We need to pay attention to the HEART-mind-body connection. Like a tree, the heart is the roots, the mind the branches, and the body the leaves. The body and brain cannot function without first having a healthy heart!!! The seat of the emotions, of love. As many say, "Have a Heart." I'd like to have the three magic words BE, "god in us." When we find god in us, then we truly have real "Love in Us," and the ability to love all, have compassion for all – then the death of hate in all.

Feeling more of the divine in me was evident in August 2000 when I masturbated and orgasmed powerfully near my vagina, the G spot? Unusual, as was the second orgasm ten minutes later, which centered in my clitoris. All I could say was, "beautiful, oh so beautiful" on the lips of my orgasm.

How often I cry over needing to <u>hear</u> the three most powerful magic words, "I love you." Like now, when I read them in the card sent to me in 1965 by my dad. But I did not HEAR them. It happens over and over again, those tears, like the keys on the piano practiced hours a day in order to find the truest expression of the feeling in the music.

Christian and I had an unusual practice session of lovemaking fifteen years after our boy-girlfriend relationship ended in 1984. I had kept up our connection through Christmas letters and occasional phone calls since then. I visited him while on a book signing tour and found him with a fever, yet looking physically robust. Enough to keep conversation going from 11PM to nearly 3AM Friday night, while lying next to each other naked. I gave him a massage, and touched him lightly all over, except his genitals, knowing he was sick and needed to be given to. Then again, on Saturday night. When I wrote in my journal that I gave lovingness without expecting anything in return, tears formed, alerting me to my child's pain of what I wasn't given: unconditional love.

Christian did hold me as we fell asleep and awakened. Sunday morning he felt much better, so I intiated lovemaking despite his initial reticence. At first, he had his eyes closed and didn't want to kiss but I persisted and eventually he was inside me. I told him that it feels good to be all (t)here with you. No doubts, no shame, no guilt, no fear, which I had plenty of when we first met. I felt very close to having an orgasm with intercourse, unusual for me until of late and if he had felt better I believe we would have made that happen. Eventually he touched my breasts, face and back and as I moved up and down on him, I whispered, "How do you like this university?" He replied with a grin, "I'm enrolled." I had a well-built orgasm with his penis between my labia, screaming tones blending with his moans.

Later, we walked hand in hand to a local diner, tears of love covering my eyeballs again, especially when I read his inscription in a book he bought for me. "I'm in awe of your luminous soul." "And look forward to our ever-connecting path, always love, Christian."

When I drove out of his driveway, I had to pull back in to say, "I know I will regret leaving without saying 'I love you,'" with tears of course. "I love you too, I hope you know that," Christian sturdily responds. I reply without thinking, "It's nice to HEAR." And that's why I cry again and again for the loss of those words not spoken (although written) by my father and not ever known from my mother.

After being with Christian, I masturbated two days in a row, when I had been self-loving once per week. I would say, "come to me" as I climaxed. Exactly what I am in the process of: **coming** more **to** know the **real me**. "The church is not where you learn to love. You know there is some kind of love there but you can't get at it…I can feel that in my gut," I sobbed in one of my sessions. Dad could not come and talk to me when I was 16 and really needed him, out of his fear of displeasing my mother, I believe. He could not say, only write, "I love you," out of fear. Learned first in his catholic upbringing, and then more of the same in the protestant born again religious beliefs. This is not spirituality. This is not the sexuality which needs to be freely expressed with love. Tears have saved me, made me more and more able to connect my spirit and sexuality together.

I was surprised to see this integration happen much more frequently throughout the rest of 2000 and 2001. A "joyful participation in the sorrows of life," as Joseph Campbell puts it, Brian tells me. I met him Labor Day weekend in the rural hills of West Virginia at a swing dance weekend. It had been a long time since I was strongly physically attracted to a man. He was a very good dancer with lots of his own creativity and splash – a lot like the way I like to dance. He danced most of the dances with me and walked me to my tent afterwards, pressing me up against my Jeep, kissing me tenderly. No aggressive tongue down the throat, which he says guys can't help when they are strongly attracted. I find the more sensitive guys don't do that. We made out deliciously and Brian wanted to be in the tent with me all night but my heart was not ready, although my body could have been. He attended a tango workshop the whole next day so I did not see him until that evening, when we danced until 3 AM. It was like foreplay on the dance floor and I wasn't surprised that Brian asked to make love with me. I was still hesitant and he said we didn't have to have intercourse. After sharing our sexual histories and health, we were in each other's arms by 4AM. Life is good and greater than any one moment…I trusted my heart to trust Brian. I found myself not rusty in the making love department, that is my juices flowed easily for a menopausal woman, and I orgasmed without intercourse. He didn't until the next morning by rubbing his penis over my labia lips. Although I had licked his penis I was caring for myself by not having him ejaculate in my mouth. I did not know him well enough. We made love again Sunday night after lively graceful dancing. I said we could have intercourse if he used a condom. But, while making love I trusted my "gut" (heart) and we were (s)kin to (s)kin, no barriers. That evening he had told me a secret which increased my trust in him that he was telling the truth about his sexual past. And then I was surprised by what happened next. I had that rare happening… a vaginal orgasm. What I describe as my first "wholehearted" vaginal orgasm where clitoral orgasm came simultaneously. It was not a vague vaginal orgasm like I'd had with Gregory; I must have negotiated the G-spot by Brian allowing me to navigate his penis as I moved on top of him. Although we looked at each other a lot and had luscious kissing, I do not remember that we opened our eyes during orgasm. And I would remember that as the rest of my story will tell.

I know that I light on any compliment that is given, especially by those who matter to me. I try to remember them. I told Brian that I felt "special" because he picked me to spend so much time with, because he was very open in saying that he doesn't dance with many women because it is no longer fun if the women do not flow with you in the dance. He's really his own man, dancing differently than others, like mixing tango in with swing. We made love again after breakfast on Monday morning. Somehow we knew this might be our last chance for a long time "to come." We live six hours apart and there was not enough love to keep us in touch☺ When we parted, I gave him my book, writing in it, "You'll always be in my heart," with my tear dancing on the page.

In my crying session that week, I did sob when I said maybe I danced with Brian in a previous life. I had cried with Brian when I told him of my previous lifetime regressions. It was another validation of the truth of those experiences because I cried when I spoke of them and sobbed in my session. The truth that our spirit exists beyond our bodies is not new, and I've known this truth for myself for ten years. And, it is the power of sexuality that owns the spark which ignites our spirit to freely letting go, in orgasm, to the possibility of expressing ourselves with childlike unconditional love. Only if we open our hearts to the vulnerability of our vital tears. The water that envigorates the spirit.

John, a dance teacher at the Buffalo Gap weekend, said I was a delightful dancer and that I have a "beautiful countenance that shines out to everyone." I had never heard that before. My countenance. Now, I do see that countenance in my clients when they cry. And realized in my crying session that I was sad that I had separated the sexual (physical) from the spiritual for way too long. The healthy whole.

It is so clear to me that I am meant to BE here despite all the painful circumstances that brought me here to this wondrous earth: the acquaintance rape of my mother, mother trying to abort me, mother nearly strangling me, surviving a fractured skull. It is clear why I name the "spiritual" to be guided by the Design of the Universe (god is aligned with religion). It is clear why my father was an astronomer, loving the stars of the universe. He IS a Star. (a moment of tears) For loving me. It is clear why I spill tears when I say to my "born-again" sister, Connie, that god would not punish the innocent – the children – and send them to hell. I cry about my lost innocence over and over, and that is what makes me know my truth.

When Connie and I went to the Farmer's Market here in Ithaca, she enjoyed the Thai food, specifically the sticky rice with mango. Boy was I surprised when I heard her say, "Mangos are better than sex." I replied something like, "You must not have had any good sex." It makes sense to me that sex is not very good when love (the essence of spirit) is not available. It makes sense that religion deadens the spirit, so many religions shame sexuality immensely, like catholics who say sex is only for procreation, and have prohibited birth control. Or muslims who cover the women, even veils over their faces, so as not to tempt men sexually. Or protestants not allowing me to dance while growing up because I would be too physically close to men and then feel sexual and possibly be sexual with them. Satan's temptation. "Sex is satan's temptation" just makes me want to puke! ☺ Throw it up and out! It used to make me really angry. My anger gauge is now down to annoyance, the greater feeling being sadness for the loss of sacred, unshamed sexuality.

After dancing for three hours in the city park's pavilion, I came home and felt like masturbating. The first time in a week as the fall of 2000 was close upon me. As I came to orgasm, I found myself saying, "Come to me, Brian," sloshed with tears. Once again I felt a past-life connection with him. As I also feel a present connection of coming home to mySelf…as my tears wash away the defenses of religion, running marathons, anger, judgment, and busyness. (The past and present connected into a whole One.)

And guess what…more humor!!!I notice more and more what I and others laugh at. So many times it is about things we feel shame or fear about…like sex. While at a workshop at Omega Institute, I was camping and I couldn't seem to zip up my sleeping bag. After several tries I walked to the café and found a stranger, Frank, to help me. He eventually made the zipper work after I directed the right zipper to the right track. The next day at dinner I laughed and laughed as I introduced Frank as "the guy I met over a zipper." Learning ways to zip and unzip. It was very funny and he played along. The sexual over (and under) tones were obvious. Laughing seems to be another way to act out or discharge feelings that we cannot speak directly - hurts of repression and oppression that lead to depression.

As my life process conveys an awakening to my true spirit through tears to douse fears, it becomes clear to me that I was born to help people out of their religious trances. It is a difficult birth with LOVE as its prize. Then PEACE. Coming in touch with my deepest pain has made it possible for me to "see the light," as it is said. The dark curtain of pain has been ripped open by the light of my glistening tears. My eyes see clearly the two and three year-old child, me, sitting at a semi-circle table in Sunday School at Bethel Grove Bible church every Sunday morning (now mourning). I have sobbed deeply about that scene many times, feeling the pain of that innocent child being told that she is unworthy of god's love, she is a sinner, depraved, not innocent. She will go to hell if she does not accept Jesus as her savior. What a damn lie!!! Look into the eyes of a baby and tell me he or she is not innocent and IS the most beautiful being on the planet. Until our ignorance and fear tells the child different.

Oh, I thought I loved mySelf before the tears flowed. I was successful in the world's eyes. That was second-hand love…from the church, or men, not from my SELF. I've been fighting to get my Self back until February 1998 when I had finally cried out enough pain that I could see clearly to letting go of Gregory and how he saw me. I feel so free in writing that sentence – so BE it!

No, I'm not totally healed, but that February was the turning point of my life, when I had more of my Self than less. I had reached the summit of the mountain where the view was not hindered and I could climb in any direction I chose. No longer controlled by fear of losing second-hand love☺ It reminds me of a significant moment at an Omega workshop, when several participants would surround me and scream out my name, "Dianea" over and over, and I could only cry. This happened for many others when their names were focused on with screams. Those lost children being validated and their spirit gaining more power and life. It is like us singing, "Oh say can you **see**, by the dawn's early light…"

A college student from Smith College once told me that her school schedules a student body scream during their final exam week where whoever wishes to assemble in the college's courtyard and scream, may. Wouldn't it be wonderful if this type of expression of grief (joy and fear) could be acknowledged on a daily basis, and not just under pressured circumstances? (Then, maybe the need to scream and yell would evolve out of existence)

Like those in West Africa where Malidoma Some, a gifted diviner and medicine man, deems his purpose to bring the Wisdom of Africa to the West. In an interview in the journal, *Science of Mind*, October 2000, Some states, "To grieve and to cry are not shameful things, but signs of strength….It's the channel that links us to the Sacred, and this is why in my village a person who is crying is a sacred person. **Tears are one of the the most direct ways of expressing sacredness.**" The spiritual connection to one another.

Sexuality's sacredness is at its very basic starting point when one says, "I'm horny." According to Webster's dictionary, horny means, "an erect penis, excited sexually and desiring sexual gratification." Or, "compact and homogenous with a dull luster: hard, callous." Sounds like when someone says, "I want to get laid." There is no love involved, it is totally a physical pleasure for oneself. Masturbation can be the seed that could bloom into a connection with our true loving spirit but gets squashed by shame to express our vulnerable feelings of fear or sadness. Expression of vulnerable hurt feelings is the soil where Love can grow. Which everybody is looking for, but "looking in all the wrong places," as the song goes.

My seventy-nine-year-old mother told me that her man-friend is "a good kisser." A new vulnerability from her, who has never talked about anything sexual with me. I don't believe we discussed what makes a good kiss but kissing is obviously an important aspect of a relationship. What makes it a good kiss? I know I have my own expectations of how that would be for me, and it is highly important to the expression of love and passion. Connection to mySelf and the other person I'm loving. Tenderness. It took some years before I could tell a man that I did not like the way he was kissing me, especially right away while he was kissing me. One risks having their spirit left and unloved if we speak ALL of ourselves. Face-to-face, eye-to-eye, "I" to "I."

Eyes being windows to the soul (spirit) is an ancient idea. The reader will begin to realize the importance of eyes being open at orgasm, the moment of love's fulfillment being truly seen in one's ecstacy of vulnerability – truly loved. I've noticed in myself as well as with my partners that the eyes usually stay closed during orgasm. It is fascinating to me as may be noticed already how our language reflects the connectedness of everything. In order to have eye contact, we must be face to face. "Ace"can mean "one that **excels** at something, or on the point of, **very near** to." And "face" can be "to recognize and deal with straightforwardly." When we kiss, we are the face to face closest we can be. We are coming close to **excel**ling at connection and **very near** to love when we can look each other in the eyes during the exquisite moment of climaxing love. When we fantasize, we are no longer with our lover or ourselves; our thoughts take us away from being present with our feelings. I am amazed to see this truth over and over again. That our feelings are the foundation to our being, which try to peek out when we feel vulnerable, like at orgasm, feeling free, no control! The time we may be most ready to say "I love you!"

As I **evol**ve (mirror image of **love**), my fantasies have nearly disappeared and my orgasms are more full, gliding, smooth as a baby's bum, and firmly intense. Echoing "yes, yes." My sensitivity, physically, heightens as I am more sensitive to my feelings. The lightest touch on my clitoris is the most exciting. Emotionally, my heart cries more easily, as it did when I looked at a photo of Megan when she was three, crying and reaching for me as she sits in the shallow rapids of a swimming hole we frequented. How could I have taken that photo as she cried out for me, her little arm reaching out for me? (tears now) When I told my grown-up Megan about my new sensitivity, she thought I was a bit "dramatic," that I knew she wasn't in danger, and came right after her. Yes, that's true, still, her feelings should have taken priority. And I also connected my tears to my own child within that had reached out to her mother, crying, many times, and had been ignored. The point being, that I am glad that I have found my lost child because my sensitivity to another's hurt is so much greater. I understand and am less judgmental.

"Only when I make room for the child's voice within me, do I feel genuine and creative." – Alice Miller, author, *Thou Shalt Not Be Aware*, and many other books

I am not so stupidly strong, like I was when I went to the morgue to see my father who had just died of a sudden heart attack in 1977. I am sure that I cried, but it was very restrained because the supervising nurse stood nearby. I know I wanted to touch my father (tears now) and talk to him, but I just stood there "stupidly strong!" It's something that I have been praised for in the past and now cry for!!!!! that lack of sensitivity. My spirit flattened like a steam roller without steam. No wonder it is said that people are "down and out" when they are having difficult times. My daddy was "down" under the ground, buried, as my feelings were trying to come "out."

They still were as I masturbated on the anniversary of my father's death, October 6, 2000. As I orgasmed I was saying, "Loving you, love you, Oh, god, yes!" Before I climaxed I had non-sexual images of all kinds of people – women, men, children, daughters, and briefly of the latest man in my life. It felt like a meaningful connection with everyone, and mostly with mySelf. That Oneness that Buddhists speak of. And the circle of complete connectedness of the planets, sun and moon. All circles.

It only makes sense that as I grieve I have more pure connections to my orgasms, therefore a greater intensity and more loving feelings. When blocks of pain are let go, no longer in the way, then pleasure and love increase, like blood flow to the heart after an unclogging of the arteries. The love connection became even clearer as I responded to my sister saying that my grieving for my dad should end at some point. I responded with my usual "Why?" If one of my daughters died tomorrow, I would grieve and cry for them often until the day I died, because I will always love them and miss them, so why should my grieving end? Love does not end! That is, real love. Again, my truth, "**One's capacity to grieve is one's capacity to love.**"

Grieving does not incapacitate, it revitalizes.

Like my beginning after 53 years to be able to say "I love you" to my mother while she cannot say it back. And more importantly, to believe that I am worth being loved by my mother. That is what is sacred, when love becomes more real and stays!

The perfect circle is: because of my father's love for me I was not able to leave my religious upbringing because he still believed it. But the crux of my ability to leave religion in 1984 was having the seed of love from Dad to begin to believe in my own truth and goodness – the result of crying out my grief over losing him as well as not having my mother's love. I smile as I write that last sentence☺

"The sublimest song to be heard on earth is the lisping of the human soul on the lips of children." – Victor Hugo

As the circle back to my true Self continues to spiral I am aware, as I am traveling on a train through the Swiss Alps, seeing the majestic Matterhorn, that there is magnificent beauty to the jagged peaks, snow white knitted caps, waterfalls trailing down like silk. When I wake up the next day in Dreis, Germany, the birthplace of my father, I cannot stop thinking about the Italian man on the moped.

Before I came to Italy, a psychic had told me that I would meet the "love of my life" as an Italian man. I had dared to meet a Belgian man in the Forum in Rome, and also eat dinner with two Italian men and two Danish women in Florence whom I met where I stayed in a small hotel.

Yet, as I was walking down the winding road from the Piazza d'Michelangelo, I would make one of the few regrettable mistakes of my life. But then again…it was one of the greatest lessons I would learn and pass onto you, dear reader.

An Italian man riding a moped had followed me up to see the statue of David, sculpted by Michelangelo. (I just realized that my father's name is Michel, followed by the word angel…my father is to be my angel of life and then guardian in death…tears cannot stop at this very moment!) Sobs tell me now, two years later, that Dad is the "love of my life" and the river of my tears are the giver of life. But in 2000, when this handsome man in a rusty yellow sports jacket with wavy black hair touching its collar stepped off his moped, and waved to me to come meet him, I turned away. I had an agenda to shop for Italian shoes and leave for Venice on the train that afternoon. I waved him away without hesitation. I write on the train, "It's always FEAR that lacks the EAR to HEAR, a greater truth than what I already know."

I cried as I wrote, "he was trying <u>to speak with me</u>; why must my heart break so many times to be able to see the truth?" I thought of how this connects with daddy….if only he had persisted in <u>speaking to me</u> about the distance between us since, I learned the truth about us at age sixteen. He tried to connect, but not hard enough, like me and this Italian man. In 2002, I return again to this same Piazza d'Michelangelo, as you will read later in this book.

Back home, I cross paths again with an old lover named Steve. We are very attracted to one another physically but cannot seem to connect emotionally enough to tackle a serious relationship. We have made love in the minor key about four times in the past twenty years, and until this meeting in 2000, I had thought he was a lousy lover despite his large penis. He was only satisfying himself and I did not have the desire to teach him how to be a better lover.

In November of 2000, he took me out for dinner for the first time, and we talked about our feelings for each other as well as caught up on our lives. We talked another hour and a half in front of his woodstove when we arrived at his home. Then, we "made out" on the sofa for another half hour before becoming naked. I knew he had changed as a lover. More time, tenderness, kissing, looking me in the eyes. We talked about whether we would respect each other if we "made love." We both tell each other "You're beautiful," appreciating our physical bodies; his muscular, broad shouldered, Greek statue-type fifty-year-old body. Not until I cried deeply could I accept that the physical body was as important as the emotional-spiritual part. Shame of the body was indoctrinated by my religious upbringing, but the little voice inside me knew much better. Our body is part of the whole. It reflects the emotional–spiritual love within. I have not read of this acknowledgement until recently in the magazine, "Spirtuality and Health," Fall 2002 issue. "Hirschfield, 38, is a teacher and Orthodox rabbi who was taught that pursuing a life of the mind and the spirit meant everything – except pursuing health, sexuality, or body consciousness. So he let his body go."

"Then, Hirschfield had a revelation: god created humans with the breath, or says the bible, and every spiritual tradition connects the breath with the divine. Yet, he was so heavy, he couldn't breathe properly…He had actually been struggling most of his life with his weight, but it wasn't until this revelation that connected his spirituality to his weight that the pounds – all 100 of them – came off and stayed off…It's about FEELING better, happier, and more grateful for the blessing of a healthy body that is the receptacle – and the expression – of our spirituality." Palmer also adds, "Getting healthier isn't about looking better." I disagree. God, or the Design of the Universe, as I choose to call the creator, has created beauty all around to enjoy and add to our happiness. Why do we need to negate any part of our being? Until we accept it as all ONE whole, we will not be accepting the total love of our spirits which is our birthright.

Steve's body is a beauty to revel in, yet his erections showed his ambivalence until I licked him and pulled him inside of me. He was ready to orgasm, so I slowed our movement and we enjoyed our oneness for many minutes. He held back his orgasm. Steve left the bed to go pee, and when he returned we just held each other, stroking each other into twilight sleep.

The next day he told me that his ambivalence is about still being in love with his previous girlfriend. I felt accepting about our slow progression toward the orgasm of love. I felt blessed to have had these loving hours, so unexpectedly good. Our communication had taken us beyond sex to making love in its infancy stage. I did not feel rejected, as I would have a few years back.

As I wrote in my previous book, *TEARS ARE TRUTH*, my health continues to improve in subtle ways as I become older, even though my health has been basically good all my life. I give credit to the deep connected-to-my-childhood crying that I spill on a weekly basis. I was aware of this ongoing healing while swimming in the ocean with my second daughter Megan, she being 26, and me 53. We were snorkeling for close to an hour, and Megan said her fingers got numb and her foot cramped. It seemed apparent that her circulation was not as good as mine. Over the past decade I have needed less sweaters and noticed that my hands don't get cold as easily. My arteries and veins have opened up, as my heart of tears has opened up, supplying freer, vulnerable, loving orgasms as well.

"*I can only depend on my tears to guide me to the deep level of truth. Otherwise I question my Self.*" – Written in my journal in November 2000.

I have also noticed how my thriving plants are the ones that are connected to thriving relationships. A relationship that is struggling, like with my older daughter, is reflected in the orange tree she planted when she was four. She is now 29 years old, and it has survived mealy bugs, neglect, and the wrong plant food. Relationships that have become very distant, like that of my last husband, are reflected in plants that have died. My Hibiscus plant that traveled from Ithaca, New York to the Primal Center in California, and had to have its roots washed at the California border as an inspection for the Japanese beetle, is now thriving back in Ithaca five years later. The orgasm of life and LOVE continues, never dies.

When I saw Steve again, we watched a movie together on the sofa. He held me close but did not stroke me while I stroked his muscular soft-skinned body. I could not help feeling disappointed, yet felt accepting as Steve was recovering from stomach cramps. He was also frustrated because he could not kiss me, having a cold sore on his lip. He didn't want to chance giving herpes to me, so I felt protected and respected, cared about. When we went to his bed, undressed each other, he was hard and wanted intercourse right away, probably not to lose his erection which I could tell was tentative. In minutes he was ready to "come" so we slowed down and he began to lose his hardness. He said, "I hate it, I hate it, that I cannot kiss you, a lot of it is in the kissing." I was glad he felt that way. He left me to take a bath, which he does every night.

Afterwards, he told me that it didn't feel right to sleep with me, because he still had feelings for Katrina, and how "hard" it was to tell me. "What do you want me to do. Go home?" I asked. I drove home feeling accepting, not taking it person-ally, which was another big sign of my personal growth. My spirit had *known* for years that I did not want to be sexual with him if he could not be more connect-ed to me while making love. But I hadn't deeply <u>felt</u> that inside. A good **lover**.

While watching the movie with Steve, called "The Only Thrill," (I first wrote The Big Thrill☺) I cried tears which I did not hide. Most tears came when an old man said to his long time girlfriend, "You are the love of my life." I thought of my father immediately. It is now two years later and I cry at those same words, now consciously noticing that the focus is not on me loving my father, so that **he is the love** of my life, but that he is the **love of MY life.** This will become clear as you read on of me learning to love my life, ME, through allowing my tears at orgasm.

In my crying session that week, I cried many tears about not being able to tell my father "I love you" face to face. We only wrote those words. How could we be so guarded when there was obvious love between us? The church dogma kept us from feeling openly, denying all the human feelings. "Pain and LOVE go togeth-er…in order to love you have to be able to FEEL pain," I speak as tears underline my words. The more I do this emotional release work, the more I notice subtle connections, like what I told to a bank teller. I write that humorous story in the center of this book…a centerfold of sorts☺ called, "It's not the Turkey's Fault." I was blamed as a child…*it was my fault that god doesn't love me*…born in origi-nal sin. That's what really hurts! God damn it! (A wee bit of anger still resides…it used to be rage.) That IS what really breaks my heart! Sobs tell me it is the most damaging thing you can tell a child!

That church dogma nearly crushed my spirit, my innocence, as I thought clearly through my tears that I probably would have wanted to kill myself if not for the love of my father. My tears amidst my writing bring more of mySelf home. I am now stopping long enough to FEEL. To ask questions, questions, questions. Like when I asked mom how dad asked her to marry him. She said that he went down on his knees. I asked where that happened. In Tarrytown. Why there?

"I was there to give you up for adoption." Dad told her, "You don't need to do that, we'll raise her." (Me, his non-biological child.)

When I told this story to my twenty-two-year old German cousin Damien after meeting him for the first time, I cried. Later, while walking with him and other family members, I was telling him about how his mother and grandmoth-er and me had cried together about missing my dad…who is their brother, and uncle. Damien replied, "I wish I had a picture of you all crying together." I spon-taneously jumped, as my arms flew around Damien's shoulders. "Oh, that's so great that you'd want that!" To remember our crying, vulnerable moments. That's a remarkable thing for someone to say, especially a man. I was so happy, and my arms flying around Damien reminded me of my arms around lovers while making love, also, wishing I could have flung my arms around daddy spontaneously when he was alive. It is all so connected, the human spirit wishing to love freely.

I've seen myself noticing mySelf as if I am outside of myself, yet it is really because I am more inside of my Self – more aware – a healthy observance, not out of paranoia. In 2000, I am still looking to see if people are watching me dance, wondering why I need the attention, and I am more relaxed with my expression of sexuality while dancing.

I am essentially through menopause, and I notice that it has not decreased my sexual desire, which is different from a need to be sexual. That was tested out with George, an exceptional dancer whom I had been attracted to for a couple of years. One night he showed unusual attention to me, and said that he was going to leave at midnight to soak in his hot tub. I didn't even think to ask if he wanted me to join him…which I would have done years ago, to have a one-night stand. I sensed we did not have much of a spiritual connection…a deeper searching of the soul, like a piece of ripe fruit, full of juice.

This same weekend, a different Steve, my friend of eighteen years, offered to give me a total body massage, which I had not had in years. His hands flowed over my muscles with much careful touch, and it didn't feel like something I needed. Steve said he'd like a massage every other day; how come I don't miss it, or need it? Because my feelings come out directly? I want to be close to my feelings first, which lead me to be close to a man with whom I can deeply share mySelf. I don't need body work to bring up my feelings, my spirit to the surface. Massage is a sweet nurturing, but I would rather have the whole body-heart-spiritual closeness.

Like how I picture the best first kiss. Lingering eye-to-eye gaze for minutes, the body's slow leaning forward until our lips are but a fraction of an inch from touching, holding there, feeling our breath exchange like a gentle breeze, eyes still open as we connect our lips like angel wings, pressing into love's beginning. It is like: a knowing you, a wanting you, a respectful feeling all at once. I felt elated when that meaning came to me. Isn't that the beginning of love, an essence that grows like sweet clover covering a field for years to come.

As Steve massaged my body which he had never touched for eighteen years, he said, "I love your body, and the only thing that shows your age are the lines in your face. If I was to meet you for the first time, I would think that god was shining down on me." Tears massaged my cheeks as I replied, "It's the <u>child (god)</u> that gives us the spirit to love all things – even rats." (His two girls loved the rat that lived at their pond) As I stepped off the massage table, Steve and I kissed for the first time. (We made love with our bodies as elaborated on in "It's Not the Turkey's Fault," in the centerfold of this book.) It was not a one night stand, not just because it was the only time or at noon time☺ It was a meeting of eighteen years of knowing, wanting, and respecting…the very integration of sexuality with spirituality…love.

As Eckhart Tolle states in *The Greatest Obstacle to Enlightment,* "**Being can be felt, but it can never be understood mentally.** To regain awareness of Being and to abide in that state of 'feeling-realization' is enlightenment." As the reader may already realize, I have a lot of trouble with writers who are so intellectual; they lose me in their tunnel of big words. Tolle says, "The thought will be the lie, the emotion will be the truth: not the ultimate truth of who you are, but the relative truth of your state of mind at that time." Can I make that simpler to understand? I hope I can.

All the unconditional feelings of love that we receive when we look into the eyes of a baby or small child, who stares into your eyes without fear, smiles widely, spontaneously and frequently, is the Being Tolle speaks of…who has not been repressed, oppressed, or suppressed by unaware parents who do not respect their child's feelings. We must cry out, grieve the pain of being told not to cry, not to be scared, not to be so silly. Unacknowledged or disrespected feelings turn into anger and unhealthy fears which cover up our true Being. We may refer to our Being as our spirit that drives us constantly to LOVE. And **Love is our true Being.** It is "god" in us. Through the physical closeness of sex, we expect to find Love. Our spirits fly during orgasm.

"Usually, such moments are short-lived, as the mind quickly resumes its noise-making activity that we call thinking. Love, joy, and peace cannot flourish until you have freed yourself from mind dominance. But they (love, joy, peace) are not what I would call emotions. They lie beyond the emotions (fear, anger, sadness) on a much deeper level. So you need to become fully conscious of your emotions and be able to feel them before you can feel that which lies beyond them," Tolle explains (parentheses mine).

And I add, that not only do you have to feel your feelings, you need to feel them in connection to the source of the emotional pain…which is usually from one's childhood.

"Real Love doesn't make you suffer. How could it? It doesn't suddenly turn into hate, nor does real joy turn into pain. Even before you are enlightened – before you have freed yourself from your mind – you may get glimpses of true joy, true love, or of a deep inner peace, still but vibrantly alive. These are aspects of your true nature…the truth is that it wasn't an illusion, and you cannot lose it. It is part of your natural state, which can be obscured but never destroyed by the mind (defending against one's emotional pain). Even when the sky is overcast, the sun has not disappeared. It's still there on the other side of the clouds," Tolle concludes.

It is my Being's spirit that continues to attract me to certain men, that appreciates their masculine beauty which compliments my feminine. Like muscular six foot one inch Chuck, whom I had met once through a personal ad ten years earlier, and now again in December of 2000. I had not pursued him ten years ago because I was turned off by our first kiss, a mouth full of tongue, which felt very invasive. It was not tender. Ten years later, I tell him about that kiss, which he wanted to talk about several times. When we do kiss as we say good night, it is sweet and tentative, innocent like a child. I did not sleep well that night, and had not masturbated in a week. My second orgasm was very intense and only a minute after the first. I said "Oh my god" about four times. Awake again at 5am, I stoked my fire into another sweet orgasm…it is very unusual for me to have more than one orgasm at any one masturbation or making love. Aliveness or anxiety I wonder??

Like I wondered when I cried the next day as I sang the words, "cross every stream" from "Climb Every Mountain." The stream of tears is what I am crossing through, making me less and less able to just be sexual because of physical attraction. Although Chuck is very attractive physically, I did not feel aroused enough to make love with him. I really needed a man who enjoys kissing and looking at me in the eyes. Then my body wants to continue sexually…I am becoming a combination of physical, emotional and intellectual connectedness.

Our culture has extremely repressed sexuality so that it is a national obsession, expressed nonstop through Hollywood movies, covers of magazines, and in lyrics of pop songs. Due to my family's repression of sex through religious beliefs, I am constantly opening the envelope with my two daughters, especially my youngest, Megan. When she was visiting me with her boyfriend during christmas 2000, they were looking through photo albums and came across a picture of me half-naked. Megan was embarassed and said it was personal and private. I asked why, as usual.

She asked her boyfriend if he'd be OK with her seeing his father naked in a picture. He said yes, which stopped Megan with surprise. There is nothing to be ashamed of, showing our bodies. It is sad to realize that we can admire naked scuptures in a museum, yet stay separate from accepting our body-Being.

It seems that in the new millenium of my life, I am being surprised about the number of men entering and leaving my life in a sexually-intimate way. At a New Years' dance weekend in 2001, I was looking to share my hotel room in order to cut down expenses. From my off-hand remark made in the elevator, Mark pipes up that he'd like to share my room.

After dancing until late, then picking up a book to read in order to wind down, Mark continues to carry on conversation about our lives, therapy, and asking introspective questions. As I shut out the light, Mark asked if he could come into my bed, to be close, that he missed being touched. I felt mixed, feeling a connection, and said okay, as long we would not be sexual. If I couldn't sleep we would have to be in separate beds. Mark kissed me tenderly, and I could feel his erection. We just held each other, and I dozed off and on, not able to leave the bed.

Mark and I ate New Year's eve dinner at a table with six other dancers, and we kissed at midnight - like an appetizer before a gourmet meal. Despite the challenge of my 5'9" frame with Mark's 5'4", I especially enjoyed dancing the "hustle" with him. In bed together, his height made no difference, we were souls that had made an intimate connection within as well as without. His broad shoulders held me at 3AM, until we became one. My orgasm came surprisingly easily for a first time encounter, his penis dancing on my clitoris. We felt the seeds of love, knowing that they would not germinate beyond friendship. I am happy that I am open to men with whom I would not expect to be. I may still be the young bird in the nest learning to fly.

The next week I watched the movie, "The Truman Show." Half way through the movie I felt so aroused that I had to masturbate, even though there were no sexual scenes. At first I could not figure out what caused those sexual feelings and one of the most intense orgasms I had had for some time. I felt tingles up to my forehead, wild and wonderful. While focusing on that question, it "came" to me that the movie is about our life being culturally scripted, and how difficult it is to be real. Being REAL is a turn on for me, more and more.

Like my client Jennifer said, "It hurts me that I can't cry." That's so Real! And during one of my crying sessions, I "came" out with "**I feel like I get a little more of mySelf back every time I cry.**"

Through the personal ads, Fred W. was next to enter my life. This Ithaca College professor of writing has endured being institutionalized as a teenager, poverty, homelessness, alcoholism, and the break up of a long marriage producing four children. He is in therapy and has been alcohol free close to a year. After a couple of weeks of frequent contact, he still cannot kiss me. He says, "You know, I am afraid of people." He's realized this since he stopped drinking. We can hold hands, I can touch his wavy graying hair, fear keeps us from developing deeper intimacy. I understand his fear to be hurt again, although I cannot imagine the fierce pain he's felt. I can leave without resentment...I am ready to fly on my own. Because, later, I cried boulders (boldly:) when I said, "We have boundaries only because we have fear"...the word "FEAR" producing the emphatic tears."

When I masturbated this week, now two to three times, I found myself saying "Oh yes" more than the usual "Oh god." Oh yes, less fear!

Next, I meet Jim while dancing at the Rongovian Embassy, a local restaurant-bar-dance spot. We snacked and talked at a late night diner, followed by passionate kissing at my car door. The next time we were together we went out for pizza, then watched a video, then made out, until Jim was pressuring me to take my clothes off. We satisfied each other manually, because I was not ready to be intimately connected through intercourse. It is like proceeding from A to C without acknowledging B. BE. I'm smiling! Jim was like the other extreme from Fred. I believe he soothes his fear by being prematurely sexual...later, I learn that relationships are "too hard" for him. So, I think to myself, you let your penis get hard instead.

That same weekend I had a dance performance with my friend Brian (see the TURKEY'S FAULT in the centerfold), eating dinner at an Indian restaurant beforehand. Brian and I have never been sexual although we have an attraction that neither of us now want to act on. I tried to articulate to Brian about my struggle to connect emotionally/spiritually with sexuality. I am wondering why I cannot be OK with the continuum toward real love, or am I, because I no longer feel guilt about my briefer sexual encounters of making love. I am very aware that, like with Jim, I wanted to look into his eyes so much more than he did – I wanted to touch and hold so much more than he did, especially once we began kissing. I feel that I am stretching more and more for Real Love, and I need to accept where I am in that process. It is really OK that I am not satisfied with how it is just physical. It is good to be conscious and growing and feeling that deeper connection of Love. Yet, to also appreciate the peaces of loving as I travel my journey. This relates to what I cried about as I watched the movie "American Beauty:"

"Sometimes I think there is so much beauty in the world – I can't take it – my heart will cave in!" I cave in when I am appreciating beauty in others, even if it is just physical, because I appreciate it in myself. I can give some love, as well as get some. Yet, it is usually me giving more because I touch more, I look more...therefore, I move on to find more real love. "The entirety of life is behind things...a benevolent force is behind all things, therefore I don't need to be afraid – **I need to remember!**" THAT the CHILD within is the most beautiful and LOVING.

I **remember with my tears** like when I told my friend, Sue, about Brian and my dance performance. My tears ran with the words, "I loved it, because I was really being mySelf."

Not caring what others thought, even the dance teachers. And that IS the CHILD inside me. Children don't care what others think of them when they are very young, and they continue not to care if they are loved well by their parents. What wonderful drops of truth my tears are!

It is a GOOD hurt, even when I am wishing not to be alone. It is not easy. I am faced with my feelings which allow me to grieve stored up pain, which seems to parallel my evolving to grander love, involving connection with the whole universe. When I masturbated in late January 2001, I visualized a man, as well as other parts of my life like mountains, along with various thoughts. It is like the universe is trying to be a part of this whole loving experience, which has become a part of the evolution of my orgasms for more than a year now. My images are becoming increasingly diverse, instead of just mountains or dolphins. Still, I did want a penis near my vagina, gently pushing inside me, a muscular male over me, kissing me, turning my nipples…turning into ME☺ As I said earlier, I've found myself saying "Oh yes," more than "Oh god" when I orgasm.

I notice that I say "Oh god" as I strain to do one more push up because I am at the end of my strength. So that is when I call on god. Or when I let go completely and it feels so goooooood that I call out "oh god." I will pay more attention to:

"Oh god, isn't that beautiful" when I see a gorgeous sunset.

"Oh god, that's awful," when I hear of a tragedy like a baby dying.

"Oh god, I cannot believe he did that; it's so out of character."

"Oh god, that's incredible" when I hear of climbing Mt. Everest.

"Oh god damn it, I forgot an appointment."

"Oh god, I'm in love"…

or as I orgasm, saying, "oh god, it feels so GOOD!" Then, "Inside me too!" as I visualize a man inside me, yet immediately connecting it with the thought, "gods inside me too!"

That divineness is inside me too! All of us!

Like in Fred C., who I've written of before, a good friend, counselor of students and great father whom I adore but cannot feel attracted to enough physically. Fred W. could not go cross-country skiing with me, so I went alone to the Cornell Plantations. And who would I meet there, but Fred C. He's shaved off his beard and looks boyishly cute! His eyes dazzle at me, and I tell him how Fred W. is scared to kiss me. Fred C. tells me that he has wanted to kiss me as soon as he saw me!

Skis on, I replied with a broad smile, "You can kiss me." He kissed me slowly and passionately, close to how I have imagined, which I told him afterwards. With skis removed, arms around each other, Fred C. kisses me passionately again, and although I am not turned on I feel delightful, like a snowflake twirliing through space. It all feels loving, and I tell Fred that I have thought of making love with him, and that it would have to be without a commitment and when the spirit moves me. He replies, "I'd like to try." So sweet a guy! After a couple years of yearning, we may have enough love to bring it to a whole union of body, heart and spirit.

When I cried about having mixed feelings regarding making love with Fred C. in my session that same week, I sobbed as I said the words "how women through their sexuality have become more spiritual people." I was grieving the loss of my sexuality, stunted through my former oppressive religious beliefs, so that I could not connect with the spirit in me. Maybe that is why I am not with any man in particular now…I have to FEEL more of the spiritual connection within mySelf, then with another. There seems to be a beginning called kissing that leads us into the deeper love of union, the intercourse of body and spirit, FEELing what is right for us to make love. I am learning to trust my deeper feeling–truth which survives under my childhood defenses. To the pain of hearing the church saying that "JOY is: Jesus first, Others second, You last." Really, it is Your feelings first healed through tears (and rage's anger), which secondly spills into compassion for Others, then, thirdly into the Joy of trusting that all is well with the Design of the Universe. PEACE.

It's really OK that Fred W. doesn't want to be sexual with me, and that I long for the man that I am strongly attracted to, that I can be "in love" with. Being "in love" is the key to unlocking the door of defenses preventing us from feeling past pain, which distances everyone from freely loving without judgment. It is like the strong attraction to one's own children…to love them, as well as to the CHILD inside each of us, dismissed so long ago! It is all ONE. The Oneness of intercourse, the Oneness of god (not divided into religions), the Oneness of Love.

Such a powerful need there is to know, and hear that you are loved. It is why religions say "god is love." But, we are used to looking outside for god, instead of inside. We are afraid of our feelings, our anger and our tears (god-given natural healers).

Again, hearing the child within is our guiding light, as eight-year-old Kyle, son of one of my clients, demonstrates when he tells his mother that people are mean "because they haven't felt their pain." Kyle had just read my children's book, *EVERYBODY CRIES*, and loved it. His insight had not been said by his mother, or in the book. He just KNEW it within his own spirit, his feelings well accepted by both his mother and father. Kyle also came up with the idea that heaven cries with snow☺ I have mused that a snow storm is the orgasm of the universe.

I rarely remember my dreams at this time of my life. In one, I do remember repeating this one phrase several times as I was in the light waking up stage of sleep:

"*He* kissed me passionately, but not on the lips."

It was Gregory that was in the dream, looking well-groomed, and acting sweet toward me. Nothing stood out about the situation we were in. For some reason (yeah sure, we know the reason), I thought that "*He*" could really be the divine (god). That part of us that LIVES, IS PASSION, and that is not just on the lips.

It is very interesting to think that one's physical passion does begin with the touch of the lips, because it our lips that forms the words we speak – so that our feelings can be expressed – BE heard. And our feelings being heard is what makes us feel truly alive, worthwhile, and passionate about our whole bodies, our whole Being!

Continuing to grieve what I had and lost, and what I never had emotionally/spiritually, is not what our culture embraces, but what the Mayan culture has practiced for centuries and continues to this day. They embrace the "irrational," the letting go of feelings of pain that continue to be our ruination through dysfunctional relationships and poor physical health.

My sexual health is now primed to the beginnings of feeling full-body orgasms reached while I am on my back, consciously in an open position, instead of on my stomach. I stimulate more of my genital area, not just my clitoris, my labia being especially ecstastic. On a February Sunday morning, my images continue to be of men I care about as well as mountains and other scenes of nature's beauty. I orgasm with "Oh, Oh, Oh, Oh," no "Oh god," nor "Oh yes." Is this again a process toward the fundamental me? The divine in all of us, similar to the chants of "om?"

I am honoring my openness: my body's, my mind's, and most importantly, my heart's, to see where they will guide me…hearing my mother's and church's disapproval and no longer heeding or caring! I will not have the guilt added to my openness, like when I had an "open" marriage. Although I have made love with a few men in the past year, I do care about them and my Self! That is my birthright and my innocence retrieved, returned…NOT reBORN. As a bumper sticker states, which a unitarian minister sent me, "Born OK the first time."

This idea is validated when near Valentine's Day, 2001, Fred C. and I finally flower our two-year budding friendship into physical union without reservations. His kisses are very passionate, tender and encompassing because his eyes are OPEN much of the time. He tells me, "You're amazing, you know that don't you?" That line springs tears to my eyes just now, although I had replied to Fred with a shy smile, "Sometimes."

I am glad that I am not turned off by the hairiness on his back as much as I thought I would be; surprisingly his butt is totally bare, soft and smooth. He kisses my clitoris with lightness and finesse, like a true love. Also, his hands and palms are so smooth as I kiss his fingers and he kisses my clitoris. He asks if I want to orgasm that way, but I like him on top of me after I am aroused like a smoldering fire. After feeling his broad shoulders and penis within me, I give him lovemaking moans and groans by licking his penis. Then, I complete our circle of love by climbing on top of him, enjoying my favorite flavor of his penis caressing my labia, rising and falling over my clitoris. We are joining in a chorus of oohs and aahs, that crescendos with my smoldering scream, a mix of "Oh gods," and "Oh Freds." I had to reassure Fred that it was OK to focus on himself before he climaxed with a mellow non-vocal orgasm. There was a sweet smell coming from our mixed juices, not needing any lubricants other than our own. I wanted him to stay the night, a sign that I had made love with him, and not had a one night stand. Although we never did "make love" physically again, I did so with my tears when he suddenly died of a heart attack two years later, March 2002.

The next day, Fred told me that our lovemaking was "beautiful, real, and honest!" Yes! And I feel the progress within my heart when I can feel and give love <u>genuinely</u> when it cannot be returned the way I wish, like with Fred W. When I see my best friend, Tanya, this same week, she tells me, "You are the only one who has given me 'unconditional love' other than Foggy, and Lucas," (her cat and baby son respectively).

I continue to have "full body" orgasms when I masturbate, now on my back, which is not as easily "come" to as it is when positioned on my stomach. I see this change as a reflection of more and more openness to my spirit, and therefore to my connection with the entire universe, instead of being so inward and protective of self. Now I am inward in an open sense☺ Open to all possibilities, even my pain. Pain grieved presents love. A gift difficult to accept. Again, it is like being in the pain of labor in order to deliver the miraculous gift of a child!

As my "Oh god" and just "Oh" build into monumental orgasms, I wonder why we extend our heads back, like an airplane lifting its nose off the runway. A metaphor for flying when our heads lift open to the heavens? The sky? The divine within and without? Unconsciously, I have noticed that I am not allowing men into my white iron bed whom I do not feel enough love or connection to. Like the two Jims, making "caring" love in the upstairs or downstairs sofa. Whereas, Steve and Fred C. I made love to in my bed because I have very loving feelings toward them, and years of friendship connection. I allowed them to BE closer to me, in the bed where I gather cozy, comforting sleep for eight hours each night.

I choose not to be with a man on Valentine's Day 2001, finding myself eye-to-eye with my mother while delivering my Valentine card to her personally. As I leave I say, "I love you, mother." She replies, "Thank you," with tears in her eyes, then mine. I felt sad and disappointed not to hear those three precious words back, but I am not crushed. I cry in my session the next day about how I am able to be with me and love me without having to depend on a man. Like I needed daddy, my lifeline growing up, as my loud tears say, "I wish I could **tell** you how much I love you, daddy." We couldn't say it out loud because of the fear that one's family might "come" before god. "Oh god, Daddy, god was in you!" (tears now) Not in what the preacher or bible said. My tears have softened my heart so that I can begin to give love to my mother and not expect it back. My father's love protected my childhood heart so that Gregory's love could open its defendedness with tear full pain. The CAN opener with the sharp cutting point. My sobs poured out of that once-closed CAN when I said, "My body is trying to rid itself of all the bad memories…all the feelings I couldn't feel or tell anybody…I had to do it on my own…oh daddy."

Before Gregory, I had to do extreme things in order to feel (recognized) ALIVE. Like the 36 marathons I ran in 36 months. How literally, I RAN from my pain those years of 1983-85. At the age of 39 I was voted Ithaca Journal's Athlete of the Year, because I had also won Ithaca's 10-mile race (for the women.) No other "older" athlete had ever won this recognition, the Journal had always picked high school or college age athletes. I thought I was in heaven, but I was still just 5'9" off the ground. My heart knew better.

As does my body on February 23, 2001, when I hadn't masturbated for a week, and I woke up with an arousal that seemed to "come" out of nowhere. I just wished to pleasure mySelf and I came with a full body wave of energy at orgasm. There was no particular verbal expression, although "Oh god" came up once during my waves of loving pleasure. I love how my body mirrors my emotional healing into truly loving mySelf, which of course sets my spirit free to be more confidently ME. LOVE.

I had just finished reading *Aphrodite's Daughters* by Jalaya Bonheim, the night before. There is an account of a woman named Naomi who, while doing body work, felt sexual energy that kept building into ecstatic feelings of being the archetypal priestess, a woman so fully surrendered to the goddess within that her normal ego identity melted away. As Bonheim states, "Christian authorities have sentenced many mystics to death for such blasphemy. In Hinduism, on the other hand, our identity with the divine is accepted as a matter of course…The real question is to what degree we *realize* our identity with the divine – not just in an intellectually, but in an immediate, visceral way, as Naomi did in this instance." We <u>are</u> this primal force, Love; it is our birthright. The unconditional love we see in baby's eyes. The child's effortless ability to commune with the spirit of love. We begin to *realize* we are this Divine Love when we cry out our connected-to-the-child-pain. It came to me with surprise that my name Di-anea is part of the word Di-vine, and that I am a vine whose journey it is to help intertwine us all together as One, through the compassion of Love. We all are on a divine journey to reclaim the innate innocence of our primal nature.

There is a true story of a wise woman named Sara, in *Aphrodite's Daughters*. She is in her eighties, and a pioneer for healthy sexuality. She had a thirty-seven-year happy open marriage which produced four children. The confidence of their love, and respect given to their primary relationship is very rare, yet, something I can't help but admire. Is it an example of an open marriage that does not act out old pain, where intimacy is not lacking? I believe I will find out someday on my own journey. I cannot help but see a full moon-circle in its last quarter.

My spiritual journey is constantly verified by my tears, such as when I cried during the movie, "Sweet November," when Keanu said, "what I live for, is to learn to love you." I know immediately that is my life mission. To learn to love you, little dianea, because so much of mySelf was hidden by religious rules, mother's rules; whose rules did not allow my feelings. I told my daughters that my new middle name is "Feel," and also that holding onto things as "MINE" is because I had so little that was mine, in feelings, when I was growing up. So I had to hold onto material things. I am learning not to hold onto men, or sex, for my feelings of love. I now need and want to "make love" when I am sexual, otherwise I AM not truly present. I cannot say authentically and deeply, "I love you."

Until Jack. I have written of several men in my life where I had hoped to love enough to feel "in love." On our first date, at dinner, I'm brave and say, "I am attracted to you, and haven't been to the many personal ad-men before you." I loved his hands, and the way he moved his hands over mine while watching the movie after dinner. When we parted, Jack says, "You scared me out of my mind." I smiled, "That's good, then, you are in your heart." He kissed me, and I especially remember the last movement of our lips as he stayed and lingered. That slow, noticing, passionate type of "being with you," instead of the fast, pressured, invasive kiss. Tenderness is a way of really caring like the slow changing colors of the fall leaves, "falling in love☺"

Yet, like a storm, our leave of caution was falling fast. The next night, Jack brought dinner to my home, and we talked long and made out long like romantics. While recounting a past life memory, I did not hide my tears as I said, "I have compassion for blacks because I've been one." Although Jack has trouble with women's tears, and it is difficult for him to cry, he doesn't try to fix it. He holds me. He may need me to help him cry, and I may need him in my journey to be truly loved for ALL of me. He says, "*Making* **love**" is one of his most favorite things to do, and I am happy that he says it that way instead of saying, "*having* **sex**." Also, I notice how "making" is so much more fun than "having."

Jack wanted to have oral sex with me, which I was not ready for, and he was fine with holding off. We took off our outer clothes (he wears no underwear), and I am wearing underpants and undershirt. We could not bare just sleeping together. Our kissing and touching evolved into me rolling on top of him, placing his penis between my legs, which caressed my clitoris. I traveled from a mini-orgasm into a full-fledged one which pleased Jack. He said, "Oh god" several times, and "Oh Dianea" in response to "Oh Jack" and "Come with me." But I was not ready for intercourse either, so he enjoyed caressing his penis between my labia, as I enjoyed watching and hearing his joy. His body shuddered like an electric lightning bolt full of love. He said he'd never had anyone do it like this to him before. I was surprised as he has had many sexual experiences as well as a long-term marriage.

We slept together, rather I tried to sleep while he snored. I had to leave our bed. And still I could not sleep until after I masturbated into a sweet orgasm where I said, "Come in with me." Knowing I meant, let's come inward to our true beings, "fearless" as he says of me. I know we will have some fear to expose ourselves to, but I have an undying desire to do so, and hope Jack will. Although I am aware of some similarities between Jack and Gregory (Jack smokes 3 or 4 cigarettes per day and wants to quit), he is not addicted to alcohol, and has a steady job which he likes. I am falling in love with Jack. He says he is tumbling and could have a hard fall for me.

Jack tells me that our first lovemaking was "one of the most powerful sexual experiences in my life!…And your sexuality is like second-nature to you." At our first dinner he had noticed that I am "centered, calm." Two days later we have dinner together again, and watch the movie video "The Kid," making love at an intermission. I had a small wave of orgasm, while Jack came with breakers, amazed, saying, "You know my penis better than I do." Another metaphor as to why he is with me…to know himSelf more…as well as me to know mySelf more. We had kissed softly before making love orally with his penis. Learning about our bodies along with our hearts.

Jack gives me his large three-ring notebook containing his novel, poems, and short stories. When we next talk on the phone Jack tells me that he is concerned that he may not be what I want because he takes his feelings inward, "internalizes" them, or writes them.

When we wake up together the next morning I experience a most incredible moment with him. He tells me, "You're gorgeous," but that is not it! We began to talk and explored what making love's significance is to us, as I pointed toward the window showing the orgasm of the universe. It was snowing outside, as I laid in his muscular arms, and said, "Orgasm is like crying, 'letting go;'" those last two words poured forth freely flowing tears. I continued to cry as I said, "The 'oh god' we explode at orgasm is BEing the divinity within us, trying to BE!" A smile pushes up my cheeks and makes my tears roll into rainbows of glistening. My mind and heart immediately ARE at one as sexuality and spirituality converge into Oneness. The compassion we have for all things because we are truly loving by exposing ourselves, so vulnerable, so real. Then, I *just* cried a few sobs into his arms. Jack *just* held me, *just* what I needed. JUSTICE☺

I remember saying during my tears that I felt like making love with Jack because of my heart's closeness to him. Later, on the phone, I asked Jack how he felt about my crying. He said that he felt fine, he wasn't scared, and it felt good that I trusted him. It IS a moment I will never forget, so special, like a double rainbow after a thunder storm.

I had taken another step into courage, beyond what I had had with Rosey, where I wasn't held, nor did I get into the meaning of my tears, only telling him that I was a bit afraid to have cried with him, yet felt OK about doing so. I didn't feel scared with Jack, it felt so very natural, safe, time stood still and soon we were making love. MAKING Love, literally and heartily☺ Jack continued to honor my desire not to have intercourse yet. I wanted to in part, as did he, but a bigger part of me knew it wasn't the right time. I kept thinking, "I want to have intercourse when I can say, 'I love you,' to him."

I had said, "I'm falling in love with you," which he also acknowledged. My journey seemed more whole, as the coming together of our bodies mirrored more of our hearts and minds – so our spirits could truly soar. I notice that I still am not totally accepting of my buttocks, or my aging skin, while wishing I had more flesh over my chest bones. I have more emotional release work to do.

The next morning, as I lay on my belly, I masturbate not just because I was thinking of Jack, but also other thoughts that were important to me and my day. When I orgasmed, I was saying out loud, "Oh god, oh Jack, it's incredible, we're together," several times. Tears rushed in as I said, "I'm coming together!" And then, I thought, I'm coming together into who I really AM!

That NEW orgasmic truth was "So cool!" to me, as the groovy talker says it. Yet, I felt so hot as I orgasmed, as well as feeling so wise. What a wonderful paradox again of how life integrates the opposites, cool and hot, like male and female.

Many people say, even Jack, "That's the way I am," in referring to some personality trait, like Jack saying how he internalizes his feelings. Yet, that is not the way Jack truly is – it is what he has learned to do – it's not the way he was born. As is everyone. Conditioned and defended.

That same day of that NEW orgasmic truth, I found a black moth-butterfly with a single white stripe down the middle of each of its wings perched on the dryer. I carefully lifted it to my hand and carried it upstairs with me as I looked for something in the basket in the loft. I placed it on a newspaper, but it didn't want to stay there. It flew around me a couple of times, then lit on my jeans. Guess where? Near the zipper of my crotch…did it like the smell of us mixed together? It stayed there for approximately ten minutes as I walked around, leaving me near the woodstove where I wrote this poem to Jack:

> A smoldering ember I am no longer,
> My constant glow waiting for your kin-d-ling
> To lie on top of me,
> Touched tenderly into yellow flame
> Fingers traveling your seasoned splinters
> Of fear and woulden vulnerability
> Kissing lips burning into red flames
> Now dancing above you
> As you pull your ember into shudddering
> Hot blue flames of open-eyed ecstasy.

The moth-butterfly symbolized the connection between everything and the energy and safety we can create between each other. The love that has no boundaries, yet limits. Like the different men I have been telling you about, how our relationships differ in feeling, and yet, bring energy and safety to heal our wounded hearts.

A day later, when Steve, the massager, interviewed me for the Ithaca Times, a local newspaper, this truth became so clear to me. When I asked Steve if he would be sexual with me again if I was free, tears freely flowed. He replied that he would, despite knowing that it was best for him to be with Andrea, his wife from whom he was still separated. I connected my tears to my deprivation of not having a real loving connection for so long. One that would be REALLY Me, because I trusted my feelings and not someone else's, like I had during my thirty-eight years under religion's rule.

Now, I was listening more often to my own little voice of my spirit that is becoming louder and louder as I wash away boulders of emotional pain that have blocked the hearing of my own truth. I ask more scary questions with Jack, like "What do you mean when you say I am the woman you have been looking for all your life, or that I am sexually powerful?" I am aware that I am a little afraid to ask, because it borders on self-praise, a no-no of the church, of course. But, I sailed through it, no longer a part of that crew.

"It's the quality I've sensed and felt, that you are very healthy physically, sexually, joyful, playful, and an evolving wonderful expression…a spiritual disrobement," Jack tells me. "How happy you are in your vulnerability, letting your tears come, analagous to orgasm, *let them come.*" He said that he liked how we were moving together in mental, intellectual, and spiritual connections besides the physical; if we were to race ahead it would not be as healthy or balanced…that the power and depth of our lovemaking is huge…that the level of intimacy with me is spectacular. He continues, "Holding back is part of the dance, delaying gratification means more orgasms before climax." Maybe it also means there is more harmonious and balanced orgasms bringing together all the parts of ourselves until we come into the climax of REAL Love, where I can genuinely say, "I love you."

"I want to understand you more before you do me the great honor of letting me inside you." I hear Jack's sincere tone over the phone. How beautiful and loving he sounds, although he did leave out emotional connection in his list of how we were moving together. I sensed that although Jack could express his present feelings toward me, that he had barely begun to connect with the hurt little boy inside himSelf. I, all too soon, found this out in an astounding way.

A few days later when we made love, Jack says he's ready in his heart to have intercourse, and I have told him that I want to be able to tell him, "I love you." He took that in without a response. When he says that he loves my leaness, I reply with a laugh, "I'm the lean, mean, loving machine." Jack immediately replies, "not mean." I reply that I know that and, "I am a different meaning of mean…full of MEANing☺"

I also relate to Jack, that I love how "TEARing one's heart open with TEARS" is a wonderful piece of unconscious language construction. Like the LOVE<>EVOL(VE) construction's meaning. After loving him orally he did not orgasm, saying that he was stuck on wanting intercourse with me. As he held me, I told him that he is the first man I have held out on intercourse within a healthy way. That he is special (and therefore I am) because *I want* and don't *need* anyone to have sex with in order to feel loved. That I can risk rejection. That this is a BIG TURNING point in my life!

No longer do I hold out on intercourse because I feel guilty, like I did with Gus, and regretted it, due to my religious convictions at that time. I feel more loving and whole, as Jack said the ways: "intellectually, spiritually, and physically," I added, "and emotionally." Jack half-smiled. I went on to say that I never saw Daddy cry, only tears well up in his eyes. I knew that he died of a broken heart because he died of a sudden heart attack. Jack asked how so? I related how dad held his pain in, and hesitated, near tears. Jack gently said, "Let them come." So they did, like the orgasms I had with Jack the night before, which were good ones, although not big screamers. But they were becoming bigger, and I was closer to having one with oral lovemaking.

We slept together and I awoke aroused, wanting to make love again. I caressed Jack's penis maybe five minutes without a response, so I masturbated into "Oh god" with Jack beside me. I felt another step into freedom with him. I even told him about it in the morning and he asked me to shake him next time, because he wanted to be awakened (in more ways than one?)

He does meditate fifteen minutes a day which he says helps to calm him. I noted how his leg moves back and forth sometimes, and told him that it is reaction to anxiety – fear. He acknowledged this and said maybe he doesn't know how to get there. Maybe that is why he is with me.

Jack's had a mild heart attack already, and an angioplasty. Now he will break both of our hearts. After we had a terrific time together while he snowshoed and I cross-country skiied, and I made dinner for us while we talked for close to three hours, we began to make love. He lifted me up in his arms onto the futon, naked. So romantic! We made snow angels and wrestled in the snow too. We made love in expansive ways, learning about our bodies together. I did not have an orgasm, and we fell apart. Jack said "I feel inadequate, guarded inside, this sense of dread." I cried, and owned my piece of it. He dressed himself and left for his house.

I tried to reassure him, and he said it was too complicated, that he couldn't be with my feelings, that he had to be with his own. It was shocking to have all this happen so suddenly. Yet, I was pleased with my calm response, and that I could sleep until 6am. Soon, I felt aroused, not from anxiety, it just felt like the right thing thing to do. As I do more often, I came to a connected feeling as I orgasmed. I said out loud, "It's for sure that I love you." And I KNEW that I was not only loving me, but also saying, "I love you, Jack." I poured forth tears like a natural spring for some minutes and made an initial connection with wanting it all to be perfect, and later in my crying session it was expanded into what I said to Jack the next day. That I felt like the child that needs to hear "I love you" from their parent, to say it first, then, together. The child's need for perfect unconditional love. Why I wanted Jack and I to feel the same desire to say "I love you" to each other at the same time.

The next day, when Jack and I stood on Geneva Street, I said, "I love you," straight into his blue eyes. He replied into my blue eyes, "I love you, too, Dianea." (tears now) I didn't really expect those words back, as tears watered my cheeks. Jack took those tears from my cheeks to his lips with his fingers.(more tears and sobs) So sweet to the taste of Love. So connected to our spirits.

Before those three precious words were spoken, we had walked and talked for a half hour, and Jack expressed his conflict over our relationship. He felt the inequality, like he was the problem and I was the wise one. He didn't feel accepted as he is, yet also realized that his feelings do go back to him not feeling accepted unconditionally by his parents. Why not have both acceptance of the now as well as growth for change? He wants that for cigarettes, he said. So, he lights up a cigarette as he leaves me, saying we are a "maybe."

The next day on the phone, Jack told me how much more respect he has for me because I came to find him, not retreating into my feelings of hurt and rejection or abandonment. That he felt "heard," as well as hearing me.

"You are very brave!" he tells me.

"It's my tears that make me courageous," I answer.

It is now March 10, 2001, there is a full moon, and Jack has brought home dinner, as well as a dozen red roses. I brought him a yellow rose with a red tip, and a poem I wrote for him called, "Full Spectrum," written on a card with Hawaiian volcanoes erupting and a man and woman under full moons. He read the poem out loud which made the feelings louder. We went outside to view the full moon, and took pictures of us under it, snow sparkling at our feet. I told Jack, "I love you," under the moonlight which warmed us in the cold *before we went inside* the house he built. Jack replied with his eyes in mine, "I love you" as he put his index finger on my nose simultaneously with the sound of the word "you." After dinner, where our words flowed freely as our feelings, we made out on the futon and slowly removed each other's clothes. Kissing estatically, knowing that we were building to that special entry of unifying our love. It was outstandingly special when Jack said, "I'm glad we waited." I asked "why?"

The answer was a bit muddled, pressed under by desire. I wish I could remember it. Jack's desire to BE all there with me felt like real-loving-respect, like one has for the birth of your baby naturally, not unaware under anesthesia, wanting to BE present with every contraction, every breath, every step of the process of this fulfillment of the loving act of intercourse where the orgasm of love gives the gift of Life.

My vagina was a bit tight at first, but Jack was gentle with his largeness. My in-Di-go boy! We MADE LOVE beautifully. Jack loved the way I gave him pleasure, saying "You're magnificent." I've never heard such grand superlatives before. When he finally orgasmed, after I had climaxed in a new way, he came and came and came. He shuddered and vocalized primal sounds powerfully full of love.

Next, we watched the movie video, "Walk on the Moon," which Jack liked because it was so "real," like our making love again, after the movie, in his bed. I orgasmed by way of partial intercourse, and then Jack orgasmed so intensely that his shudders and sounds lasted for several minutes. Finally, he said, "That's the most intense orgasm I've ever had," except when he made a baby. (He has two daughters.) Yet, the best part came while lying in each other's arms, when Jack said, "This is the best part, the contentment and feeling of Love," after our culmination of physical pleasure. Jack's words made the word "beautiful" insufficient to describe the largeness of my heart.

Jack read three pages of his novel, *Meteor* before our second round of lovemaking. He described the male sun and female moon (Diana is goddess of the moon) as exquisitely complimentary in their differences! " 'Oh god' is not sufficient to describe all the greatness of this man," I write in my journal, with tears echoing those words. Why? Is it about me, Jack, and Daddy all rolled into one?

Jack and I are together again a couple of days later, after he asked on the phone for me to think of how I would fantasize the best lovemaking to be, and to tell him when he came over to my home. This is what I wrote down:

"Slowness – waiting inch by inch, into my lips; to appreciate every touch, every look, every cell of (y)our skin

Passionate - lingering kisses, with eye contact ever present, intermingled with the need to be with oneself.

Moving to oral sex only when I cannot stand not having it, because so many loving kisses, hands and fingers stimulating my nipples have led to irreparable fireworks. Like I have to beg for it.

Tongue light as a feather on my clitoris – back and forth like a hummingbird – and fluttering down my labia occasionally.

Me giving your penis kisses and touches of ecstasy so that you shudder, then me, lying on your back, stroking my clitty on your butt –

Then you, doing something new, lying on top of me, facing me, your penis between my legs, rubbing my clitoris and labia until I am coming and then you enter me gently and wildly. As if I was the only one you could ever love so fully! And you come with me to paradise – eyes open to each other."

Our lovemaking mirrored much of what I wrote, adding "I love you" to each other. The best part. I had a top notch screaming orgasm after being on a wave of orgasm for a long time. I could not fully scream because my housemate was upstairs. I felt at times that I was trying too hard, which I realize keeps me from having potentially more ecstasy. That fear that I am taking too long. Jack wants me to be inside him – my finger in his butt – which makes him go wild with groans and moans and muscle contractions, sometimes while stroking my silky hair.

After Jack first arrived at my house, while sitting on the sofa, we talked for a half hour or more, and he said, "I love you, Dianea," adding, "I want to be the first to say it, to have us more equal." I am glad that he is aware that I usually say it first and more often, and that he wants as much equality as possible. Balance.

When we made love again in the morning, and were holding each other after orgasm, I said, "I love you incredibly," and began to cry. I cried for a couple of minutes, a letting go right after my orgasm of love. It was a very spiritual moment for me, and I said so to Jack. He was silent while he held me, and brushed away my tears with his gentle carpenter hands. We had had more light on when we made love the night before, and Jack said it was his error not to have had more light during previous nights of lovemaking. Yet, it seems fitting to our process, to begin in dimmer candlelight, and grow into greater light as we learn and know more about each other.

I asked Jack again what caused the huge conflict over us to change from a "maybe" relationship to a clear "yes." He reiterated that he had felt "heard," and that I didn't try to defend or change his feelings of fear that night he left so abruptly. He had no reason not to trust me. He said that my openness and honesty were key, not mentioning my vulnerability of tears, or me saying "I love you" for the first time.

Because Jack had only certain nights for child visitation, we didn't see each other until two nights later. We could not help but make love, and Jack continued to orgasm with intensity, while I experienced smaller orgasms. The next morning Jack wanted to make love again, and though he comes wildly, I am satisfied without orgasm. He seemed disappointed and a bit distant when he left for work. He said he is not good at goodbyes, and came back to kiss me. I felt really sad when he left; I had not heard "I love you" when we made love this last time. At dinner the night before, we had talked about his previous girlfriend, Kate. He said it was hard to see her struggle alone, although she had left him. I replied that I knew the feeling in watching him struggle alone with his feelings the night that he felt "dread." And had to leave, to be alone.

Only two months ago they had parted ways. I felt a little scared when I thought about them possibly getting back together, then, I thought about how Jack had said that he had waited 44 years for a woman like me. And how the night before at dinner, he had told me that it was special how I had thought to wear a red thong under my long, cotton spaghetti-strap blue nightgown that is designed in an innocent girlish style. The contrast was beautiful. Yes, that whole child-adult beauty. Jack had said something like, "I've been with many beautiful bodies, and none rate next to yours." I was embarrassed and blushed in disbelief! I couldn't remember his exact words, and I was annoyed that my old emotional pain – growing up with shame of my body – got in the way of my memory. We had talked for three hours before making love, me massaging his sore shoulders and back, after Jack lighted three candles…one was not enough for Jack.

Like religion is not enough for me. Jack told me about when he was eight years old and couldn't sleep for two nights because he was scared of not being able to see god. He called a Congregational minister who reassured him that he would be OK. But I have never been OK in the slavery of religion, which dawned on me in a significant way, again, while talking to Jack at that same dinner, where tears rolled as I said, "I love you Jack." I hesitated and waited for the connection of my tears to my old emotional pain…that of not being able to say those words to my father, or hear them said to me, although dad had written them many times. Also, I was connected immediately to the most significant conversation I ever had with my father. I was sixteen, and in our kitchen; I can see my dad walking up the cellar steps, and me telling him, as I leaned on the kitchen table, how I had just realized that I was this separate being, able to express my own individuality, how special that feeling was to me. And also, to be a person born out of one of a million sperm and one egg coming together. Those last words prompted tears reflecting my lack of recognition of my specialness because of how the church made me feel unworthy of god's love. A true slavery of the spirit! Jack was fine with my tears; he beckons them.

Yet, after dinner he walks outside to have his favorite cigarette of the day. He knows it pains me, as well as his daughters. I cannot entertain the painful thought that we will not make it together. His email the next day tells me that he has to slow down, that his emotions have not caught up with his attractions. I am understanding. I may be the one who is dumped into the gopher hole if the horse travels too fast. I know that I must learn to love as though I have not been hurt. I feel safe to cry with Jack, to be so real, and I know that the pit of my stomach needs to cry more, I could feel it! This I need to do alone, or in my crying sessions with Susanne, so that **I can love as though I have not been hurt**, where defensiveness and fear cannot rule.

Interestingly, the same day of Jack's "slow down" email, I receive a letter from Fred W. apologizing for cutting off all communication with me. "Too many triggers, and too much unresolved anger and grief," he writes. "I'm trying to work hard in AA, exercise, better diet, therapy, to grow and become a better person." I hope Jack will do the same.

Two days later, Jack and I talk about our relationship. He says we are "too different," surprising me by telling me that I'm, the "light-hearted" one, and he the "gloomier, denser." I am pleased that he sees me this way because I am the one who does all the crying. He continues, "It's coming from my gut feeling; we're not balanced, I'm afraid you're already way too attached. I am not as emotionally available as I advertised myself to be." His heart is still with his previous girl-friend, even though he gives no hope for a return to that relationship.

Tears parallel my words, "Does this mean you are dismissing your love for me?"

"It's not logical, my guts tell me. I feel guilt and reservation after being with you. You have tremendous energy and power and I get swept up into it…I'm pre-tending to be free when I am not. I am still attached to Kate, and thought I could abide both, but I was wrong. Because I care about you, I don't see anything but hurt down the road for you. It's not easy for me to back away."

With tears shaking my words, I say, "Why would you walk away from some-thing so good? I am okay with the hurt."

Jack goes on, "The more I know you, the more I see how wonderful you are. There's no reason not to fall head over heels over you. It's about my feelings. I am not ready to be a patient."

"How about being patient?" I reply. "It seems you put up walls before the foundation is built." As I am writing this over a year later, I begin to cry in read-ing Jack's mail, "the more I **know** you, the more I see how wonderful you are." This is the whole spiritual process of which I am writing. **Know**ing my inner feel-ing's source, the divine Love all babies are born with, which had been taken away from me, whose pain I had locked away as a child, the massive heavy door of reli-gion making it most difficult to enter my true heart's spirit of love for mySelf, then others.

Before we hung up, I told Jack, "These are GOOD tears, I hope you find yours!" Alone I cried maybe twenty minutes, feeling and seeing my connection to my pain with my mother. She threw away a good thing…Me! Although I am learning to feel more and more of my pain while alone, at times it helps to receive support from an understanding loved one. I called my daughter Megan, who lis-tens and feels sorry well. I told her how much I appreciated her love and tender-ness.

After calling Megan, I called my dearest friend, Susanne, who supported me with love for maybe ten minutes. Then, I picked up another friend, Adriana, to attend a dance benefit for a man with cancer. I had fun dancing…yes, I am "light-hearted," because I let spiritual tears flow.

When we talk again, Jack says that the big difference between us is my drive to improve, and that he is more self-satisfied. That he trusts his fear, forty-four years of "instinct." That therapy is "self-centered."

I counter with an email the next day, "If we find more REAL LOVE in Oneself, it naturally turns into compassion for others, and as you know from history – indiviuals with their heart open are the ones who change the world. Anyway, if we are really honest, everything we do is for the Self. Even my giving cheap rates to my clients comes out of making me feel really good, so in giving to others, I am more self-loving, and self-satisfied.

"Also, I'm surprised that you don't value therapy's huge contribution to this world's exposure of physical, sexual, and emotional abuse, even moreso to the possibility of healthier relationships, more Love, so that this 'self-centered' work only contributes to the good of others. Yes, it is painful, like the nail striking the wood – but there is a difference between nailing the coffin, and the nailing of the heart, by allowing it to split open, letting the tears fall like rain onto a parched earth.

"You say, you wish you hadn't said what you said to Kate – but you trusted your feelings then (good for you), to say what you needed, and it didn't turn out as you needed. So which 'gut feelings' can you trust?

"This has been my work, and others, to separate out the feelings of FEAR that we have built up as a result of our experiences of not being loved well – and therefore defend against with all kinds of addictions and busyness – and the healthy fears against true dangers.

"Why wouldn't you want to do that for yourself and your children? Except it is too painful? Yet, with support, it is the path to freedom!! To be that indigo boy full of innocence and joy! As building a house is a process (probably the trees cry as they are cut down for limber), so is breaking open our heart to REAL LOVE. One hour a week is not much in the big scheme of things – you are worth much more than that!...

"What's in it for me? Our relationship is a crucible of Love for which I am forever grateful. Thank you for allowing us to fall in love, it is the seedling to bigger and greater Love, and all its possibilities. It allows me to cry out more pain, and free up my cells to love more☺ (Tears now of course☺) Yes, our differences in emphasis may seem very great at this point, but as you say, 'the universe gives us what we need.' Let's take advantage of it – don't you miss our wonderful love-making? Let's MAKE more Real Love!! You are a very special man! I hope you have a safe and sunny trip to Texas and into the warmth of our love – Dianea

P.S. I give you all the room you need, that does not include giving up."

The night before, Jack had become annoyed when I gently asked about why his side carpenter jobs were so important. He had replied that he needed the money to put his two daughters through college. I said, "But if you don't take care of yourself, you won't be able to take care of them. You've had one warning of a mild heart attack."

Then, Jack ended our conversation with an angry tone, "This is getting boring. Good night Dianea." I felt strong and more settled even though I was sad, because it was clear that he did not want or dare to do the emotional release work necessary to move our spirits closer to Real Love.

The next day Jack emails, "Let's talk when I get back. I think you are an extraordinary person and a remarkable lover. And yes, I'll miss that. Jack."

So, the first day of spring brought an ending, not a beginning of a love desired. Yet, I signed onto another beginning, a lease for an apartment on Gray Road, because I had finally sold my house after it being on and off the market for six years. I was aware that there was more and more *gray* in my life, but until recently, I had not liked the color gray. It was too blah and drab. Now, I was glad that I was moving far away from my "black and white" religious upbringing: one way to god, one way to think, one way to dress. One way to feel. I was glad to be in the "gray" zone, and it was reflected outwardly in my life as well as inwardly.

In 1994, I was shopping for a used Jeep, and the one I found in the newspaper was gray. Shucks, but the price and upkeep were right! Even though gray is not a beautiful color, it does allow other colors to shine, like the thin rainbow stripes I had stuck around the Jeep's middle. In December of 1999, my daughter buys me a gray bathrobe for Christmas! And when I read the word "princess" embroidered on the back, yes, you guessed it, I cried tears that shone with love. And since June 2001, I have lived at and loved 4 Gray Road, where I have a gorgeous view of a long valley of trees of many different colors, and am next door to a state park full of splashing waterfalls. GRAY is now special to me, lightning the darkness of this world.

I just noticed that RAY is the largest part of the word "gray." A RAY of light that is so wide that my sexuality can arRAY itself alongside spirituality like the two people laying next to each other making love with the intercourse of conversation and the intercourse of the body finally becoming one.

And my body continues to heal itself in small ways, like the pigmentation moles from too much sun exposure falling off of their own accord. And my body desiring to stay healthy in its form, by being a healthy weight with good muscle tone. I wish to represent this childlike body…retrieving the innocent unconditionally-loving child again, who is the foundation for an adult body and soul to become fully responsible for healthy loving. Could there be a fountain of youth from my fountain of tears?

In my crying sessions with Susanne the same week of Jack leaving me, I was crying about how I used to be so strong outwardly, so competent in repressing and suppressing my feelings, and now I am in such a better place of BEING with my feelings… "I want to FEEL." The word FEEL brought forth intense tears, like a waterfall in spring.

I went on to cry about how hard it is for me to say or write good things about mySelf because I have been a religious enslaved soul. "Pride comes before a fall," the Bibile says. You cannot be proud of yourself. My tears said, "I have to speak out more and more about listening to our own spirit, and not believe what others tell you. I will not shut up about that! I'm coming out of the religious slavery in order to be a spiritual Being.

It is difficult for me to write what an astrologer told me, "You are a virtuoso on the keyboard of Love," in 1996. Or, in 1999, another astrologer said that Iam going my own way and others' advice is not going to be all that helpful. I see an astrologer every two to three years, to check in with another way that the Design of the Universe may be helping me along my path. As the tides are connected to the pull of the moon, so the planets and stars have their meaning in the inter-connectedness of everything in creation. I will embrace and heal mySelf with my truths and my tears. My tears validate the truth *that religion is slavery, and feeling is freedom of my spirit…to really Love.*

I ask myself, "Must my heart be broken over and over again so that I no longer hurt and only love?" As Mother Teresa says, "I have found the paradox that I love until it hurts, then there is no hurt, only more love." I cannot imagine mySelf to be like Mother Teresa, yet, I can imagine feeling less hurt, and loving more.

After Jack left my life, I missed making love, being close, feeling the beauty of a man. These shorter connections with men that I have told you of are not bit-ter, but sweet, like the smelling of roses in the garden. Not just walking by and noticing their beauty. And it is because I like/love these men. The smarter thing to feel! I am reminded of something that a male friend, Davide, told me one night as he drove me home from dancing. He surprised me when he said, "Women are smarter in every way than men." I didn't want to accept that at first, because I do not feel we are better than men. This does not mean that women are superior in value, spiritually. Yet, a well-known anthropologist, Ashley Montagu, who wrote several books, one being *The Natural Superiority of Women*, (first edition 1952, revised 1992) agrees with Davide. I do sense that women are leaders in the emotional/spiritual arenas while men are leaders in physical strength. It is why I am aware of the crux of our behaviors even in orgasm.

Like the orgasm I had soon after Jack told me to move on. I had not awakened aroused, and was spending my usual thirty minutes or more lying in bed, think-ing creatively, which has happened increasingly in the last few years where I am making time to be more aware. When I finally orgasmed, while lying on my stomach, I said, "Oh Jack, Oh Jack" knowing I was close to my spirit in feeling, spontaneously adding, "Where is the Love?" which spouted tears. I immediately thought of Daddy and wondering when I was sixteen whether he still loved me after hearing my mother yell, "He's not your father." I felt so close to LOVE with dad, and then it was quickly taken away, like what happened with Jack.

When I cried about this orgasm in my session with Susanne, and said, "Where is the LOVE?" I responded with ,"Inside of me." I was sobbing as I continued to say, "Open your own heart, Dianea, to find the love." And that is why I am with these men, like Jack, to trigger my old pain, grieve my childhood of inadequate love which opens my heart to truly LOVE. And BE LOVED. In this process I am more and more aware of how severe the trauma of that sixteen year-old event was for me; how alone I felt with my painful feelings. Immediately, I feel more sensitivity for other's pain, *compassion*, and thereby understanding and non-judgmentalness.

And, also I understand why dancing plays an important part in my life. It is where I am more of my Real Self than anywhere else. I am connected to a partner, and uninhibited on the dance floor. "Feminine, frilly, and free," or "sexy, sensual, and showy of my body."

Grieving shows me how to understand the difference between a "gut" feeling to follow or not to follow. Jack said that it was his gut feeling that he needed to leave me. He did own that it was his fear, but not knowing really why. Our gut feeling of fear is many times from repressed past painful experiences, and therefore we act them out in our behaviors. Like I was almost willing to act out sexually for Gregory so that he would not leave me. But, as I continued to feel my rage and sadness, I felt a big growing conviction to say NO. I will always remember that day of self-confidence. Fear no longer owned me...although I felt sadness for some time. My conclusion: **my spirit is alive when my capcity to grieve is widened, making my ability to Love deeper!**

It is a slow and gradual process that needs regular attention! My journal has been my most effective way of meditation to healing awareness. Our bodies need regular attention – exercise and good food. Our minds need regular attention – reading to learn. Our heart-spirits need regular attention – crying, expressing feelings. In summary:

DANCING is how my body expresses the Real Child's Truth.
CRYING is how my feelings express the Real Truth.
READING and WRITING is how my mind expresses the Real Truth to others.

And, dear reader, you have noticed how I love the interconnection of language with our truths. Another came about for me in answering a personal ad voice mail. I was so spontaneous that I said, "Oh god" while thinking *out loud* of something to say, about something *good* to say about myself, laughing, of course. (We laugh many times when we are afraid, anxious). Isn't it interesting that GOOD is just one OH from the spelling of GOD☺ I'm smiling again!

Because there is also a connection to GOD DAMN IT! Which is an anger that I feel less and less. One day I was triggered by one of my clients who is forty years old and very afraid to tell her mother, "Stop telling me I am wrong!" Her mother had discounted Sharon's feelings all during her growing up, as my mother had, and I had worked several months with Sharon to feel (face) her fear so she could learn to trust herself again. I was losing patience because I needed to feel more of my emotional pain. Later, when writing in my journal, I yelled out loud at my mother for telling me that my feelings and beliefs are wrong. (My mother is not present at this outpouring). I added, "God damn the disrespect of parents to children's feelings," with tears of hurt. "God damn it, you're not always right, mother! Just love me for who I am! Oh god."

As usual, anger is a cover up of our fear of hurt feelings, but what is interesting in this discussion is that we invoke 'god' when we are feeling FEAR or anger that covers the fear. Or, at the other extreme, when we feel incredible joy which is the face of LOVE. Like at orgasm. The opposite of fear. And when we feel helpless, very vulnerable, is when we are most conscious or unconscious of needing god. The divine within. Out **comes** "Oh god."

If only we could be free to express all of the divineness that we are born with, seen in the eyes of babes! So here we are again, aware of the united spirit(uality) of language that helps make the "oh god" of orgasm of love most meaningful. I am told that I "press" people too much to ex "press" their feelings, when they are sup "press"ing them, causing de "press"ion. This was graphically illustrated in a conversation with my thirty-year-old Erin, when she asked why Jack and I broke up. The easiest illustration I could come up with at the time was to tell her how while we were making love, Jack up and left because I wanted to hold off on intercourse. Erin said that she did not want to hear about my sex life. Yet, the conversation was not focused on our sexual behavior, but on Jack's fear, re "press"ed childhood pain. And, what I understood to be Erin's repression of her childhood pain from my expecting her to become a "born again" christian while I was still enslaved by it until she was twelve. She was brought up with a similar shame of sexuality although much less than what I have experienced, but it still prevails, sad to say. Sexuality and spirituality still have tracks that are far from crossing each other.

The lack of crossing paths with men who will risk being deeply vulnerable is why I continue to have short term relationships and to be alone a great deal. The men I have been *in love* with, Gregory and Jack, leave and I am alone. I don't like it; I cry and sob about it sometimes, and say, "Hear me out there? I know the lesson, but I don't have to like it!" And the lesson is that when I am alone, I am more sensitive to hearing my own feelings, than others who have been alone a great deal more than I, loved less well. Still, I know I have family and friends who do love me. I am truly trusting that the Design of the Universe, "god," has something better for me, and I have to go through this "sensitivity training," grieving, to get there☺ This training has given me greater immunity to illness, less anger, and above all, expansive orgasms of love.

Like the orgasm I had another morning because I was being desirous of giving myself pleasure. At orgasm, I'm a lovely one, I said, "Why can't you come along with me?" while thinking of Jack. The tears appeared when I added, "I know you are scared." Like I have been in the past, to ex "press" my vulnerable feelings.

Jack and I did get together one more time to have dinner and make love. It blew my mind, OUT. I finally had the screaming orgasm I'd wanted with Jack. Before now, I could not let go enough, I tried too hard. I did have to be persistent, Jack's penis between my labia and he tuning in my nipples with the gentle twist of his fingers. Sometimes I worry that I'm taking too long, but Jack was patient, and later said that he enjoyed my pleasure a great deal. He was not in a hurry to have intercourse and licked my clitoris with less pressure as he had learned to due to my communication of what I needed. As I have become more sensitive to my painful feelings, then, letting go of them through tears; I've needed lighter and lighter touching of my clitoris in order to reach orgasm. The harder pressures dull my pleasurable sensations. I don't NEED much pressure to FEEL!

I love this new found sensitivity of my body, heart and spirit! As Jack walked into my house that evening, I knew that I would look into his eyes steadfastly like a baby does, and wait for him to passionately kiss me. I relished his long gaze, his slow lean toward our kiss, his large hands cradling my head and chin. Lovemaking had begun with a long kiss. Our eyes open.

LIKE LOVE IS. After our incredible orgasm, I said, "There's not much that gets close to the experience of making love," as I thought about childbirth. Then Jack said, "Childbirth!"

"Yes," I added, "Playing with babies; receiving their unconditional love." That is what making love is all about – what we are all after – unconditional love. After Jack's first orgasm I said, "I love you, you know." He didn't reply this time, and I didn't feel like crying. I was making another step toward being able to give love without expecting it back. We held each other for many minutes, and made love again, although I was very satisfied. He had a huge orgasm again, and said, "Come with me." I was close to another orgasm with shivers throughout my body. I was satisfied that I had such an intense effect on Jack. I knew I was special to him. Out of the blue he said, "You are an outrageously spectacular lover." I asked, "How do you feel that?"

"Your passion and freedom." He liked that I touched him lightly too. I really am the light-hearted one. We held our hands at the end of a scrumptious dinner at the Boatyard Restaurant. He touched my hand smoothly and tenderly, fed me cake off his fork before he ate some. I toasted to "more love of life."

Jack was wise to leave me so that I could meet Gare through Match.com. That's how I feel as I gain trust in myself: more acceptance and trust in the Design of the Universe. "I have waited so long" for REAL love, is why tears flow every time I sing those words from, "Maybe It's Love," by Trisha Yearwood. I am continually on the search, tears leading and lighting my path. And my body reflects this healing again in the smallest of ways.

For a week or so in April 2001, I developed a rash around my belly button. In my weekly crying session, I connected those symptoms to how my mother never loved me from the time I was in her womb. "I've waited for so long," for love, like Gare, an unhappily married man for thirty-six years. Like my father who was not loved by my mother. Mom admitted to me that she cried on her wedding day because she no longer loved this man whom she had fallen in love with.

So, here I am again repeating the family patterns, but with a new twist! My spirit is connecting my awareness with my innate ability to grieve and let go of these past pains in order to find Real Love! As I sobbed in my session about feeling so unwanted and unprotected in the womb because my mother had seen a doctor in order to abort me, I connected those feelings with what I felt when I did not hear from Gare over the weekend. I was worried that he had changed his mind about getting involved with me, and would not want me. It is the antithesis of orgasm!

"I am coming. I'm coming. I'm here. Welcome me!" I want him to SEE me when I am having an orgasm. Look into each other's eyes. Not waver. Like with babies, looking into Gare's eyes will be a rush…of life! A wanna Be of Love.

Gare contacted me from Spokane, Washington, and I did not want a long distance relationship. Surprisingly, after reading about him, envisioning his strong, muscular, 6'2" body with brown eyes, mixed with other important commonalities, I could look past his status as married. Interestingly, just now, I thought of how my father was legally married when he met my mother and declared his love for her. He did divorce the woman whom he had married because she had threatened suicide if he did not marry her, then married my mother four months after my birth.

The only way I could entertain a relationship with a married man was to expect Gare to tell his wife about me. She found him emailing me, and so the truth of him not loving her came out. He said that therapy would not help him love her again.

Maybe I was trying to give Gare the love I was not free to give my father, or mySelf. A few days before I flew to Spokane, I awoke about 3:30AM aroused to orgasm, thinking of Gare's strong, big body and brown eyes. An hour later, unusual for me, I was aroused again and felt a full-body orgasm, smooth shivers, while saying, "All over me, all over me." I wanted him to envelope me, like the womb. To feel protected, because I did not feel that way inside my mother.

My first orgasm that night "came" with "I want you with Me." I felt some sadness as Daddy "came" to mind. Then mySelf love that has been left behind. I am forever grateful for this body of mine. Especially for the tears my body pours forth like when I connected in session with sobs of how my body has been fiercely shamed. Religion's oppression. I am beginning to say good things about my insides and outsides when I orgasm. My spirit no longer contained in the black and white extremism of religious walls. I am a blend of spiritual rainbows and clouds of gray.

I am connecting more with my own GRAY matter than with what others (or bible) tell me to be true. My newly purchased second-hand red Jeep has a **GRAY** interior! How fitting to have the brilliance of color and the uncertainty of gray. I can go my own way. Tears to let go of fears.

Now, I touch my clitoris lightly and my spirit will respond with the sensitivity of pleasure which re-"press"ion of emotional pain has denied me. Being able to tell an old boyfriend, Carlo, "I love you," as I leave from his home where he and his wife live. He laughs and does not return those feelings. I had stayed at their home the night before my flight as they live two hours closer to Buffalo's airport than I do. I was a bit disappointed not to hear those three words in return, yet, actually was glad that I could say them and not expect them returned.

For a reserved guy, Gare had no trouble undressing me in our room at the Ramada Inn, next to Spokane's airport. Twelve red roses bloomed on the bedside table as I blushed forth a stupendous orgasm. It was with his penis between my legs, caressing my labia and clitoris, which Gare had never experienced before. He was an incredible lover considering he had only been with his wife and one other lover, for a short period during his 37 year marriage. What was so magical was how he touched my breasts and nipples without me giving any direction. So lightly that I was delighted and electrified. I did show him how wonderful it is to put off the orgasm, to draw it out like ocean waves coming into shore. Gare was amazed how often he could become soft and then erect again to feel the building waves toward orgasm.

He, also, had never experienced oral sex, which happened two days later. Again, he surprised me with his beautiful touch, with his tongue so light, so on target. We had built a strong month-long intellectual/emotional bond that made two hours of lovemaking as amazing as the beautiful view of the lake and mountains outside our motel window. Our *long* lovemaking was a reflection of the *long*ing in our hearts to be and feel loved.

When I called Gare from the airport to say goodbye, there was a silence. He said, "I love silences too." That made me cry, and why? Maybe because it is those spaces that give us the opportunity to be truly ourselves...our inner being that feels so much and is usually run away from, by filling in with words, and busyness.

Gare and I had a major disagreement over the use of guns. He said, "I love you, and you are just out of reach." The same thing I felt about my father, and my tears came rolling as I knew our love for each other was "just out of reach," that there were too many feelings locked inside of us. More than once I felt I was feeling about my father while I was with Gare.

While we were hiking I was thinking how lucky we were to have found each other, like Daddy and I, and consciously thinking of how I was giving Daddy and myself what I couldn't give us while he was here on earth. I cried when I told Gare how I wished he'd cry with me, like I wish Daddy had. And when Gare said something like "I am perfection," making my heart swell with pride and sadness with the recognition that the church said I was just the opposite, I cried again. My spirit feeling free to BE more of itself, while with Gare.

I was taken aback when we went out to dinner our last night together. Gare was wearing brown pressed pants, a light stonewashed green long sleeve shirt and a brown belt. The shirt and pant's colors were almost exactly of those that my father had on when I found him in the morgue after his heart attack. And a brown belt too! The only difference was that dad's shirt was short-sleeved. I sobbed when I wrote those words in my journal.

I cried again when I said, "Don't give up your dreams." Isn't that the spirit speaking? My dream is to find real love. I cannot do anything else. I am accepting my journey to that end more and more, silencing the judgments of how that journey "should" go. Or is to "come?"☺

I had to tell Gare, "I love you, but it doesn't feel quite right," which was difficult to do. It is hard to hurt another's feelings, but we hurt them more, as well as ourselves, if we are not honest. He understood, and it feels so good to say one's feelings so *clearly*. It's like I have to have a "perfect love," working toward, that is. I wrote that in my journal nearly two years ago, and now in 2003, I have met a man named Brad, who has been an astrologer for thirty years and has recently told me that my astrological chart says that it is my life goal to strive for "perfect love." I FEEL that☺

And I wish for the body to reflect that inward perfection that we are all born with, baby's innocent pureness of ability to unconditionally love. Yet, it is still a bit scary to ask for that from a man I am dating…abandoning the conditioning of my religious upbringing to the dump. "The outside doesn't count, but it does" I cry with deep sobs in my session. Then I say how Gare has everything I want in a man, yet I am not physically attracted enough, "What else could I ask for?" I kick the mattress and cry "God, that's stupid! And I KNOW it's not! But it FEELs crazy."

Now, I easily connect to the "craziness" of my religious teachings. Don't trust your feelings, only "god." Yet I am more and more confident, as I cry out my emotional pain, that my feelings are what guide me back to my spirit (god or divine within) that has been silenced too long. I am on the journey to align the mind with the heart-spirit, the knowing (thought) with the feeling, no longer separate, like a river merging with the ocean.

Like the merging of my masturbation "Oh Gare, Oh Gare, I want you in me," with my full-fledged orgasm saying, "Oh Gare, Oh god, oh Gare, oh god, make me love you!" I am more and more aware of this whole process having the focus of learning to love mySelf fully, (I hear the 'you' as being me) so that I can fully love others. Yet, I need all four parts present…like one sings: soprano spiritual (supremely sensitive), alto emotional (fully feeling), tenor mind (tender thought) and bass physical (beautiful biology).

My journey continues to be surprising as portrayed in the continued awareness of the synchronicities in my life. It was amazing how I had one of my orgasms at 3:33AM a day before I reserved Gare's airline ticket to come see me in Ithaca. Originally, the ticket agent told me that the fare would be $362 dollars. Then, when I called back, it was $333 dollars!!! WOW! When I told this to Gare, he said, "Oh my god!"☺

We are both facing our fears of whether we are receiving enough love. I do know I am receiving enough love from Gare, as he is head over heels in love with me. But, do I have enough love for him, which means am I giving enough love back to mySelf? That is the amazing circle of connection that makes the circle of love complete. The journey we are all on…

To heal disconnections like the one written of by Betty Dodson in *Orgasms for Two*, pg. 104. "In ancient Ireland, the Gaelic word for masturbation meant 'self-love,' but with the arrival of Christianity it was changed overnight into 'self-abuse.' I am aware that I am *working out* (like the gym for my body) more feelings for my heart-spirit about Daddy and me through Gare as well as with others, like my daughter Megan. When I wrote to her on her birthday card that my tears are the only way to show how much I love her, no words will ever do, I meant that for my Self as well. It's a well of oneness that I smile about now as I write this sentence. The oneness of LOVE that I feel as I cry in watching a video where a black woman says to the Ku Klux Klan member who killed her son, "I've already forgiven you." The oneness of my eight-year-old granddaughter's eyes looking up at me with acceptance as I tear. The oneness of my tears as I sing the words of songs saying, "You are so beautiful to me," and "I love the way you love me." I love that I can cry for mySelf and my Daddy, the two truest loves in my life! I cried as I said to my best friend, Tanya, "I am conscious that I am giving back to Gare what I couldn't give my dad when he was alive, <u>the love without fear</u>. And, wishing to have no fear to show mySelf fully, by crying at orgasm with a man I love. It is so clear to me that what I am doing with Gare and any relationship…is working through my emotional pain into healing love. And, in so doing I am giving more love to them." Tanya was amazed how easily I made these connections. I realize they come with my deeply connected-crying process.

In a crying session in May of 2001, I also made the connection of being with Gare in a previous lifetime, being in the same area as Spokane, Washington. I imaged myself as riding a horse (which we did when I visited him in 2001), falling off a bluff, and dying. "Gare has been waiting for me all this time," brought deep sobs – no wonder he feels so strongly about me. I saw him lying on the bluff, crying and crying, thinking of killing himself. It felt like I was his daughter then, and maybe that's why he stuck with his present family for thirty-seven years, because he lost me. He still has those cowboy boots and hat, and a huge gun collection.

I have a sense that we have to grieve and relive this pain because we as humans are not sensitive enough to our true spirits as yet. Our vulnerable feelings are too suppressed and repressed. Our true heart-spirits need to learn to be really sensitive to Love.

It is curious that as I progress I am meeting more men that wish to cry with me while making love. Gabriel said that he'd love to, because it would make him feel so "connected and erotic."

The next time I masturbated, I thought of dolphins, and the Grand Tetons briefly, then of Gare, his touches, his muscular body, him kissing my breasts and I orgasmed with "Oh, oh, oh, oh." I thought of the musical sound "Oh" and not "Om" the universal sound many speak of. Babies don't say "Om," but "Oh." "Oh" has this quality of "naïvete" to it that was spoken of in one of my client's sessions as a wonderful quality. "Naïve" means to be "marked with unaffected simplicity, ingenuous, meaning showing childlike innocence, simplicity, candidness, lacking craft or subtlety." In other words, very REAL.

Yet, as I have matured, after learning to pay attention to the not so subtle, such as my feelings☺, I do love the subtleties of paying attention to detail that I now have more attention for: detail in art, nature, my chosen words of communication. This was marked by a comment of a friend that observed me dancing. Sue said something like, "You are a beautiful dancer," and along with "thanks" I replied that I can't see myself, and would like to sometime. She replied that I should, and it is the "subtleties" of my moves that make an impression on her. How wonderful to express the subtleties of maturity along with the unsubtleties of childlikeness. Again, the oneness.

I tried to assure Gare of this truth when he was telling me that he gave up his dream of being a wildlife conservationist so that it would be easier on his parents financially. He choked up in tears and was silent for a moment. I said, "Are you crying?"

He said, "Yes, darn!"

I said with intensity, "It is wonderful that you can cry and share that with me!"

"I want to cry together," I added. Gare replies, "That will happen." He compliments me on my ability to imagine and visualize possibilities as sensitivities toward all things. Maybe I am like a photographer who develops his own images (of Love), sensitive to the lighting, the contrasts, the clarity of the photo.

I was reminded of that fact when I drove my mother home from brunch, and she noticed that her butterfly pin had fallen off. She reminded me that I had given that pin to her years ago, and now it was a pin I didn't like, too many fake jewels in it. She said that I had given it to her "when you loved me." I was surprised by that and replied that I had never said "I love you" back then, and do now. But she felt it more back then because I "pretended" of sorts...my being a born-again christian made her feel closer to me. But, I am much more genuine now, and she can't feel that. So, I was feeling really awful and amazing all at once.

The gap between religiosity and spirituality.

After leaving mom at her apartment I went to dad's grave, to honor and talk to him, saying the "I love you" that always brings me to tears. Too many years of no "I love you Daddy" grief! (God damn that FEAR, the demise of everyone's spirit.) Genuinely spoken and felt, even now I spring tears, because he is truly the mother I never had, emotionally speaking. I laid two sprigs of lilacs, a half-eaten apple, and a kiss on the bronze letters of his name. I think it is smashing that I was there on Mother's Day!

I think to myself, I may be the mother Gare never had. I know Gare is in my life to carry on and beyond where my father left off. I want to cry with you Daddy. Give Gare what I didn't give Daddy. Gare says, "You are a leader in honesty." I enjoy the silence.

And then Gare told me two stories during our hike in Treman Park. First, when he was 8 years old, after going swimming he found that a centipede had wrapped itself around his penis. Second, when he was sixty years old, while at his cabin on the lake, a hornet got under his swim suit and stung his penis, so that he had to jump up and down, trying to kick off his swim suit, running naked to his cabin. I was laughing so hard I gutted tears, and actually I am laughing out loud as I am writing. I was bending over on the trail with tearful laughter, and although these are painful story-moments, they make one laugh because they sound so funny. A paradoxical fear? I just had to share how tears come at painfully funny moments...again the oneness.

To finish the story, after the hornet stung Gare's penis, an hour later he had an erection "non compare." Way to go Gare☺

One evening, before retiring, Gare finished giving me a full-body massage that he had begun on a previous visit, where my whole backside felt cared-for. Now, he was massaging my toes with slow strokes, as if time was there to serve us. Then, my feet, legs, abdomen, waist, arms, hands, breasts, neck, the final act being my labia and clitoris. The lotion covered me with gentle waves of ecstasy. I, then, massaged his penis with my hand, and then his penis massaged my clitoris until I came, and then he came inside of me, easily and strongly. Later, he told me that it was the most intense orgasm he has ever had. In his 62 years he had never experienced how prolonged making love can be.

In another session of our lovemaking, Gare had some trouble holding his erection, and was surprised to find out that it did not concern me. I explained that a softer erection could reach into crevices that a hard erection cannot, like being able to slide up and down the walls of my labia and over my clitoris with tenderness. He was surprised how understanding and accepting I was, especially when I can be so rigid about other things, like my principles such as: no slavery, no racism, no smoking, no abortion, no guns. And hopefully, eventually, no need for religion. I explained how emotional release work increases understanding about relationship issues so one can change, whereas principles are not as flexible as feelings. Again, an illustration of healthy rigidity (no slavery) versus unhealthy rigidity (religion). The sun and the shadow.

I hoped that Gare would pursue his shadow-tears that clearly healed him in a small way while in front of me. While we were driving to Buffalo to catch his plane, he was telling me about his friend Chuck, and their tradition of smoking cigars after the hunt. He pointed out the tear in his eye. How sweetly vulnerable! When I asked how he felt toward Chuck, first he said a thought, which I cannot recall. I said again, "How do you FEEL?" Gare answered, "I love him," which trickled tears that were wiped away with his hankie. Earlier, we had stopped for a chocolate nut frozen custard ice cream cone, and he'd felt an allergic reaction afterwards, stating that walnuts have caused such reactions before. The tingling of his tongue and lips disappeared right after he cried, and Gare observed that connection for me!

I noticed that I continued to leave "god" out of my orgasms while with Gare, knowing that I was not "in love," although I do love him. As I said in an email to him, I know that he loves me "dearly," but not necessarily "deeply." A reflection of mySelf. Our word choices are important as reflections of Self, "not just words," as he said at one point.

So, when he said that maybe he ought to bow out as soon as he got in, I felt very hurt, that I am not worth the hurt that we may have to experience in order to achieve real love. In my session that week I cried, "Oh god, it's all right to hurt and share and let go…Are you willing to have your heart broken in order to love?" I could immediately connect my hurt to my father, how he avoided talking to me about how I felt at age sixteen when I found out he was not my biological father. "It kept us apart!" Emotionally and affectionately distant. I needed my father to come to me and tell me he still loved me. "I NEEDED TO TELL YOU HOW I FELT!" Sobs. So many swallowed tears…is a greater hurt than if we had talked about the hurt of that day's painful revelation. I wanted and needed to cry with you Daddy! That's a *good* hurt. I need the whole of Love. The sun and the rain.

When I masturbated the next day, I only wanted the physical sensations of pleasure, even though I thought of Gare's "cowboy" hat (his penis) between my legs, because it has a brim that makes my clitty sing, and his lips on my nipples are so pleasing! I said, "Oh my cowboy" when I orgasmed with pure pleasure, only connected to me. Just loving Me. Not *need*ing another? Yet *want*ing someone to give entirely to me. Yet, "I do" also want to give back if I really love the man. I was concerned about my lack of passion for Gare on the physical level although I had a huge heart-connection. But like I cried the night before, I need the whole! I want to feel as Gare does, such strong passion that I drive him crazy☺ I felt aroused as I thought about his great love for me. That's the RUB…the eternal truth! I need and want to love whole-heartedly. MySelf. Then, I can truly love others!

The home I live in is a metaphor and reflection of my internal heart growth. I sold the house where I was surrounded by trees, where I cut down more and more trees in order to let more light in. It was a home to protect the Self. Now, I live in an apartment, which is a renovated chicken coop.☺ Less and less am I being a "chicken" to express my feelings, my truth. My apartment is not owned by me, just like my heart is freer and freer to be connected to the whole universe through compassion for all living things. And, it sits on top of a hill overlooking a long valley of a diversity of trees, with a state park of waterfalls as its neighbor. There is expansive light surrounding me, as I open my eyes every morning to the sunrise shining into the two windows at eye level with my double bed, from which is a view of the universe. Stars and moon are shining bright. I do not own a home, but I have a home inside my heart!

That is why I can no longer abide the use of the word "fuck" in my family or friend's vocabulary, like I would not use the word "nigger." They are abusive violent words. It's not that I cannot swear, because I say "shit" or "damn" when suddenly hurt. But those words are not connected to people, like "damn you," or "shit you." Fuck is always violent and usually used like "fuck you" or "you motherfucker." Or, even during sex, "fucking" is all about mechanics, the physical thrusting, not about loving tenderness.

During an emotional release workshop with John Lee, I was triggered by his use of the word fuck in a "lighthearted" way during the discussion/lecture. I had some individual time with a workshop leader to release my feelings about my third husband asking me to say "fuck me," and my fourth husband liking me to be his "whore." I wept many tears and was somewhat angry, but not so much that I wanted to hit anything. I felt sad and yelled, "You can't do that to me! Or anyone! It's not loving or respectful!!" Some belly sobs escaped with my tears as I became clear about my truth that my sensitivity to the use of those words is like not using "nigger." It is our evolution away from anger and disrespect, and toward Love.

It is with **LOVE** that our human **spirit** is truly free at **orgasm** - *sacred*, not *scared*, angry or violent. Like when I say at orgasm, June 2001, while loving myself, "come inside me, inside me."

It is the spirit of Love that I wish to "come inside me."

Not like the repressed feelings that Gare tells me about from his time in the Marine Corps, where you are bonded to your leader and each other with a suppression of your own instincts. They teach you to scream and "it brings out everything in you that there is." "An anguish as a robot, reserve," Gare's tears say, "you don't expose him to be all alone."… "I need to talk to myself and there you (Dianea) are!" Sadly, the screams are not connected to the true spirit inside us all. It is an act out. Unlike: "You're a great, great listener to hear and feel what I've felt and I never would have shared this with anyone else. Thank you." Gare continues with more great questions.

The next morning at breakfast Gare told me that he likes being "vulnerable. It gives more flavor to life." When we made love the night before, Gare had an orgasm before me, so I asked him to lick my clitoris. He created my orgasm. He said that it was the first time he had ever done that for a woman. He enjoyed it. He had a fine gentle touch, unusual for the men I have been with, and what surprised me more was my belly laugh (I had written *life* instead of *laugh* interestingly) as I slid off my orgasm. For minutes. Am I creating joy now that my emotional pain has dissipated more and more? I finally felt like holding Gare's hand as we walked down the street…but was still not "in love."

We visited the British Columbia Museum where we viewed a film called *The Dolphins* on a huge IMAX screen. I was tearful near the end when the narrator said that we connect with the soul and heart of the dolphin in becoming more conscious of how we connect to and understand them. And my tears would add, connect and understand our selves.

More importantly, I cried during a conversation with Gare regarding my curiosity about having a ménage a trois. He asked, "Don't you know that I would be hurt by you telling me this?"

"Yes," I replied with empathy, "but you need to know more of who I am!" It was a bit scary for me to say, yet, I felt calm. It challenged his "adequacy" and "monogamy" issues.

Gare concluded, "I thought I had something different, and now it's not there." Tears connected me again to my sixteen-year-old memory when I learned that my father was something different than I had known him to be. I no longer knew him to be my biological father. That traumatic day, he was not there to comfort or reassure me, nor did we ever talk about it in the ensuing years. I lost trust in his love because he did not come to me to talk about what that all meant…how he felt about me. It created a distance that we never resolved before his death and that I continue to grieve, now appreciating even more his not-so-perfect love for me. Many tears fell as I lay next to Gare. Then, he held me. If only I had had that with my Daddy: cry with him.

Gare clammed up when I asked him how he felt. Then, he told me that he felt "frozen, and had a pain in his chest." I related that to his old pain, which he understood intellectually but had not felt as yet.

That evening Gare sang in the German Sangfest, where groups from all over the northwest meet to sing in German. It felt good to be a part of this German cultural tradition, since my father was born and raised in Dreis, Germany until he was seventeen. I thought of how dad had loved to sing, and was surprised to hear the German national anthem sung to the same tune as "Be Still My Soul." No wonder dad had played that song on the piano so often!

After the concert, there was a big dance, where Gare tried out some of his swing dance moves. He also danced with the woman who taught him, and so I was able to dance with other singers as well as the soundman. His name was Martin, and we had an instant connection as he said he hadn't danced so easily with anyone before, and waved me back for another dance. I knew I could not pass up our energy and asked for his phone number, knowing he lived in Victoria, Canada. Martin became the knife to cut through Gare's and my teetering relationship.

Gare asked me many questions about *The Warrior's Journey Home*, a book I gave to him that he was reading while we were riding the ferry. His desire to grow emotionally and spiritually made me want to try to make us work, but there was not enough physical attraction. I was clear at this point that he wasn't a life partner. As we rode through the North Cascade National Park and Forest where sky meets pointed mountains, I was moved to tears, many tears, near Washington Pass. The peaks were so magnificently dressed in white, peaks facing me with sun-magnified eyes piercing my heart's door, to the room of pain of the lost beauty of my inner child's Love. It was as if I was falling into those mountains that wanted to welcome me home.

I asked Gare to shut off the music, that I wanted to be quiet for a while. Later, he asked me what my tears were about. Wunderbar! This kind of moment is where I felt I loved Gare, but I didn't feel like saying, "I love you." I had cried like the snow melting off those mountains because of missing my connection with Daddy through nature, as well. I said out loud to Gare what I knew in my heart, "I know WHY I am with you…to give you what I couldn't give to my dad." And to my Self. I am so very conscious of it, like a fly landing on my leg, or a soft breeze brushing my cheek.

During my crying "therapy" session that week, I cried heavy tears, sobs, as I said, "my spirit comes alive when I honor even my sexual feelings…follow my heart…let myself be curious and free…to find mySelf." My tears are the true story of my life!

The next morning I had a self-loving bombastic orgasm where I said "Oh god" six or seven times (must have been seven as the orgasm was so perfect☺) I saw no images, just pure connection with Me. Oh god could be me?

It is the first day of summer 2001 when the contrast of positive light of the longest day of the year meets the negative lessening of light as the days now become shorter and shorter. Always the two, night and day, shadow and light, and we must incorporate them both in order to have the whole. Like the whole day of our birth. My birth spiritually seems to take years, but if time is all one, a day is as a year, eh? That's all fine and good, but practically we can't understand that mystical concept of timelessness. If we know that we have many years of repressed feelings in our bodies from not being allowed to cry, only crying once a week in the deep way that I describe means that it will take time to let go of all those years of hurt unreleased, stored in our body's cells. It's a journey no matter what time says.

Next, came the email from Martin, which felt like a tailspin. He told me that he is married – a happy marriage – with two daughters. Still, he wished to pursue a relationship with me. He had an open marriage and his wife was turned on by his encounter with me. I feel torn. I kept thinking about Sara, the woman in her eighties who had an open fifty-year marriage that was happily loving, birthing four children. Could I have an open marriage that is not acting out? I am curious as to why the Design of the Universe has brought these people into my life.

After making love to myself that morning, saying, "I want you, I want you," several times as I orgasmed with thoughts of Martin, I also wondered if I was "wanting me" when my mother couldn't! The connections back to that pure child, Diane, come more and more readily, like the dawning sun on a clear day. It is clearer and clearer to me how I am creating situations in order to bring up my past pain – in order to heal it – to let it go.

I notice my memory is improving as I grow older! That I could allow my arms to move in opposition to my feet, remembering the dance step sequences better than my younger partner. This coordination ability was new for me. It makes sense that I am opening my body's circuits, with less pain to carry.

During this strained time, Gare continued to appreciate my uniqueness and specialness in how much he was learning from me. When we talked again, he raised the monogamy issue, and although I was not looking to be non-monogamous, I wanted the choice. I cried with my sister about recognition from Gare; how I am the one who is greatly giving the guidance toward greater love and how he is the first to truly recognize it for its worth. He is truly special…I called him a "Love Warrior."

I cannot help but notice the Design of the Universe's escalating care for me. As I wrote earlier, I'd moved to an apartment that I knew of because my best friend, Tanya, had lived there a decade earlier. It was vacated the month I needed it, and that same month my landlady was trying to evict me because she did not want my clients to come to my home-office. At first I was annoyed, and knew it would mean more money spent to rent an office when I was trying to save for publishing my books. She would not relent, so I found an office that would allow my clients to scream, be there part-time, lowering the rent $100, and was two blocks from a beautiful waterfall. A hairdresser was on one side of my office, a diner, on the other side. Many needs could be met because a Laundromat for one's "dirty laundry" complimented my work on the same block☺ Surprisingly, or not so surprising, was that the office was unfurnished, except for a desk and comfy desk chair. Then, Tanya told me that she had a 9'x6' rug, rocking chair, sofa and double mattress in her barn ready to go to the Salvation Army. Those are the exact four items I needed for my office! Tanya tells me, "Tears make her feel closer to god." The DoU (Design of the Universe) as I call it! An IoU for my tears?☺...An awesome spiritual journey!

And how does that story relate to sexuality integrating with spirituality? Because feeling "sorry for myself" in this deeply connected way to my child's spirit is what increases my trust in the Design of the Universe to provide what I always need. **I learn to trust my Self's spirit, so that I can trust the DoU-god, and thereby trust that when I fall "in love" that I will regress back to that angelic child inside me,** so that I can be more conscious of the PAIN that keeps us all from deeply really loving. Crying pain out in the connected-child way that we were not allowed to feel as children, to let it go. I am tired of so many books and tapes saying to "Let it go" when it is not something one can do by thinking it. It is like having a light bulb without a connected plug. There is divine light when the child's feelings are re-connected to its naturally loving spirit.

When I made love to myself again, (not "masturbate," which means "pollute with one's hand" in old dictionary's) rising to a beautiful orgasm, I thought of Gare, then Martin, saying, "Take me Martin, fill me with your love." TEARS came too. Because that is what we all want when we have intercourse, is to be filled with love. And, now through my grieving of my childhood pain, I am filling my Self up with love, by emptying out my pain!

When Gare emailed me eight questions about monogamy, I answered that honesty and openness is more what I trust than monogamy. Gregory was monogamous, but lied on several occasions. Monogamy can help us face our fears of intimacy, but it does not ensure intimacy by any means. I will follow my renewed heart, my new-birth sexuality, and trust it...not like I did in my open marriage to Reid. I have cried many tears about my past, when I was so far away from my true self: my vulnerable feelings of fear and lost love. My whole experience with Gare was about helping Daddy and myself to be able to Love better, without fear. I sobbed when I said that last sentence in my session. I wanted to give something back to Daddy, who is the leader to my soul-spirit. Sobs underlined my words, "Daddy you are mine; I wish I could have appreciated you more and loved you better." Now that my tears have opened my heart to its vulnerable pain, there is more of the true Me to trust...to follow my heart where I act <u>out</u> less, and act "<u>in</u> love more." Then, we can act <u>on</u> our true spirit's ability to love all of creation. Deleting judgmentalness.

It seems that I cannot say it often enough. When talking with my friend Gavriel, I cried freely as I spoke of how religion nearly killed my spirit, affirming religion's oppression as my <u>core pain</u> that runs as deep as the ocean. Cried out enough so that in 2001, I finally do not feel guilty when being lovingly sexual with the men I care for and connect with emotionally. It feels better and better to be able to trust mySelf, to face Gare's disapproval, like I couldn't with my father by leaving our religious beliefs. To trust myself carries over to being able to trust more in the bigger picture of the Design of the Universe, the spirit of LOVE.

I have felt repressed sexually and spiritually, all mixed up together, while growing up. And it was all tied together in another weekly crying session when I sobbed as I said, "It's like moving from darkness into the light!" What an incredible connection between letting go of one's painful feelings as a child (darkness) so that we can reclaim the divine spirit of love (light)☺

I can now say I love who I am!

I am still a work in progress, one who can hear hurtful anger spilled out at me, like Gare's when he heard that I would see Martin and his wife, to explore the possibility of a healthy open marriage. And not return that hurtful anger. After he calmed down, and had received an understanding reply from me, he told me, "I am surprised that you took my venom in such stride." It proved that <u>in</u> feeling my old pain, I don't have to dish it <u>out</u>! I felt really loving and powerful all at once.

When I masturbated days after Gare's angry outburst, my intense orgasm chorused "**Oh god,**" once, and "**Inside me, inside me.**" That's god, isn't it? It is like thinking about Martin coming *inside me*, as I pulsate my energy into him, and then he into me. That connection of energy is very special. And can be love if we so wish it to be, when expressing and letting go of the pain that barricades out the love. I continue to feel sensual and sexual; there is no decline although I am in the declining stage of menopause.

Gavriel, a professor of Russian Literature at Cornell, became my lover for a brief time, as he kept persisting, saying, "I am crazy about you." Although we talked well together, I could not summon up those electric feelings of "in love" for him, and I found myself being with my Self during orgasm although I wanted him inside me as soon as I was climaxing. I have accepted now that I must experience these partially-loving relationships until I find the one I am deeply in love with, wanting commitment. Gavriel needed a lot of guidance to learn how to be a gentle-sensitive lover. Sensitivity continues to heighten my orgasms…sensitivity to my old feelings has contributed to my body being more sensitive to touch…needing less pressure to feel intensely. A wonderful paradox; like my mother's surprising statement when I arranged a professional massage for her birthday.

"I don't know who I am," popped out of her mouth as I drove her to the massage appointment. My mother was turning eighty years old, and clear in her thinking. Not being an introspective person, she would still surprise me with lucid statements…if only she was conscious of how true her statement was! I am on the path to know more of who I am by tears melting away the fear and guilt that produces judgments about my self and others. Like my mother's church dogma does, where who she IS is hidden and what I cry most about, my lost-hidden-child-self. Like I did when triggered by my friend Sue's judgment that "Sandy can't change." And my tears that resounded when I said, "I hope my mother someday will love me." It actually feels good to cry, to let go of repressed pain. Because this is what really matters…care of the soul…so your spirit can fly free!

Dad's or Gare's disapproval will not hold my spirit back, or down, or flat.

I flew to Bellingham, Washington, where Martin picked me up and drove me to his and Carolyn's home in British Columbia. I met his two daughters, played with them in the pool, ate dinner with Martin and Carolyn, danced with them, and asked questions like, "How do these extracurricular sexual encounters enhance your thirteen-year marriage?" At first, Carolyn replied, "I haven't thought about it that way." It was difficult for her to put it into words, "into a higher level." She didn't use the words "love" or "intimacy" which I later asked about. Carolyn added, "I love sex."

I answered with firmness, "There has to be some kind of connection emotionally for me, I couldn't have anonymous sex." Even if it was just a couple of days with Martin and Carolyn, several emails and phone calls with Martin connected us before "making love." Although I would have preferred to have Martin alone with me, Carolyn wanted to be involved even if it was just to be close by. I went along, they knowing that if I was not liking what was happening in this ménage a trois, I would say so, and possibly leave. Carolyn did become involved by touching Martin while he was primarily kissing and having intercourse with me. We tried several different positions where I felt very good, but I didn't feel like having an orgasm, or that I could ask to do exactly what I wanted, although I did have his penis between my labia for a few minutes, my favorite. I realize it takes time to learn what each other likes in touch and kissing, yet I nearly made Martin come with my mouth massaging his penis, but I did not want his semen in my mouth, not knowing him well enough. I did not bring him to climax orally, which disappointed him, yet he orgasmed intensely with me on top of him during intercourse. I am glad that we were facing each other. I was looking at him, but he was not looking at me, which says something about the lack of connection although it was better than me looking at his genitals. I did talk to Martin a couple of times, saying that we felt loving, and he replied with a yes. He didn't talk much and said he usually does during lovemaking. He knew that I did not like the word or action of "fuck," so he was probably cautious. We both said, "Oh my god" several times. Do I wonder why I say 'Oh god' when I'm finishing my thirtieth pushup after my yoga workout too? I will follow up on that connection further along in this book.

When Martin woke me the next morning, I was naked, and asked him to lie down with me for a moment. It felt good just to hold each other. As it does to continually be more open with all of me: not afraid to share my intimate feelings.

The conversation I had with Martin and Carolyn after our "making love," was during our ride to the airport, and added more substantial beauty to my soul. I asked how they felt about our sexual encounter, and Carolyn replied, "fine." Even Martin said that response drives him crazy. I was surprised a bit by how open I was about my own experience. He had wanted me to come with intercourse, "I want that, I like that." I told him that I do not come easily with intercourse and it is rare. That I like having his penis between my legs, touching more places inside and out of my clitoris and vagina. That I like the long-drawn-out arousal, and the subtleties of all kind(ness)s of touch. It felt good to be taking my openness to a greater degree of detail.

Martin told me that he could not have sexual encounters with other couples if they were using it to try to make their troubled marriage better, or if they were jealous. That seemed to be more mature. They shared some of their experiences with others, saying that it is harder to attend when there are four people, like when with another couple. In the past three to four years they told me that they have had approximately 45-50 encounters with 15 other people. I was impressed with how stable their marriage appeared to be, and it was obvious to me that they loved each other and respected each other's feelings.

It also felt healthier because getting to know me was just as important as being sexual with me, maybe more so. I liked them a lot.

The next day, when alone in my motel room, I masturbated before sleeping, with my focus on my own sensations rather than on flashes of Martin. It was a very intense orgasm, felt in my feet as tingling, while I said something like, "It's beautiful," despite the unbeautiful way that Gare ungreeted me with an empty motel room. He admitted later that he had not resolved his hurt and probably wanted to punish me. Later, he admitted that I have this effect on him to make him emotional, teary, which he doesn't feel when he is alone. That I spread "radiance." Which I believe to be the spirit in all of us, and that continues to awaken us by diving into the river of our deserted, dried-up childhood tears.

Gare spent the next week with me on a group raft trip down the Klamath River in northern California, after canceling out once. The trip was led by Barry and Joyce Vissell, an over thirty-year married couple who have written books and led many emotional healing workshops, several of which I had attended over the past decade. When we were invited to share our intentions for the trip, along with twenty others, I was surprised by my spontaneous words and tears as I said, "I love Barry and Joyce, as if they are the parents I never had" (emotionally speaking).

I expected healing into friendship with Gare while on this river, as I do for my soul from my own river of tears. Tears have made me more sensitive to nature's subtle beauties, like when rolling over some big and gliding smooth rapids I commented to the raft's guide, Sequoia, that they looked like fresh-blown glass. Sequoia appreciated me for noticing. She said many never comment on them, and it is the only place on the river where she has seen them like that. I know my emotional healing leads me to enhanced "natural" awareness. I can slow down and notice.

My heart is *not-ice*(d) anymore.☺

Although Gare and I shared a tent, I was uncertain as to whether we would make love of any sort. I was fairly neutral in our kissing, yet liked his muscular body, and his exquisite touching of my nipples, the best nipple-touching by any man with whom I have ever been sexual. And he liked his penis between my legs; I didn't write "labia" in my journal. Or "vulva." And why is that? Not close enough to the real thing…Love? That I can be accurately unembarrassed by speaking the truth of my sexual parts? I voiced, "Oh my god" a few times to this 62-year-old man, and to the universe under the stars.

I especially noticed how I am becoming more generous as I emotionally heal, when in contrast, Gare did not want to share the knowledge of the blackberry bushes behind our tent with the others, or to help a man who needed a jump-start just before we had to leave camp. I encouraged him to help the man, he did, and we made our destination just fine. I am struck at times how open I am to being with men that I am not fully attracted to, but hope to be because they seem to be open to being vulnerable emotionally.

I am looking to find more Real Love, like the river finds its way through ragged rocks, stubborn stones, lounging logs, making its tears sound like bamboo in the wind, a percussion of constancy, making bubbles into pearls, so perfectly round that I find no end to the ocean of Real Love.

For pain is our friend, the river says:

It smoothes rocks into roundness,
Smooth as kisses from a lover's lips –
Kisses from a parent to child
Kisses sweeping up tears
Into arms of
river rapids blowing rocks into glass bowls,
reflecting rough edges worn down.

Blocked hearts worn open by pain –
The river refreshed by rain –
Rotating hate's strain,
Washed down river, into the sea –
Ocean's wide heart of Love
salty as tears,
Reversing our fears,
Growing Love in ongoing years.
RIVivER

On the last day of the river trip, while unloading our gear, I struck up a conversation with a woman, whose sweet singing voice I had heard accompanied by the river's lapping. I asked what her jobs were, and she replied, massage, then surprised me by adding that she strips two nights a week in order to make enough money to develop her singing-acting career. I asked her many questions about stripping, and especially wanted to know how she felt about helping her clients act out their emotional pain. She said she struggles with that part. I asked why she had chosen only me to tell about her stripping job. She answered, "I felt you would not be judgmental." I was touched by the realization that my heart-healing has helped her feel safe with me, unbeknownst to me. This is another example of how the spirit within can revive its ability to love unconditionally. I know in the past, as a religious person I would have been judgmental and expected her to quit her "sinful" ways. Even though I want better for her, I know the openness we created in trust will be more of a healing balm.

As I continued to talk with Gare about his *heart-break* in being disappointed about me not being his life love, and trying to hear his *heart-voice*, by letting go of inner child pain, where he would be less reactive and judgmental, I cried as I said, "I'm transmitting and saying to you what I couldn't say to dad – from a *deep-heart* place." Gare put his arm around me as I continued tear-laced words, "Daddy's death broke my heart, and that's a good thing although I miss him so much." I love him more now, as I did Gare when he replied, "I need to get the (hurt) little boy out of the way, so that I can be more able to allow you to BE." (WOW! Wonder of Wonders)

He could not join me on our second planned week together, backpacking in the Grand Teton National Park. He said it wrenched him too much to attach and detach from me again. "It's too painful! It's much easier to be distant and angry."

Gare and I made love one last time, and I came close to climax with him inside me with me moving over him. But, it was best for both of us with his penis between my legs, sliding over my clitoris, he enjoying my orgasm before he had his own. He told me that my lovemaking is exquisite, and I enjoyed his body that felt like a mountain with smoothed rough edges. My orgasm was "Oh god" with threads and puffs of tingles down to my toes, like the clouds dancing fluffily on top of the mountains: white for points of intense exhilaration and grays of drawn out penetration of skin's sensitivity to love. All those uneven edges of the clouds are felt by the sky, as I felt Gare's penis lather the crevices along my clitoris, labia and vagina…a river of love flowing through me.

It is comforting to know that eighty to ninety percent of women do not have orgasms with just intercourse, as most people believe should happen. As Betty Dodson states in her 2002 book, *Orgasms for Two,* "Although sisters Jennifer and Laura Berman state in their book, *For Women Only,* that 80 percent of women do not orgasm from intercourse alone, I suspected the number to be closer to 90 percent if we factored in the women faking orgasm. The clitoris is the woman's primary sex organ, with eight thousand nerve endings, and the vagina is the birth canal."(pg. 40)

Because this is the reality about women's sexuality, making love becomes more fluid and creative, because there is an admiration and respect for how miraculously our bodies provide pleasure to our lovemaking. So too, came respect from Gare for telling him the truth about Martin, although at first he wished that I had not told him about our sexual encounter. Gare, before I left for the Grand Tetons, told me, "I admire you for telling the truth!" So true is our spirit, for surely the "truth shall set us free," to BE our true loving being. Sex meets spirit! in truth! "Rather than love, than money, than fame, give me truth." – Henry David Thoreau

I continued my love affair with the Grand Teton National Park by visiting a fifth time, my first to hike three of its canyons. My first night there, I found myself sitting on a log at Leigh Lake, looking up at a sliver of moon, feeling sad, missing Daddy of course, the astronomer of my heart, his profession. How easily I cry for him, how good it is to be sensitive to this Love, to feel a mosquito lighting on my skin, or a wood fly, before they bite me. It is not easy to be alone, nor to brush aside my feelings of heart for which I am more and more grateful! Grief for my father is more than a brush with true love…it is the painting!

Of the big picture! Where I see and experience evidences of synchronicities with growing frequency. While at Jenny Lake Ranger station and bookstore, I bought gifts for family and friends that totaled $77.77! The perfect number in sequence. That morning I had asked the time from a fellow camper who told me 7:11am. Was I in the seven eleven store? No, but I thought of it as I sat down to pee☺ As my story progresses you will read of many more synchronicities that make more love connections with the whole Design of the Universe.

Like me meeting Rob at a dance in Bozeman, Montana, where I stayed overnight on my drive back to Spokane airport, from where I would fly home. It happened to be the night of the big dance of the Festival of the Sweet Pea. Most everyone was dressed up in formal attire, while I wore casual, a red-white-and blue polyester pantsuit that I had made for America's bicentennial. Red cut down cowgirl boots danced my feet. It was like the peaceful co-existence that I had experienced in Grand Teton National Park, where I met a brown bear on a canyon trail, or a huge bison with its calf lying peacefully near the paved road with cars driving by.

A shoulder-length blond-haired cute guy with bright blue eyes, three inches shorter than me started up a conversation while we waited to buy drinks. Rob and I danced and talked throughout the evening, and decided to drive to a cowboy bar nearby when the dance was over. I wanted a taste of the real Montana cowboy. There were maybe thirty people there, dancing to a country band. Rob and I danced very sensually, and our mutual attraction steamed into this summer's clear night.

He was a mechanical engineer with broad shoulders, as well as a muscled teacher of Tai Quan Do. As we talked at the bar, he really hooked me when he said, "It *breaks my heart* to see that older couple dancing." I told him how much I liked hearing him say that, but cannot recall what he meant by it. I was too much into the feeling his statement arose in me. I felt that we understood the sensitivity of that statement to mean the love he saw shared by that couple. As paradoxical as it seems, a broken heart is one that can be opened to LOVE and its spontaneous sharing without fear.

Gare could no longer make love with me because it hurt too much. He had too much old pain to defend, held inside, preventing a healthy sharing of pleasure because we did love each other to some degree. It is good to avoid pain that endangers, like drugs and sexually transmitted diseases do, for momentary pleasures. Like what could have happened with Rob, because I did not know him for more than several hours. I expected to drive him home, but somehow we reached my motel first, having talked past where he lived. I told him that I did not want to be sexual with him, and he replied, that we could just cuddle. Sure. With our attraction?

As I suspected, the cuddling did not last long before we were removing each other's clothing. This was unusual for me; I had not had a one-night stand in decades. I didn't want to think of it as that because we did have more than a physical attraction. Still, was I going to trust my feelings? I had to stop our kissing and ask about my sexual diseases concerns. He promised me that he was healthy and that I could trust him. That he is "harmless." My heart was more trustworthy than ever before, so could I see this brief lovemaking encounter as that?

More accurately, could I *feel* it as that?

The next day when we were talking at breakfast I said, "I want to trust you," and tears appeared with surprise. As I wrote in my journal then, and still a year and a half later, I cry because I wanted to trust my father's love for me, his desire to know me, my feelings, especially after the 16-year-old painful revelation that he was not my biological father. Both of us, too afraid to talk about it before he died 25 years ago.

So, I had trusted, and felt Rob inside me, connecting with me in a sexually intimate way, with communication to lighten the firm touch of his hands, and he learned quickly. We gave to each other orally with ease. Our lips kissed passionately in between kisses of our most intimate parts. I was still tentative about putting his penis between my legs, whether he would like it or think it strange.

I told him he has a beautiful body, which I was disappointed not to hear in return. He had said so on the dance floor. I had not been drinking, and he had maybe two beers. We looked into each other's eyes and I told him how much I liked that. Eyes open reflect openness, like windows without curtains letting in the light. And as I let go of my pain in tears, I feel lighter. More able to trust my spirit's flight into the night shadows of old pain preventing me from fully loving.

By Rob's sighs I could tell he liked my vulva and clitoris caressing his penis, and although I came close to orgasm, I did not, and gave him the go ahead to have his climax. He did so with grunts of pleasure that made me think of a satisfied sculpture carved out of beautiful wood. We kissed afterwards, and held each other alternately throughout the night. It seemed that he wanted closeness as much as I did. Not just sex. (Rob had not been sexual with a woman for seven months and said he was fine with that.) Tears reverberated with that non-sexual closeness that I had wanted with my father; we could not trust enough to be as close as we wished. The wall of fear was too great.

When Rob and I awoke the next morning, he rolled his leg over my pubic area, which rubbed my clitoris and turned my warmed up body into flames. I felt a denser sense of excitement throughout my labia, and with a gentler lover, being in my favorite position, I vocalized a loud "Oh god" a couple of times before feeling a fuller, deeply intense orgasm, not popped but fuller like a balloon fully inflated. I had to keep my eyes closed while climbing to orgasm, fearing I might not make it, or take too long. Not room enough or time enough for me is what many of us have experienced as children.

At orgasm I opened my eyes, as I have wished to more and more with the men to whom I make love. Love is open, and connection is through the eyes of our heart-souls that have nothing to hide. I also liked seeing Rob's beautiful muscles define as he felt the pleasure of his coming. Into our own? Heart of love? Isn't that what orgasm is all about? So beautiful, so vulnerable, so free of control…so free to Love if we can connect to the unconditionally loving spirit born to us all. No longer hidden when we can freely **tear** away the repressed emotional pain with our healing **tears**. Then, sexuality becomes intimate with spirit.

Later, at breakfast, Rob became tearful as he related how much he grew with one woman with whom he had had a long-term relationship. With me, he was a very young looking 39 and never married. He thought I was 41; I was actually 54-

years-young. Both young at heart? After three more hours of sharing our lives as we ate breakfast, we sat in his driveway, where I asked questions I would have been too scared to ask a year earlier. I asked, "What was your sexual experience with me like for you?"

His first word was "Passionate!"

"And how was your experience with me different from being with other women?"

"Your sensitivity."

"What attracted you to me?"

"You ask questions☺, listen, are easygoing, and good conversation is a real turn on!" WOW went my heart. I was happy that his answers were more about feelings than about my body. I had to ask, "What about me physically?" He laughed as he said, "Your long legs, I am a leg man." I appreciated him relating to my spirit more than my physicality because that meant we had made a heart connection that was more loving than using. He had laid his hand on my leg while we were talking in the car. I am enjoying my sexuality joining with my heart's spirituality more and more. I wondered how many more such encounters I would find before finding my true love. It is like picking up a special rock in the canyons when I was hiking, and bringing it home with me. Read on, dear reader, and December of 2002 may reveal that secret☺

I slept very well the night after I left Rob, and remembered dreaming about acquiring an important position, being recognized along with another woman who reminded me of Janet Reno. We hugged and congratulated each other. I looked for my family members to hug them, but just wandered around them. It was a warm feeling, but lacked closeness. Then, I opened a door to welcome a handsome man who was small like a boy, with an old man's face. He said, "I'm glad you are home." And where is home in your heart?

Then, I felt aroused to masturbate into a fine orgasm, saying "Oh god" a couple of times, then "I want it." I laid quiet long enough to ask myself, "Want what?"

"Love, of course." And of course, the tears coursed down my cheeks with thoughts of Daddy and how **he gave me a taste of love, so that I could go (come) for more!**" Could return home to Real Love, our birthright. Look, no, st<u>are</u>, into a baby's eyes. There you <u>are.</u>

As I drove back to Spokane, I was listening to the radio and heard a song I hadn't heard in years. "You Light Up My Life" caused me to be awash in tears, remembering myself waiting at the window for my daddy to come home and light up my life. Lighten it up from mom's abuse. He kept my spirit alive.

When I returned home, I kept my appointment with 68-year-old Dr. Glass, who practices homeopathy after leaving traditional medicine. I have always been in good health, looking to improve it in any way I can. I made an appointment with him because I have bruised easily below my knees for many years. I cried intermittently during the interview when talking about: mom not wanting me, missing my father's love, and how my spirit was nearly crushed by religious oppression. Even though I have cried for close to a decade about the hurt of hearing from the church that I am not worthy of love, I am still amazed at the depth of this pain, and it is one of the major reasons I am writing the books that I do. And why spirituality and sexuality can be integrated when shame, fear and guilt given by religion is let go through out body-heart's tears.

Dr. Glass remarked that he had never met anyone like me, and recognized my "vitality" and "childlikeness." When he said I am "extraordinarily beautiful and lovely," all I could do is say thank you and smile away my embarrassment. I am still working on feeling truly comfortable with such big compliments, as I was taught not to say good things about myself, which is what I am doing as I write this.

Spirituality connects us to all of creation's ability to love, to help, not separate or judge. Why I am open to astrology, psychics, homeopathy, past lives, yoga, etc. as compliments to tears' natural healing through grieving repressed childhood pain. Dr. Glass is distrusting of the medical model and told me that my cholesterol of 259 is really okay, although the normal limits are below 200mg, not 300mg as it used to be. I had felt that to be true in my heart-gut, but couldn't quite trust it.

Like I finally do now, to swim nude at a local waterfall called Potters. Not only to show my birthday suit without shame, but also to swim with the snakes and the fish. Peaceful co-existence until the city ranger arrives to tell me to put on my bathing suit bottoms. A couple years ago, we had to have the bathing suit top on as well. Now, women have won the right to have their tops off like the men. Our evolution is leading us to trust that our bodies will be appreciated and not be violated. Religious shame is losing its grip as our hearts open to real feelings of love.

Which I feel when I am with my granddaughter Denali as she makes comments and asks questions that make me smile. Her questions and observations are simple, unwrapped, forgotten by adults because we are too busy or shut down. She even noticed the small wasp's nest outside my bedroom window. What I notice most is how much I love to hold her gaze.

And I've found I write often about looking into each other's eyes throughout the recent decade. It is the strongest connection I know of, and have missed. The child-spirit to LOVE.

My love was limited when I opened the Blueberry Morning cereal box and found a colony of ants invading. Mosquitoes and ants cause me to say out loud, "Sorry, I have to kill you," and then I feel some satisfaction eliminating them. Will I ever love them?☺

Or love my mother enough to have her love me back?

By the summer of 2001, I was beginning to appreciate my mother's new interest in me. She asked several times to visit my new apartment. I drove her to my redwood renovated chicken coop, where we shared take-out Thai food. I joked and said, "Isn't this romantic?" as we sat close on the sofa eating out of the same aluminum container. In some subtle way I felt my mother's admiration of me, which she could not express with an "I love you." I bought her a birthday card that said those three magic words for the first time in print. Wasn't I coming closer to the spirit of love?

When I next saw my best friend, Tanya, who lives with her verbally abusive husband, she admitted that she would like to strangle him. I wanted her to return to therapy, and when I said it took so long for me to listen to the little voice inside of me, tears ushered in like an echo of a huge truth. The truth that "the little voice" is my pained spirit: not listened to, or trusted for many years. I am glad that I can now cry easily about past hurts because my tears point to the truth about what needs to change. Not only to what I have lost. But also to what is true!

Sadly, Tanya feels no desire to be sexual. Her spirit feels as if it is "crucified" she has said, being in a very unhappy marriage, and fearing to leave even when her husband refuses to go to therapy. She is an example of the interface between sexuality and spirituality in an obvious downward spiral.

As I continue crying sessions every week (a form of meditation), I am profoundly aware of how greatly my father's love has affected me as the saver of my spirit from the oppression of religion that he taught me less rigidly than my mother. I sob as I say, "He was the light of my life who made everything okay, the only real light in my life." I am aware that I am closer to being able to give love without it being returned from my mother and oldest daughter. It is very difficult to tell them "I love you," and not hear it back.

My journey is not about sex; it is about learning and wanting real love. More tears arrive as I ask myself what I was doing with Martin and Carolyn. Sobs underlined my words, "I am exploring how I feel, what is love, and what isn't. Honoring that journey and my feelings – my real feelings about what is true and what is Me and trusting that truth…**my feelings are the leader of my soul!**"

In the past, I down deep sensed that my feelings were not healthy when I was acting them out with Gregory, or other men. I was too afraid to make love with a boyfriend of twenty years ago, Gus. I was a born again Christian then and felt too guilty to have intercourse with him, even though I felt love for him. It is so sad, because those feelings were not truly mine. The guilt and fear had been drilled into my heart by the brainwashing of the church and my mother. I had to wade through all those unhealthy feelings in order to find my own. Open my own eyes, like how I want to open them when I am making love with a partner. It is when I feel most loving, face-to-face, eye-to-eye. OPEN-hearted. Fully SEE. See, and want to be seen.

…I will raft to the great wide-open ocean to sea –

...where salty tears turn into deep love –
...fresh water of divinity.

In August 2001, I was conscious again of how I have less and less pain in my tears and sobs, my head is no longer stuffed up when I sob. And I sob less often. And, I trusted that my sexuality would drive me deeper into real love. I welcomed my cleansing journey as I continued to self-love once or twice a week. More and more often I would have fuller body orgasms, intense, with several "Oh my gods" and shivers up my trunk, tenseness in my legs down to my toes, and incredible humming in my genitals. Sometimes there is a man's image; sometimes it is all about me, and my feelings within my body.

As my body and spirit become more united, so do other parts of my life like noticing, "I *write* to become more *right*." Right - in the sense of becoming more healthy and whole in my ability to love. Limited by the lack of awareness by my parents of their own pain, which arises now in me as I well up in tears when I read my daughter Megan's inscription in a book she bought for my birthday. "Love you lots," in many situations makes tears ooze from my eyelids. Although I felt love from my father, it was still limited, and not what I am destined to be satisfied with. Even my astrologer friend, Brad, says that my planetary chart draws me to find "perfect love," or what I'd rather name as "real love."

And to more concrete realizations, that everything is connected in the most unrealized ways by most people. That I was a black boy in a past life, therefore I am connected to the black race now with a white face. That laughter is connected to pain just as often as it is to joy. How often do we laugh when someone is falling down and getting hurt? Or when someone is being put down, like when made fun of because they have zits on their face? Or when one hears a "dirty joke," because they are afraid to talk about sex. All very sad scenarios. Yet, we laugh to dispel our fears, our pain. Our spirits cannot yet be REAL.

I cannot say enough how glad I am to be so sensitive to my tears, which I find uncover the loving spirit I was born to be. As you are, my travel-along reader. This was graphically exposed to me in the realm of nature, as I was blueberry picking with my grown daughter Megan. She remarked, "I wonder if the blueberries left behind misses the blueberries we picked?" What a sweet, sensitive thought, which at the time made me smile. But, when I wrote about it in my journal, sweet tears blurred my vision, and clearly made me love her (and automatically my Self) more. My tears connected me to the pain of how I have not been sensitive to my childhood painful feelings of being inadequately loved, and therefore not capable of being truly understanding of other's pain until the past decade.

It is why I cry when saying goodbye to Megan, or enjoying a firm hug from my brother as he leaves. These are sweet, sweet moments of love being realized, and why more and more I need to have sex and spirit connected in order to be intimately real with Love.

Our true nature then becomes more sensitive in and to nature.

Like noticing a snake eating an insect outside my kitchen window, or two squirrels chasing each other around the trunk of the big black walnut tree. The sound against the tree bark is what drew my attention. I have noticed the textures of trees' bark more and more of late, as I like to BARK out my truth☺ (Just cannot make this only a sad book because crying makes me happy…have I said that before?☺)

By summer 2001, my heart had softened enough so that when I jumped out of the cold water at Treman Park's waterfall swimming pool, I landed on my mother's lap, whose extra padding was pleasantly warm. She loved my coolness; I loved her body's warmth, cooled by my water, like when unwanted-in-her-womb. Now, she wanted me to cool her off, so we laughed and I placed her arms around my waist, as she would not have done that on her own. That was sad, but I was glad that I could feel good about wanting to be on her lap. I couldn't, when I was little…it wasn't safe no matter how much I needed it. My spirit of love was coming alive again so that I could give love knowing that I could bear the pain of not receiving it back as I needed. Because I was feeling more Love, I was gradually expressing it more physically with my mother, like I continued to experience more crying with orgasms. Spirit and sex becoming One.

Isn't it fascinating that fast running water becomes white, like that of waterfalls? And, that as tears fall fast they make us more pure of heart, like the color of white? And open light?

Everything is connected into Oneness, only if we can feel deeply, which roots out our pain, leaving more room for Love. As my healing continues, I am deeply convinced that being "in love" serves the purpose of sticking to a spiritual journey in its most advantageous way: mixing the best ingredients to make the soup of Love. Hope for Love all in an attraction, both inside and out. The whole.

"People want so badly to have a connection and don't know how, so they remark about other's disconnectedness," I sob in one of my crying sessions. My brother, Eric, had recently said to me that he was miffed at my daughter, Erin, for not answering his repeated phone calls. That she was "emotionally distant." I replied, "Like you, Bro," and we both laughed, because we both knew he was from me and other family members. I had deep sobs with kicking feet as I said, "I tried so hard, Daddy, I tried so hard"…I didn't know how to get through our fear of painful feelings when I learned he was not my biological father. I couldn't make it across that barrier at age sixteen, even though I knew I loved him, it wasn't enough love to overcome our fears of those painful-vulnerable feelings. To talk and to cry together.

Now my tears have given me enough strength to not give up on hearing my daughter Erin or my mother tell me they love me. I continued to show them my tears of disappointment and sadness from their rejection, requiring us to face true loving. I cannot give up trying, like I did as a child. I will free my spirit to love more fully, even as I no longer wear a watch, except when I am with clients. It is rare that I use an alarm to awaken me. Time no longer rules me like a slave. My spirit is freer.

Maybe tears **are** Love.

I am still taking in how I am no longer in need of sex to fill up my loneliness, as I could have had sex one night with Gavriel, a Cornell professor who is crazy about me, but I chose to self-love. "Oh gods," with myself were better than being with someone who I cannot fully Be There with. Maybe if I knew Gavriel was a great lover, like Gare, but Gavriel is a bit too rough, not my kind of great lover. Maybe that says it all, "BEING a great LOVER"…a metaphor for the possibility of Love! So the lover of mySelf is more and more "coming" into "being." Being with one(s) she really <u>wants</u> to be with – not necessarily <u>needs</u> to be with. So it is with orgasm, which we call "come"…so I wish to BE-come the most loving BEing I can BE.

Like how, I cannot keep myself from saying "I love you" spontaneously to my clients at certain moments. Why make or say love when my whole heart is not there? Even though Rob and I had only one night to make love in Bozeman, Montana, I felt good about it afterwards because I acted out of feeling love, and not out of need from the body. It was not the traditional one night stand, as was proven by Rob contacting me a year later when he was in Montreal on business, wanting to be with me again. Sex was connecting more and more to spirit, as it continued to do so with Christian, who had been my boyfriend in 1983-84.

One of my outstanding memories with Christian is facing him in his shabby rented room, standing near his desk, hearing him say, "Can't you just have some compassion?" I cried about that fifteen years later when saying, "I am sorry, Christian." Even though I had fought for him not to be labeled or discriminated against as a mental health inpatient, I was clearly not hearing him at that moment in 1984. It is clear to me that I did not have real compassion back then, as I have never forgotten Christian's statement. Having cried in my sessions about it has washed me with compassion for mySelf, automatically creating a desire to apologize to Christian. Creating deeper Love.

Which continued as I laid next to him while we talked until 3am one August night of 2001. We were naked, as Christian held me, and I stroked his body lightly. I wanted to make love, but he did not. I found out why the next morning after talking for another hour. He said he was becoming emotionally committed to another woman; "I'm a one woman man." I understood in part, yet asked why not make love when he is not committed. He replied that I should value the fact that he told me, because it was hard for him to do so. And, why did I need to be fully sexual? Weren't we "making love" in our conversation?

True, but that does not make our experience **whole**. We love each other. Tears scooted down my cheek, into my ear as I heard myself say, "I'm glad I'm crying." The more I cry, the more whole I become, and **whole** is the word that propelled my tears in conversation with Christian. <u>Whole tears</u> make us holy? Spiritually speaking?

The next day, when I left Christian in his driveway, and was turning to get into my jeep, after hugging goodbye, Christian waved and said, "I love you." Without hesitation I exuberantly responded with "I love you too." I was so happy that he took the initiative, and not left those wonderful words to me, as usual. I knew we had some real Love, the kind that lasts over time.

That same weekend I was participating in a dance workshop where I met James, known as J.T. There was a lot of chemistry, and as we talked more intimately about ourselves, it became clear that we would make love the second night we were together. This does not usually happen to me at the several dance weekends I have attended yet, it seemed to be happening more often. We made love in his hotel room, which he was sharing with a friend, who interrupted us twice near orgasm. But, that made the pleasure last even longer, as we hid under the covers like teenagers.

Although I had a smaller orgasm, it was the way I enjoyed it the most, with his penis between my labia, sliding over my clitoris. J.T. orgasmed right with me in this position and he was especially pleased by that. We enjoyed touching each other, and he looked into my eyes more than most men.

It was very easy to cry while with James. He usually responded by listening and leaning over to kiss me when I became silent. There were three significant times where I cried while with him that first weekend, one being while driving in the car, expressing my excitement about the changes in me, and my clients. My voice became higher in pitch, intense as a crescendo in music, as I said, "Tears have brought back my spirit and real love." My *excitement was joined with **tears*** in an intense and quick way that I had never experienced before! It validated James and my understanding that separateness and connectedness meld into oneness. All the paradoxes (excitement<>tears) bring us into the oneness of connectedness. For me, that last sentence is a clearer expression than reading that we are all one. Like crying makes me happy. We are unique individuals, yet the same whole of being human…because we are so interconnected to the rain, food, and sun that all feed us into life. I wished that I had recorded that "bawl of yarn" conversation between James and me that happened in bed the next morning. We were so responsive to the other's perspective, like we were a well-tuned tuning fork. We no longer needed the polarities of evil and perfection…just knew we were part of the glorious continuum of **evo**lution toward Real **Love**.

James exhibited a special newness for me as he experiences the energy of kundalini, which I was not familiar with until meeting him. His energy had made lights go on and off, as well as kept computers from working. He had been a highly paid Wall Street investment broker who had tried several different healing modalities. We both felt that it was a gift to meet each other and want to converse about spiritual/emotional issues. He was 38 and I turned 55 in two days.

My second crying episode that first weekend with James happened while preparing dinner of salmon and salad. I took issue with his statement that "insects are like machines." It is like people saying that a beautiful view looks like a postcard. The truth is that the insects and scenic view originated before the machines and the postcards, that the postcard looks like the view and the machine works like the design and ability of the insect, not vice versa. When I said that the postcard does not show the depth of the beauty seen in nature…guess which word produced tears. **Depth** tears. It was easy to connect it to the lack of depth in knowing myself. I was astounded by that connection! And excited about how everything we do seems to be connected to a feeling☺

The third cry was a sobbing with James, in bed in the morning. He told me about his dream about being excited to steal out of this safe that had many complexities to unlock. I asked him what he thought it meant, and without much of an answer, he asked me what I thought. Maybe, that he felt excited to find the path to the "safe" place to release his feelings?

He said that he felt safe right then, and asked if I did. I checked in with myself and said I might be a bit scared to tell him how I felt about the word, "fuck."

He had said something like "keep fucking me baby" the night before. I had replied, "I'm not fucking you, I'm making love." I had felt a bit annoyed (hurt), but not enough to distract me from feeling continued pleasure and an orgasm that was close to exquisite. "Exquisite" was the word James used to describe how I kissed and caressed his penis, and that I was intuitive about how I did it without direction. My orgasm was intense and drawn out with several minutes of being high before my vocal explosion. I had said, "Oh god" several times as I approached orgasm and had such presence that I asked James to open his eyes and look at me. He did, as he touched my nipples, accentuating my orgasm. I wanted him inside me immediately, and placed him there as he had already climaxed. Then, it was easy to say, "I feel love for you." A few seconds later, he replied in kind.

When I told him about my fears of alienating him if I told him how I felt about using the word "fuck," and that he'd leave somehow, and how that connected to my mother not wanting me, and how I say "I love you" to her and do not hear it back, I initiated sobs. I felt safe and accepted as James held me. Kissed me as you would a child. A very special sharing of loss of love tears. **Grief** tears.

My spirit was coming home. Now in the intimate safety of making love. As I let go of the pain of not feeling loved for my feelings in the past, I allowed in the feeling of being loved more for my feelings being shared. It is the privilege that I feel when clients are vulnerable – crying or angry — when with me. And the understanding when they say, "I *know* something to be true, but I don't *feel* that way." The issue of being able to change deeply through one's thinking, instead of through the feelings, continued to be a difference between James and I, and I was glad I could stand by him in love, not having to convince or persuade. Debating does not work to change one's mind; I learned that well while with Gregory's broken heart. These feeling changes within me demonstrate the main reason we are not in tune with the loving spirit with which we are all born. When there is this dichotomy between the mind and feelings, our spirit of love cannot be whole (in its expression).

James and my relationship felt the most balanced of any relationship I had been in as far as give and take. I was firm in my position of feeling being primary, and flexible in seeing my lack of gentility in the way I expressed my opinion where he could feel validated. Still, he admitted that he needed to take some responsibility for how he felt as well. Firm and flexible: how I like men's penises to be. I felt so genuine in this interaction even as I said "I'm sorry if I hurt you." (Not sorry that I disagreed.) We took equal responsibility. I felt good that James confronted me. And I felt good that I could clearly sense what's mine, and what's not…unlike when I tried to persuade others to be born again christians.

I am very glad that my truth inside my heart is no longer dressed in a doubt-ful feeling inside my heart. As I am glad that I can sob in my session on my 55th birthday, as I say the word "birthday." It is the confirmation that my spirit was already feeling hurt by my mother not wanting me, so the day I was born was not a happy birth day. Mostly, glad that my tears enlighten me to a deeper FEELING of love, not only for my father who did want me, but now also that I want to be who I AM. A deep-(w)hole of Love for all…no anger…no judgment.

The love of my father, who kept mother and child together, is the love that fosters my desire not to give up any of the material things I have that belonged to my father when he was alive. My most "spiritual" possession might be the Sunbeam toaster that he gave as a wedding gift for my first marriage over thirty years ago. It worked for thirty years, and now serves as a planter, with a plant in one slot and a glass statue of a mother holding her child up in the air, in the other.

James and I had engrossing conversations about healing into Love. Once he said that feeling love all the time would be "boring." That surprised me, although it is understandable in our finite experience of love. Yet, the changes or growth in our ability to love involves limitations and expansions of the Love feeling, so it never gets "boring" in our imperfect awareness. I can't imagine what it would be like to love with perfection.

Maybe I came close as I cried with James when he shared my fantasy about crying with orgasm, that expansion to feel joy and sadness all at once. It is very loving when one can look into the eyes of another at that peak moment of sharing! Being SEEN, truly, is the word on which tears burst forth. The pure vulnerable gift of whole Love.

And, the best gift of that birthday weekend was my dream of Daddy where we hugged each other! I couldn't remember the last time I had dreamed about him, it had been many, many years. I walked over to him and held him, and although he was reticent, I felt him hold me. I feel sad now as I write this in February 2003, because not feeling safe to be held is a fundamental loss of love. I wish he was still alive, even though I know his bud of love is inside of Me. A spiritual connection for Me.

James called himself the "cuddle monster," as he likes to hold hands and hug a lot. Fine with me, as are our hikes in nature, like to the top edge of Taughannock Falls, cascading downward 215 feet. What an energetic pull I felt while looking over the edge. The edge I find as I cascade toward an orgasm, fearing I might not make it to the roaring scream of the most satisfying orgasm with lovers. I thought I would scream, while standing up making love in the living room, when James came to Ithaca to spend a weekend. But it didn't happen; instead I felt the thick resolution of a calmer orgasm like one floating on cloud nine alone. I did feel an "Oh god" during the build up, but not at orgasm. I knew I was not "in love" with James; maybe I could not connect with the "in-Love-spirit" that comes to bombastic orgasms like I had the following day when I masturbated. Yet, still no screams when I masturbated alone. So far, it seemed that I was not able to scream unless the "I love you" feeling came while making love with my lover? Then, I am fully there. Present. A gift. Of supreme Love.

My masturbation orgasm prompted "Oh god" as I approached climax, then, "Oh yes" over and over again as I came. Is "god" conjoining with me as my spirit becomes freer to be expressed?

Like the *sad* tears of my six-year-old granddaughter, Denali, who called me when she was visiting her other grandmother in California, so that I jumped for *joy*? Because she felt free to call her mother in Baltimore to get my phone number in Ithaca, to tell me that her grandma Ruth had sent her to her bedroom to cry. "What was the big deal?" Denali said to me. She asked me to tell her grandma Ruth that it was OK to cry, and that she didn't need to be sent to her room, to be shamed for crying. I am nearly convinced that there are no tears of joy, only that I can jump for joy that Denali embraces and honors her spirit by expecting her sad tears to be respected. Truly SEEN for her WHOLE self.

Or like, my best friend, Susanne, who after three years of weekly sessions to free-up her tears of love lost, told me that after a particularly deep crying session, she had gone home and masturbated to a full-blown intense orgasm, something she had not found possible for several years, with a lover or alone.

Or, like the poem I wrote:

I WANT To CRY With YOU DADDY

It is the pain that has kept us apart,
distance between two love-stifled hearts.
I visit your grave on Mother's Day,
permitting my tears to mold the clay
holding my spirit as it finds its way.

Mom pregnant, wished "me" to abort,
five months along; she thinks to adopt,
dad writes his name on my birth certificate,
mom's unloving, then he might stop.
Not 'til I was sixteen did I finally drop…

Into the well with a stone high wall –
Mom yells "He's not your father,"…became so tall.
My heart had to love you as a faraway star –
To your hugs, I pushed up a bar
Could I dare?
Ask, "Do you still love me?"
I was unaware.

Chorus:
I want to cry with you, daddy.
Don't leave me alone
Come to me, daddy
Tell me, "I love you,"
So my heart no longer roams.
I need to hear, please dare.
Letters are not enough
My heart is too unaware.

You played badminton often without gravity,
Typed up my utopian junior theme.
I hold the whistle you whittled from a willow tree,
But I needed "I love you" to be said to me.

"Our heart looks everywhere to find our soul-spirit," says Martin Prechtel, a shaman, who believes we need the grief ritual in order to get to the other side with our ancestors.

I could not find the side of myself that could fall "in love" with James, which became more evident the next time we made love at his apartment. I talked with him about how I like to kiss, and he told me that sometimes kissing is a distraction to finding his orgasm. I felt sad that at 2am, he wanted me to have a really good orgasm, approached me from behind my buttocks, while touching my nipples, without kissing. Not kissing face-to-face kept me from feeling as connected as I wished to be. Despite the distance, I felt like giving to James, and enjoyed him entering me, giving him a big orgasm.

At breakfast it was especially intimate to be able to talk of our sexual union, where he said his orgasm was unique, raw, animal-like. It felt very good to him, but where was I? He said sometimes the kissing is too intense. His energetic fields go up and down a lot, which I cannot fully understand because of lack of experience with the "kundalini energy" he spoke of, and I read of later in *Living with Kundalini*. I wondered about him taking the medication, Wellbutrin, an antidepressant, to help even out his energy. He had not cried with me.

I felt good that I could ask questions that I was apprehensive to ask, and that I cried a pile of tears after watching "All the Pretty Horses," when I said, "I did not know the truth because I was not in *contact* with mySelf, my feelings, for many years. Due to the lies of religion. The word "contact" had intensified my tears, because without contact with my heart, I could not *really* love.

Then we discussed with the intensity of locked antlers. James would say that at any one time, one's experience is their truth. Like my experience as a born-again christian? That was my experience but it does not make it a "truth." We looked up the word truth in the dictionary, which in its archaic form allows for sincerity, but more presently represents a factual experience. Not just anyone's experience. A good example is a psychotic person who experiences hallucinations, which he or she may believe are real, but in actuality are not a truth. I would not want someone to leave me in that lack of reality or truth. I am glad people, such as my ex-husband, Reid, argued with me, and helped me out of my religious delusion. James became very frustrated (helpless) saying, "You don't give up do you?" I retorted, "You don't either, do you?"

My truth has come from carving away: the untruths, the conditioning, the repression of my feelings, which tell me the truth by me crying on certain words. Words like my "birthday," in telling how I spent part of it with my dad at his grave, because he'd be the one who would want to celebrate my birth day the most. (My eyes are misty now.)

James was very good at hearing my tears, although his had not shown up. Yet, he seemed distant as we climbed the stairs to bed. When I asked how he felt, he said that he felt good physically, but didn't know what he felt emotionally. I sensed a wall to feeling his feelings, although he could talk about them. He said he needed to be with himself and I was proud that I accepted that even though I was feeling aroused and sensual. We cuddled and went to sleep, until 2am when he pushed his erection into my buttocks, and although I did not feel resentment, I felt disappointed that we could not be face-to-face kissing. It made sense that he would act out his distant feeling.

Two days later, I drove my rented *gray* Chevy Cavalier home because the day before a woman had lost control of her car and slid into my red Jeep, making it unsafe to drive. On route 88 I enjoyed the fog interplaying with me, as I wrote notes for a poem, "I Disliked the Color Gray," while feeling sexually aroused as the crotch seams of my black Capri pants bounced on and off my clitoris. I began to touch my nipples, and was very aroused for more than an hour. I wondered if I should stop and masturbate to orgasm. I was surprised I had all this sexual energy as the night before James and I had made love, and although we did not kiss, he did not rush me after being inside my vagina from the rear, allowing me to move on top of him with his penis between my legs, he still not wishing to kiss even in the dark. He did moan with pleasure and because I slowed myself, and rubbed just the way I liked it, I built to a fine orgasm with a muted scream of "Oh yes, oh yes, oh god," and it was easy to push him inside me just as I climaxed. He then, turned me over and thrusted himself into more vocal moaning than I had heard before.

I had given him a back massage beforehand, when he told me that he is more vocal with a massage than with orgasm. Now, that makes more sense to me because again he has no distractions from himself, and therefore can gain more pleasure. A love unshared? He appreciated the massage I gave because he didn't take on any negative energy from me, but had from another woman friend who has given him massages. That was good for me to know, as it validated my capacity to give more love than negative feelings.

Later, we had another very fruitful talk about his $8000 exploration into various medical modes of healing in order to help his myo-facial difficulties. Nothing really helped, so I encouraged emotional release work as he also had noticed how much better my circulation was than his, despite my being 17 years older than him. We discussed how humans have lost (or not found) the ability to grieve. How the polarity of the pendulum swings throughout history, from conservative to liberal, is trying to find the balance experienced **"in Love."** It does appear that the extremes of violence and religion are lessening through the consciousness of becoming in touch with our feelings. James said, "It makes sense."

As it did again, when I felt tears and mild anger as I talked about the Danny Williams case, where the criminal system wants to punish a 14-year-old for killing instead of rehabilitating him. My tears said, it is not okay to punish a child!

When I arrived at my office, after coming out of the cozy fog on my drive back to Ithaca, my first client told me that the World Trade Center in NY City had been hit by airplanes, as well as the Pentagon in Washington, D.C. Two hours later, I found myself masturbating on my office sofa, releasing the built-up sexual arousal during my drive home. It was a very intense orgasm coming with the words, "Here it comes" four times, followed by "Oh my god," four or five times. Beauty devastates suffering, even on the day of the historic 9/11 terrorist attack carried out by muslim religious fanatics. I am more committed than ever to devastate religion, which unknowingly murders the soul-spirit that wishes to bring us all together into Love. I was shocked by the 911 tragedy yet, felt calm inside, knowing this was another wake-up call to look inside our true heart-spirits – to be more conscious of our feelings. To be spiritual, not religious.

Feelings are much more gray than the rigid rules of religion. Gray is the balance between black and white thinking. James says that I am balanced, as I am okay with my beautiful red Jeep being dented in an accident so that I can be less car-vain. James acknowledged that he is overly vain about his $40,000 Land Rover, with its many gadgets and obvious cleanliness.

I have also noticed my five-year yoga progress in relationship to my sexuality. When I arrived home on 9/11, it was very easy for me to roll backwards (a yoga position) where my knees can touch the floor. It is usually difficult for my knees to hit the floor, and after being in the car for over three hours I wasn't stiff, and wondered if it was my sexual energy flowing, contributing to my enhanced flexibility.

9/11 forced people to come together to help one another and care, as it did my oldest daughter, Erin, who called me from Baltimore to see "if I was alive." I was surprised by her caring as I live four hours away from NY city. She thought I could have been visiting, yet, when I ended the phone call with "I love you, Erin," those words were not returned, as had been true for fifteen years. My spirit felt calmer than in the past, but still hoped for those three magic words. I am becoming more trusting in the evoLution toward more Love through being more vulnerable to my hurt feelings, connecting them back to my childhood, or past lives. In regard to Erin, her love-change toward me will be revealed later in this book.

The hoped-for change to the "in-love" feeling for James did not occur, yet we had an in-depth friendship that enjoyed the expression of physical love-in–the-making. That had occurred with George and Gare, to whom I had much less physical attraction than to James, who had a beautifully proportioned muscular body and a boyishly handsome face. Still, he had not cried with me, as the others had, and although mentally stimulating and open to exploration of feelings, James and I would not connect deeply enough. To the Self we all leave behind in our repressed-feelings childhood.

When I attended Martin Prechtel's workshop on grief rituals, I found mySelf crying as we sang, "Please do not forget me, please remember me," which I immediately connected to Daddy as well as to little Dianea inside, her spirit-feeling forgotten for thirty-eight years. "We can talk about the emotions, but where are the feelings (shown)?" carried many tears in my crying session. This superficially-deep paradox reminded me of the wisdom that tears gift me.

On September 13th (my lucky number) 2001, I realized it was the tenth anniversary of my fractured skull surgery. Out of my brain and into my heart decade!☺ I even dreamt of my first husband, Chuck, kissing him and looking into his eyes, which I had not done in twenty years.

Wanting to renew our communications despite his resistance. Love always wants to connect, which is why I will always love my husbands, because we have connected more than physically. Most definitely, because I have felt tears wash away fears and anger that would prevent me from continuing to love. MORE.

Even loving mySelf in masturbation with "Oh, Oh, Oh," and thoughts of god, as well as saying out loud, "Oh god, oh god," or "Oh _my_ god," as has become more recent. Am I able to be with _my_ true Self more and more? Not needing to be united with a man? To feel loved? As my Self is united more with the divine than with a man? It seems so. Still, I am attracted to men in order to trigger the feelings that bring me closer to my emotional pain that is a barrier when not fully felt, (grieved) to loving fully. What a wonderful way to evolve into Real Love!

My sexual energy seemed to be flowing like a fresh rain as my spirit flew freer and freer with "Tears for Fears" as the rock band is named. Jack Kornfield, trained as a Buddhist monk, who now teaches around the world as a clinical psychologist, agrees in his book, *After the Ecstasy, the Laundry*, when he writes, "One Sufi master told me that in his tradition it was taught that masters become sexier as they become more highly awakened. He did not mean simply sexual, but more full-bodied, awake, and alive." (pg. 182)

"The key to this open and free heart came to the Buddha after years of fighting against his body. He wandered through India for six years fasting and undertaking extreme and arduous ascetic practices in a battle to overpower all bodily desires and fears. Finally, he found himself exhausted, close to death, lying on the earth. Spontaneously a memory arose from when he was a boy seated under a rose apple tree in his father's garden. He remembered how there had come to him on that spring morning, all unbidden, a wondrous sense of wholeness and stillness, his heart at rest and at home in the midst of all things. Amazed, he realized that his whole spiritual quest for liberation had been misguided, a *fruitless fight against his body* and the world.

"With this vision he discovered the middle path, an inner unity that neither struggles against the world nor becomes lost and entangled in it. He opened his heart to the suffering and beauty in life as it is, and rested in peace." (pg. 185)

"The emotional wisdom of the heart is simple. When we accept our human feelings, a remarkable transformation occurs." (pg. 215) My question always is:

How does one accept our human feelings so that we can heal into Real Love?

Morrie Schwartz, who taught social psychology at Brandies, is quoted by Mitch Albom, author of *Tuesdays with Morrie*, in the midst of the agony of Lou Gehrig's disease as saying:

"Take any emotion – love for a woman, or grief for a loved one, or what I'm going through, fear and pain from a deadly illness. If you hold back on the emotions – if you don't allow yourself to go all the way through them – you can never get to be detached, you're too busy being afraid. You're afraid of the vulnerability that loving entails.

"But by throwing yourself into these emotions, by allowing yourself to dive in, all the way, over your head even, you experience them fully and completely. You know what pain is. **You know what love is.** You know what grief is. And only then can you say, 'Alright, I have experienced that emotion. I recognize that emotion. Now I'm free to detach from that emotion for a moment'...

"I know you think this is just about dying, but it's like I keep telling you. When you learn how to die, you learn how to live." And when you can live, you begin to be able to really LOVE.

The big question I keep coming up with is: how can we allow our selves to dive into the ocean of tears, which brings us the wisdom that Kornfield speaks of?

"As the first scales and gowns of disguise are peeled away, we begin to learn what is underneath the contraction of anger, judgment, and wanting. Usually we discover a new layer of hurt, loneliness, fear, and grief.

"This is where offering a tender heart becomes essential. This is the place of cou*rage* – the *cour(heart)*age to hold in love the hardest pain, our deepest sorrows and greatest fears. It is here that trust and surrender are nurtured. The awakening of this *spirit* of mercy and kindness is like the visitation of the angels. There comes an energy to forgive, a new softening and receptivity of the heart.

"My teacher Ajahn Chah put it like this:

"If you haven't wept deeply, you haven't begun to meditate."

The grief and sorrow that arise when we begin to open are both personal and universal. Many teachers say they had not expected such grief to *come*, but the heart has its own logic. One respected Zen teacher remembers: "I grieved for all the conflict and insecurity of my early years, the hurt of lost relationships, for the ways I'd misused my body, for sorrows, for the death of my father. Only then after two years, did my sitting open to an immense and deep silence.

"The dragon skin of our unshed tears covers the sadness and longing that connect us with the realm of sorrow in all of life. Sometimes our sorrow is the result of a particular event: the death of a parent, a family history of alcohol or abuse, a major loss in our life. Other times it is the accumulation of a thousand moments of **being unseen, unrecognized, unheld.**" (pg. 33-34)

There are few books that support this courageous process of feeling our feelings in connection to the source of our emotional pain. They are recommended at the end of this book, as well as groups that support this process such as Re-evaluation counseling, or Co-counseling, as some call it. I will continue to show you my process as you read on, in hopes that you will find support for healing your own heart, dear reader.

I believe September 11th was a wake up call for all of us to feel more of our hidden pain of losing our way in how to love. A new sense of caring developed as people came together to help in this 9/11 tragedy. People cried more openly than ever and talked about their sadness and anger. A few days after 9/11, I was driving my mother to her appointment with a massage therapist, a birthday present I had given her. She had just turned eighty years old and had never experienced a professional massage. She was excited about it although she told me that she had cried a whole Kleenex box full of tears that morning as she watched the tragedy on television. As she cried with me, I could only respond with my hand on her knee and to say, "It's good that you can cry about it." I wanted to say more, what I've told her before. That, as Elizabeth Kubler-Ross, well-known researcher and author of *On Death and Dying,* and other books, said

"When you cry, you always cry for yourself."

When I picked my mother up after her massage, I asked her how she liked it. "It was OK, but I felt a little nauseated." I know that nausea is one of our body's reactions when fear comes up, so I took the opportunity to relate her feelings to her past pain, which not surprisingly she denied, like most of us do. Still, I was happy that we did not argue, and felt good that again I had made a universal truth known.

A couple of days later it *came* to me as to why I had shed few tears in watching the attack on America by Al Qaeda's fanatical muslims. My well of pain is smaller because of the seven years of regularly crying out my deeply-connected past childhood pain. I am much less triggered by other's pain; I am now connected to my own. I did have tears when one wife said, "I've lost the love of my life." Which for me indirectly is my father, and more directly is for little Dianea.

And when I heard the song's words, "and the home of the brave," tears told me that my heart is the home of the brave – to show my true Self-feelings – which was scary to do as a child. And that is sad!

Like my Lindy-dancing partner, Brian, telling me that he likes kissing Nancy, a new lover, but had backed off kissing Megan, his girlfriend of three years, because he feared entrapment. He admitted that his parental relationships have contributed to his difficulties with intimacy. Brian is working on himself in therapy and is a sensitive man who wanted to paint a portrait of me. He is a very gifted artist, making his living painting all types of scenes and people. After he painted my portrait, I suggested that he change the yellow that he'd painted the whites of my eyes, to white. Others had commented on the lack of white as well. I believe my eyes are wider and brighter as white, which in real life, they ARE. He did repaint them before he left without me even thinking about him actually doing it. I was so pleased by such a seemingly small thing! Maybe, because it was a portrait of me and I wanted it to be as true to my spirit and my beauty as possible.

As long has been said, "The eyes are the windows to the soul" (spirit), and I wished them to reflect my wide, bright openness, which seeks to connect to the openness of Love. Why I wish my lovers to open their eyes while kissing me, and at orgasm. Why kissing is so important to creating intimacy, as one is facing the other's face and eyes.

I cried as I told Brian about my recent dreams of Daddy and my first husband, Chuck, and while telling I made the connection of how Chuck was the *first* man I loved in a romantic way, and Daddy in a parental way; that *first* loves are FULL of vulnerability, as was also true of my love for my *first* born child, Erin. It is so like our spirits when one is *first* born as a baby. So pure and innocent, full of trust and unconditional love. Therefore, it makes sense that our spirits are desperately trying to rediscover or uncover that divine-god-spirit we are all born with by falling "in love." It is the *first* and best love that opens our hearts, then our eyes, wide!

I did not have to ask James for open eyes the weekend after 9/11, when James and I spent the weekend at my home, three hours from where he lives. One of our activities was to attend a Jung Society event, where drumming was part of the speaker's agenda. I wondered why drumming rituals had never spoken to me, but I made a connection while discussing it with James. The drumming arouses feelings in the chest, around the heart, a rising in adrenalin, which increases the heartbeat's rate, making one feel more energetic and alive. This in turn makes many people more emotional: joy for some, sadness for others, a sense of belonging. There is a very primal connection with drumming and chanting. A feeling of the Self because the heart is aroused?

But, it is not an enduring connection with the Self or other, which I continue to find through my spiritually-connected tears, allaying my fears to be fully open with my sexuality. Another step toward this union was that Sunday afternoon drive with James into a meadow near Treman State Park. James rolled out his full-size sleeping bag onto the meadow floor, flannel mallard ducks lining its insides for our bodies to comfortably lie down on. Tall Golden Rod, and purple Beebalm flowers embraced our lovemaking circle, matted down like a deer's bedding. The clear blue sky was a dynamic blanket covering James and I as I viewed pine cones aroused on the pine boughs overhead. We kissed more, we eyed each other more than usual, until I screamed a wide-full orgasm into the open air. The orgasm felt more real than others with James as I screamed out "Oh god," yet sadly no "I love you," followed. I had experienced more closeness with eyes open and lips meeting as well as being touched the way I needed to be. I enjoyed James' non-verbal vocal orgasm even though he did not look at me. I climaxed by sliding my clitoris over his smooth penis, my favorite way, after we had joined with the intercourse of lovemaking while James' fingers rotated my nipples. And although it was a special making love, with great intimacy of sharing afterwards about the process of each of our orgasms, I knew in my heart that it was far from what it could be with someone with whom I am "in love."

When I followed up with homeopathist, Dr. Glass a couple of months after our initial meeting, I had not noticed any changes in how I bruise easily below the knees, and he said that I would feel differently emotionally/spiritually speaking as well. I did not with the Ignatia he had prescribed, so he prescribed phosphoric acid and again said that he had not met anyone like me amidst his 1,000 patients. "You are charismatic, having a wisdom and cosmic intelligence that most do not have." He emphasized my unusual ability to love, be sensitive and compassionate. Even though I still feel a bit uneasy (fear) to say these positives about me, I say them in hopes that the reader will find more credibility in my words. And I am grateful for the validation from others who do not know me well and feel this love emanating from me. This is my hope of hopes for you!

In the fall of 2001 I woke up, my clock reading 3:03AM, another time 7:07 AM, and during the day similar numbers appeared more and more frequently. I sense that it is happening because as I heal emotionally, my spirit is freer to become synchronous with the Design of the Universe's plan to Love with all its heart. My legs kick and my eyes cry tears in my crying session over the barrier I had to put up to protect mySelf, even from the father who loved me, limited and inhibited by religion's fear. The fear to be vulnerable with our hurts, express them to each other. No, we were to take them to "the Lord" and leave them there.

I am glad to "Cry like a Baby" with Casey Chambers, an Australian singer/songwriter, because my tears are uncovering the spiritual being I am as that baby, and can BE as an adult. It's like a daily shower. My body and soul becoming the free spirit! We all are born to BE.

Wouldn't it be great if we could see tears as sexy someday?

Like tears that spilled out at the Farmer's Market when telling my son-in-law what a great person my friend Steve L. is. He is alive and loving, unlike the greatness lost in so many of us, feeling unworthy of (god's) love. And the child's laughter lost I'm finding more and more, like when James said how he is "absolute that there are no absolutes"☺ except that things will change. I laughed and laughed! Isn't it great to say things like "I'm absolutely crazy about you?" And thank god or the DoU (Design of the Universe) there are absolutes like the sun rising and falling every day?

Until blue Monday, September 24, 2001. I was looking at my blank computer screen in disbelief! I press back, click upward, downward, my ninety-some pages of this book are gone! Yes, gone! As are my defenses. I am screeeeeeeeeeeeeeeeeeeeeeeeeeeeeeeeeeeeeeeeeeemmming! Tears ran with anger at the fastest speeeeeeeeeeeeeeeeeeeeeeeeeeeeeeeeeed I had experienced since 1998 after leaving Gregory.

Besides, AAAAAAAAAAAAAAAAAHHHHHHHHHHHHHHHHHHHHHHHH-HHH, all I could shout was "stupid, stupid, stupid!" It was the first day I had not printed out hard copies of pages I had written as I went along. I had written five pages of the best writing I thought I had done in a very long time. I was crushed like I was under a spring waterfall. I tromped around my apartment with tears trailing. I cried again as I told James, "I loved what I wrote and was so happy how it was all coming out, and now I can't get it back!" I had a flash of Daddy and little Dianea.

Helplessness. I was the baby again.

I connected to the loss of Self, my words, my expression, which felt so deep, asking "Oh god, why?" In my weekly crying session I sobbed like an unattended baby as I related my loss of Self due to my mother's religious teachings and conditioning which crushed my spirit. There I was condemned, and then felt my gut tightening, letting go of old pain as I said amidst my sobs, "How much I want to tell the world how bad religion is – how it makes you feel depraved and born in sin – it took away my innocence."

"As a little girl I was in TERROR of going to hell, instead of recognizing my goodness. We are all born worthy of love, and innocent! I am so glad I can let go of my pain – my heart is open to my tears – it wasn't for so long…Thank you Daddy for the seed of love you gave me.(sad now) I wish I could put my arms around you, that's god right there. Loving you and missing you is so much like how I've missed my Self, little Dianea, for so many years.

"Our hurt (vulnerable) feelings are our thread to the soul, not anger. I am not angry with the terrorists, I feel sad for them and me and my mother even. I know I am meant to feel this so that I can feel true compassion for others, relate to them in a loving manner. It felt good to be unloaded from all that anger that called me "stupid." I needed to be dunked in my tears☺

I was reminded of Kevin saying to Erin that same week, "Maybe someday you will open your heart to your mother so that you can say that you love her."

I also noticed during that session that although my gut was tight, I did not feel the pressured pain over my heart that I had felt a few years earlier when I first began my deeply connected grieving. And by the way, I no longer have any shoulder or neck tightness, which I had intermittently until sometime in 2000.

Another change is my ability to accept compliments and not diminish them with some negative response. More recently, I am beginning not to hang onto compliments by not writing down as many of them in my journal. These examples of acting out compensations for emotional hurt are again evidence of how much the church emphasized diminishing the Self. James captured this truth when he said, "Really?" after I told him how cute his face was in that moment.

I am glad that I describe my idea of god as the Design of the Universe (DoU) as an energy consciousness (spirit) that directs us toward the perfection **in Love**. "In Love" there is no polarity of bliss and shadow, or male and female. Love has no need for polarity when it is perfected. Love has no fear. Love is perfectly whole in peace.

I have not experienced real or perfect love, but I can envision it, as my <u>tears</u> <u>tear</u> down the defenses and conditioning which are not the true me or spirit of me. Yet, I feel the spirit ever pushing me forward in an EVOLution toward more LOVE.

I was with James the next weekend, at Bailey's café where live music mixed with my *hearty* laughter when James told his story of his eyelashes being caught in a plaster mold. I was near to a belly laugh at hearing someone's pain. I ask my self, "Can pain be so closely aligned with joy?" Previously, I have written of their close nature when laughter defends against fear and pain. Now, I wonder if this is healthy laughter. Yes, James was telling the story in a jovial way, still, I find these states of being so incongruent. I again, come up with my helpless feeling...I can't imagine laughing while his eyelashes were stuck and he in pain. Yet, I would now?

In all of that laughter, James shocked me when he said, "You love me, don't you?...I feel you do." I was dumbfounded. I did not know what to say except "I'm shocked and surprised."

"I love you, you know," James shocked me more. I knew I could not say those words back because I did not feel that depth of feeling. Finally I said, "I feel loving toward you, and you must feel that."

"Why do you feel shocked?" James inquired readily.

"Because it seems from your behavior that you keep your distance, like: not calling much, short succinct emails, not looking at me when we make love, unless I ask for it."

"It felt like a demand," James responded.

"It was a request, so call it a demand although I did not say you must," I acquiesced.

James had no response after I shared the importance of feeling connected and close to him in our union of lovingness. Also, his kisses were not freely passionate. I felt the slightest bit guilty for not saying, "I love you" back, knowing it would hurt him not to hear those three gut-desired words. But, I was glad I remained my genuine real self! Yeah!! I wrote in my journal.

So, here I was again being told I was loved more than I felt back, like with George and Gare. A change from the cycle where I was the one who felt more love for the man than I felt in return, like with my last two husbands, Alain, and Gregory. It is an interesting parallel to my ongoing emotional healing.

Yet, even though I am the one told I'm loved, I still feel I give a lot of love in showing others the way to more capacity to love. An example of this happened on the phone with James, when he asked if I had called on his 800 number (4.9 cents/minute), which I had not thought of doing. I asked him if he wanted me to. He replied that I could and then buy him an ice cream cone. I said, "that hurts because you tell me you love me, yet there is little behavior to show it, other than our relationship equally pays, each for ourselves."

"That's a balanced relationship, right?" James stated.

"But does that equality mean love that wishes to give, be generous and keep an account of every little thing that is spent? It does not feel loving that one feels owed or obligated to keep things exactly even," I answered.

"I said it in jest," James counters.

"We say things in jest that have a bit of truth underneath them, you know."

"I was used in previous relationships, so I am more careful now," James admitted.

"That's fine, but that does not mean that you can't be generous because you FEEL like being! That's old pain curtailing the present ability to love. You spend money on gadgets for your Land Rover, even if is only a few dollars, don't I matter as much as your car?" I wouldn't have felt so strongly if I had not heard him say "I love you" the night before, in a public restaurant, not in a fit of passion. Otherwise I could have accepted an even-handed lover-friendship with him. I won't accept that Love which pales, and it is my growing edge to know and feel that.

A couple of days later, at home, I awoke to see a maple blasting orange and red into the window across my bedroom, and then turned to see a wash of long green valley topped by a white halo out the window next to my bed at eye level. I became aroused; I wanted to share the beauty around me with the inside of me. It was one of those easy, expansive waves of arousal, no frustration of wanting, just *know*ing I would come, yet wanting the pleasure to last because it was so intensely present. From my anus, to vagina, to labia, to clitoris, where it was most intensely felt like when one reaches the summit of a mountain revealing a 360 degree view. Complete.

I felt the waves throughout my body like a warm blanket keeping out the cold. My head tilted back – an image of openness. "Ohhhhhh, then oh god, oh god, you are so beautiful, here I come." Another vision of how we need to come into our fully god-loving selves. Where did that expression come from, "I'm coming?" for orgasm, for love, for joy?

As unpleasant as it might seem, when my anus is being pressed by a rectum full of feces, my orgasms seem to be more intense. There is a pressure on the vagus nerve that enhances pleasure, like an old boyfriend would say, "like a good dump." It is a present metaphor for having one's shit right at the surface, near expulsion, and "shit" is a common word that my clients use to call their pain. They say, "That's my shit, or stuff coming up" when their "buttons are being pushed." So as I unload my shit (emotional pain) there is more and more pleasure of love in life.

I noticed how I don't think to ask James for oral sex or 69 either. Am I becoming less interested in that expression of lovemaking because I am more interested in being connected to the other person and mySelf, more than with the physical body? More than pleasure, I want Love! This parallels my desire to be face-to-face, and eye-to-eye as well as lips-to-lips where passionate love is crystal clear between lovers. There is no hiding. Like making love de-light-fully with candles, instead of in the dark where neither can be seen. Unseen, like when our parents could not see who we really are by not allowing our feelings to be respected, especially with our tears.

The last weekend in September 2001 I attended a second workshop with John Lee who does expert emotional release work. In one of my groups, I focused on my fear of hurting others, and how I don't want to feel badly for <u>telling my truth</u>. Those last three words spun tears down my cheeks as I once again connected my pain to my mother's and church's oppression of my spontaneity, to say how I think and feel. People in general dig me because I am direct, even "pushy" with my truth with kindness, so then I liked when Justin, a co-workshop-attendee told me that I am "sassy," whereas in the past I would have interpreted that name as a negative characteristic.

Another workshop exercise had participants who usually give, receive touch as they wished it to be given. I asked Marjorie to place her hands on my cheeks, and as I looked into her eyes, I felt tears hold my face, wishing that Daddy could have touched my face, not accepting the church story that it was wrong to be so close, because one might become sexual. Many tears washed away more pain-grief over being shut down to showing each other love in such a basic and GO(O)D way.

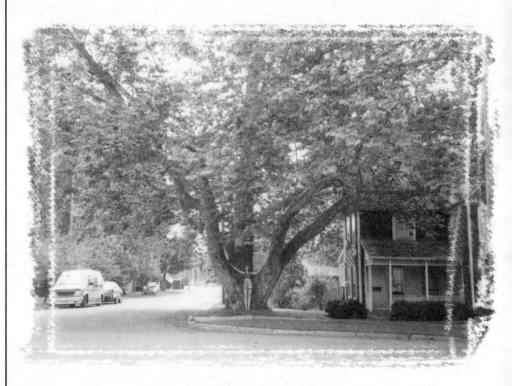

Sycamore tree, corner of First & Adams Streets, Ithaca, NY.
How big can your heart Be?

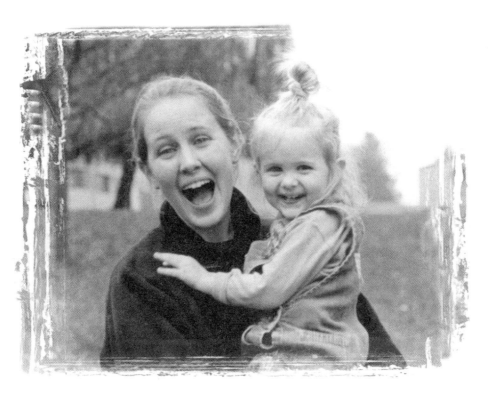

Author's daughter Erin holding her daughter Hannah Denali.
How big can your love-joy Be?

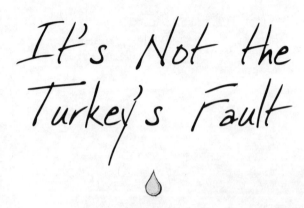

It's Not the Turkey's Fault

I sit alone in the Cornell University's movie theater, waiting for "Love and Sex" to begin. I've been without a boyfriend, partner, spouse, for over two years - something that is good for me, but tastes like spinach not well-washed, without any dressing.

Yes, I am an attractive woman; people say I am a Faye Dunaway look alike, but that doesn't usher in the "love of my life."

I've always enjoyed sex, despite being deprived until I was 22, a virgin for my husband that I'd hoped and been duped to believe would be my one and only. Like I am the only one in this movie theater – until just now, one middle-aged couple chooses seats four rows behind me. Then, a fortyish woman drops into her cushioned fold up chair by herself, and now two college girls. All delicately spaced throughout the rows, as if trees competing for the sunlight. Who comes to a movie like this at five in the afternoon?

I asked my friend Steve to come along, but he had things to do. He's been a friend for eighteen years; we weave in and out of each others' lives like nightlights, plugged in, or pulled out. When my two daughters were in elementary school, they would come with me to Cornell's Teagle Hall, where I would lift weights, and Steve would mind them while he handed out towels. They loved Steve "Teagle," as we called him, a jokester, and lover of children. But I had to turn down his offer of romantic love back then, because I was not physically attracted to him, although I loved his spirit.

I've been to Steve's house for parties, run with his blind friend, bought his children's book, seen movies with him. He's written newspaper articles about me. He's helped me with self publishing. We've had many talks about his or my marital difficulties, and shared his children's friendship with my granddaughter. Once, our naked bodies met in a hot tub at a friend's party. My hand found his erect penis underneath the water, others not suspecting our playfulness. Our eyes met, but never our lips. Just hugs of appreciation.

Summer 2000 changed that. Our paths crossed again, this time at the annual

June Ithaca Festival. Only his daughters were with him, he being separated from his wife for two years, like me from my husband. Steve was still trying to revive his marriage; I was not. I danced with Steve on the soft green grass, helplessly noticing how his biceps and pectoral muscles had filled out. The glimmer in my eye now reflected his, which had not been reciprocated in the past. I began to wonder what it would be like to make love with this man, whose great heart I'd always admired.

In August, I saw Steve again while I was dancing on the Ithaca Commons, outside in the sticky air. It was near my birthday, and he offered to give me a massage for a birthday gift. I, laughingly, took him up on it for some future date.

My heart was softened again, as I read his Thanksgiving Ithaca Times article about his two daughters, and how they taught him to cheer for the rat's survival on their farm. I smile as I write, thinking what a rat I'd become, causing Steve's focus to swerve from his marriage, conflicted over what was his responsibility, and what was mine. I knew Steve was not "the love of my life," and that our honest friendship could stay just that.

The day before Thanksgiving, I was depositing money at the bank, and as I left I told the teller, "Have a great Thanksgiving." She replied, "I will, and I'll probably gain ten pounds **due** to the turkey." Without hesitation, I came back with, "It's not the turkey's fault." We laughed, and she said, "Well then, it's the pie's fault."

It's a Sunday December morning when Steve arrives at my glass door with his massage table in hand. He finds the space in front of my wood stove an ideal place for bodies to be born naked to the tender firm strokes of his farm-worked hands. I had not known until now that he went to massage school back in 1979. I hadn't had a full body massage in years, and hadn't particularly felt the need, but the almond oil of human contact from a dear friend was welcomed. We talked for the hour of his laying of hands to my body. I felt Steve's respect of not only my body, but also for my person. His touch was not sexual in any way. I felt my heart connecting to my loins as we explored where each of us was in our relationships. Deep things. He said there was an unspoken agreement between him and his wife that they could be sexual with others while they were separated, waiting for each other to change. Waiting for his wife to find therapy as a way to salvage their marriage, as Steve continued his. I wondered again about my responsibility. I've always been too responsible for others, my needs lagging behind like a toddler trying to walk as fast as its parent.

Steve became so warm near the end of the massage that he took off his long sleeved sweat-shirt, revealing his bare chest. I wondered again at what is happening to me. I would go with my heart. Like a cherub, I rose off the massage table, and I hugged Steve a big thank you that has no words. Our hands held each other, my head to his chest, his hands up and down my back. The almond oil brought our bodies together where there is no separation of oil from vinegar. My head bent back, and our lips met for the first time in eighteen years. I wondered at their wideness. After a minute of consensual kissing, I asked, "Are you all right with this?"

"If you are."

I was. I took his hand like a child would, and led him upstairs to my white iron bed, where my one remaining piece of clothing was removed. And his. I was all at once amazed, accepting, and comfortable with what was happening. I was trusting my heart to become whole. We felt our skin meld into each other's like long-lost kin. I felt the ocean waves rise and fall as he so tenderly wandered my body. I looked up at Steve and said, "Since this summer, I've wondered what it would be like to make love to you." He replied with a smile, "I've wondered that for eighteen years." We laughed. We returned to the waves of our souls, closing our eyes to feel the center-delight of our bodies. "Afternoon Delight" played along as our fingers played. I opened my eyes to say, "Look at me," and his blue eyes and John Travolta mouth reminded me of my brother's face. I felt connected again. I now felt attracted to this man physically, as well as to his heart and mind. I told him so. "This is (w)holy."

"Well, we are in church," Steve grinned as he has just entered me. "The Bible says our body is the temple of God." Holy Spirit, I thought to myself. I chuckled as I said, "Yes, it is Sunday! What a great way to know the Divine, it is truly what church is!" I laughed **heart**ily because I was happy to have made this greater connection to the divine love in us all through this man who has seen it in us for 18 years. And my tears were for the sadness of not seeing the goodness in myself for all my growing up years. Not until I was 38 years old! In 1984. When I left the organized church…

And opened my heart, like I do deeply in my weekly crying sessions with Susanne, where I have come to experience the critical healing that tears provide. Even my male Bangladesh client says, "Crying makes me happy." After ten years of this heart-opening work, it has become easier for me to connect my irritation to the hurt child walled off and defended by the anger, because the tears spout only when specific words roll off my tongue. Sometimes I surprise myself as to when my tears spontaneously appear, like when I spoke the exact words that I had said to the bank teller: "It's not the turkey's fault." I began to cry as I spoke those syllables, and immediately I connected this seemingly off-the-cuff statement to how I had always felt, feelings hidden in the crevices of my heart. From age three on, every week, I heard in Sunday School how "it was my fault" that I didn't deserve god's love. I had been born in original sin. Through my tears, I've had the image (several times) of me falling off the small chair I sat in close to the Sunday School table, where we gayly sang, "Jesus Loves Me This I know." The knowing was in my brainwashed mind only, not in my heart, where tears tell me my truth - that I am loveable, and so sad not to have felt that for so long.

Now, less than four hours after my "church" experience with Steve, I'm waiting for "Love and Sex," to begin. The lights are dimming, as the movie splashes the big white screen with color. Just enough light to see a slightly built man about to sit down four rows in front of me. "Ken," I say, full of surprise. He immediately comes and folds down the chair next to me. It is another one of those synchronous moments, where Ken's and my life intertwine, meeting at the most auspicious times and places. As if energy of certain colors flies together like those of the rainbow after a storm. Ken, like Steve, is another friend with whom I've connected on an intellectual level, without the physical attraction crystalizing in me. We figure for about sixteen years. And like Steve, our paths cross every few months. My surprise is doubled this day, because it is Steve and Ken meeting me on the same day!

After the movie, Ken has forty-five minutes before an appointment, so we meet at a nearby bagel shop, where he buys lasagna, and I ask for a cup of hot herbal tea. I leave it up to him to pick the flavor. While he orders, I find a table where we can sit. He tells me he ordered vanilla almond. My mouth flaps open. "Unbelievable," I gasp.

I tell him about the almond oil used for the massage I had that day. About the four almonds I eat every day to ward off body toxins. There is no reason for either of these men to know that I like almond. Almond, I later notice, can be split into al-mond. Mond comes from Latin, then French (monde), and Italian (mondo), meaning world. So almond can mean all-of-the-world. So today, have I connected with all-of-the-world?

Or all of me? Or at least most of me? The divine source of me? Is it no longer my fault, that I am unworthy of god's love? I can still play by memory "I Am Not Worthy, the least of his (god's) favor," on the piano. Out of five years of piano lessons, it is the only song still committed to memory.

The following Sunday, Brian, my platonic friend of eight years known mainly as a dance partner, has dinner with me after our practice. I think about the "turkey" as I eat my chicken breast dressed in its Mexican spicy black bean sauce. I tell Brian about my synchronicity with Steve and Ken during our mouthfuls. I forget to tell about the almonds. The waitress asks if we would like dessert. Brian asks what are the choices. She lists: chocolate decadence cake, flan, almond nut pound cake, Mexican ice cream and raspberry torte. I tell Brian to choose.

"We'll share the **almond** cake."

12/2000

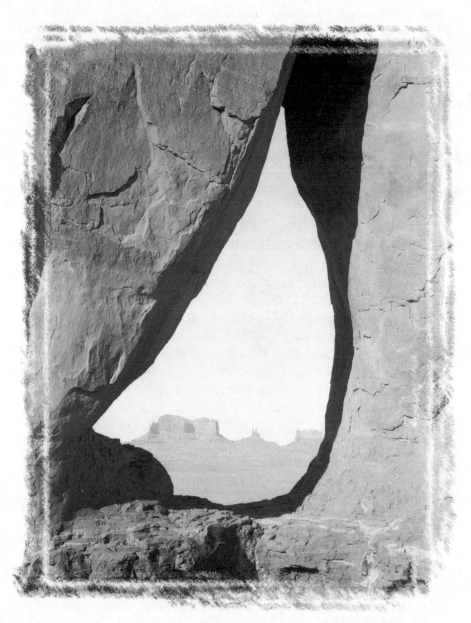

Tear Drop Arch, Utah. Henry W. Farnam III, photographer.
How big can your tears Be?

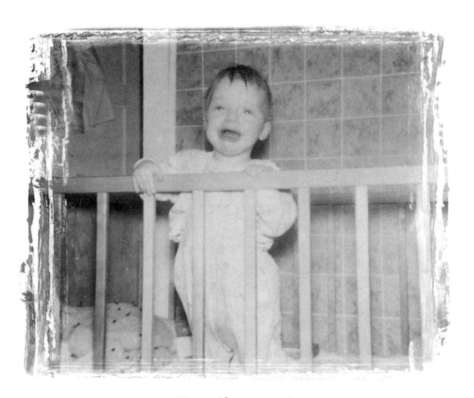

Karen Olsen, now 46.
How come we photograph our child crying?
To BE? (or not to be).

part four

◊

EVOLution of an Orgasm as the Harvest Colors of God-in-Us

The SEASON of FALL...2001–2002

What happened to the knowing of the three magic words, "You are go(o)d," which U.S. Andersen writes in his book, *Three Magic Words* (parenthesis mine). All I can think of is that my path is to learn to Love without needing it to be given back. Tears immediately underlined that truth☺ That kind of love is a more real and deep love, it is true – but so hard to manifest when it comes to one's own daughter or mother. My tears are falling into more love, filling a reservoir of Love within me.

The reservoir of Love is found in the very child we are born to be. And was especially vivid in my daughter Megan when I cried with her on the phone, as she lives in Boston, six hours away from me. I told her about losing my book manuscript off my computer, and how my screams of tears were connected to losing the reservoir-of-love-child inside of me. Her response: "GO(O)D for you!" Before saying goodbye, we easily said to each other, "I love you!" Not love ya, not see ya. We are solid in our love. Not afraid to express it in words. Like children can. As the bible says, "Suffer the little children to come unto me, and forbid them not: <u>for of such is</u> the kingdom of <u>god</u>." Mark 10:14

And it fascinates and supports me that Lewis Carroll, author of *Alice in Wonderland*, uses the metaphor that we can cry and cry until we find ourselves, like Alice, afloat in a pool of our own tears, adrift in a <u>transformed</u> world. (My middle name is Alice, which means the truthful one.)

Historically, we seem to waffle as to how we perceive tears. Miguel de Unamuno, Spain's most influential philosopher, states in *The Tragic Sense of Life* (1913), "Yes, we must learn to weep! Perhaps that is the supreme wisdom." Then, instead of listening to our own tears, Tom Lutz notes in *Crying: the Natural and Cultural History of Tears* (1999), that one can find on the internet a quote from the New Age guru Baba: "The spiritual path is closely connected with feelings; that's true. However this does not mean that inner passion should be exposed through an outer display, such as the shedding of tears… Nonetheless, someone with a "pure and sensitive heart" should weep spiritual tears; they should "weep within continuously." Baba's advice to never cry and to weep internally is another summing up of our age's double vision." (pg. 302)

"Whatever it takes for an individual to vent and release stress is essential to our emotional health," says Jodi DeLuca, a neuropsychologist who studies crying at Embry-Riddle Aeronautical University in Daytona, Florida. And crying seems to work well: one survey found that 85% of women and 73% of men report feeling better after crying. DeLuca continues, "We are genetically programmed to cry, and denying that impulse damages our physical well-being."

And therefore, it endangers our spiritual being, which I find especially connected to the physical feeling of orgasm. It came to me that my need to cry at orgasm is a small window or vision of how one can learn to Love fully or wholly-holy. Orgasm is our body's natural response to the demand for Love. Whether it is to create the unconditional love of an unborn child, or to look into the eyes of our lover and see the Beloved in each of us. We must SEE Love in all of its exposure of vulnerability, the **light**ness and wonder, which happens when we are out of control at orgasm.

James said that I could not demand Love. I say I can! I cried telling him that I will not repeat the pattern I had with my father, where we were both afraid to press each other to FACE our pain of not being able to be physically demonstrative of our love by hugging or kissing. We were both too scared (not sacred) to lose our "love" for each other, which had been scarred beyond repair by oppression of our feelings: a great deal due to religious dogma. (Notice: dog-ma: "ma" for mother who has the most intimate tie with her child, and "dog" is god backwards, as religion leads us backwards from our spiritual being.)

No, I cannot force my daughter or mother to love me, but I can demand a response, a responsibility to move forward by responding to my tears. I love enough to not ignore, or to coast. I felt powerful in expressing this truth through my tears, and James responded by calling me "The Love Warrior." I smiled as tears sparkled "thank you" scribbled on my cheeks. What do I have to lose? I have every Love to gain, as the reader will find out by the end of this book.

James and I then discussed the use of "fuck" as I have written earlier, when he tried to defend the positive use of what he concluded was an "animalistic" way to "make love." Animals, of course, do not make love; they copulate in order to reproduce their species. They do not face each other or have a love connection. James could only think of one example where I "demanded love." When I asked him, "Look at me."

James and my lovemaking continued to improve by being more drawn out in time, feeling good intercourse mixed with clitoral satisfaction without any oral sex from him. I felt long waves of soft orgasms, maybe two or three? Many "Oh gods" spontaneously flowed from my mouth without "I love you," although I did tell James, "You have a beautiful body." When James climaxed, he said, "Oh god" once, new, and said afterwards that was interesting. "A long release instead of the big bang." That was how it felt for me, enjoying all the sensations for over an hour. Our.

It was not meant to be that James and I would fall "in love," yet we made more love each time we were together through our growth in honesty and openness, challenging each other's journey toward a Love we both longed for. I am grateful for each male-lover-relationship as I travel toward telling my lovers, "I love you," with all of my heart-spirit. It is so easy to say those three grand words at my father's grave, as tears fall hard…like I wish to with a man with whom I wish to stay. Wish to kiss without reservation, troublesome with James. I talked about our kissing again, and he said that smell and touch could greatly affect his desire to kiss. I asked him to be more direct about what he needed: me to brush my teeth, or touch him differently. He applied some oil to his lips, which felt dry and cracky. Kissing enhances intimacy because we use our lips to say what we really need in order to connect, to be intimate.

My two daughters and I kissed thousands of times as we grew up, but those precious kisses do not make up for my two ears needing to hear "I love you" in the present from my mother and my oldest daughter Erin. I continued to press them for a response, even enlisting Erin's partner Niki in support of this needed healing. After receiving an email from Niki, giving her support, she also stated that maybe I should focus on the little bit of progress Erin and I have made in becoming closer, and not on what we have not achieved. I wrote to Erin, which helped me feel another significant piece of grieving into a Love that would manifest sooner than I had expected.

My body continued to express its pleasure of being alive in making love with masturbation or with a partner once or twice a week where images seemed to be less and less a part of my experience. The "Oh god" continued with "How beautiful, you're so beautiful" falling from my lips. I would feel my orgasms in various parts of my body, my head tipped back with openness to the universe. It seemed that tears had taken a breather from my orgasms, as I continued to have insights during conversations with James interspersed with welcomed tears of wisdom.

I never wanted to be seen as arrogant as some authority figures who called themselves healers, and came to see that I could learn from others while not taking advice from them. I smiled as I saw advice broken in two…ad-vice. It would be a "vice" to "ad"(d) or heed others' direction instead of listening to my own inner voice of wisdom, which I can hear louder and louder as I cry away the ear muffs of past repressed pain. To be a "Love Warrior" I needed to heed my own heart's voice. Trust my Self- the god in me. (Take away the o in voice and you have vice. The "Oh" of "Oh god?"☺) I love to see how language is ever connected with the Design of the Universe.

Even with music, which helps people cry. One of my last times with James, he played one of his favorite CDs, "Ascension." As my hand laid on his leg and hand, my eyes on his tears and shivering chin, I felt tearful hearing the low sad tones of the music. No connections, thoughts or images came to James. Yet, it was good to share our vulnerability. As I continued to read *Living with Kundalini*, I found depression to be tied to the experience of kundalini, along with not allowing oneself to cry. I was quiet, hoping James would take up more emotional grieving.

My weekly crying sessions, where I go much more deeply into my grief, sobbing, is where I feel and know my spirit thrives. Not only are the main themes of childhood pain revisited, but also new ones like crying about the use of the word fuck. Fucking is thrusting hard and rough, beating one's penis against my birth canal does not feel loving. I am glad I feel this way because I do not want to hurt my body in order to feel pleasure, or enable what some might think as love, "fucking one's brains out." Their only way to get the mind out of the way of the heart?

Are you drinking from the well of pain in order to Love well? Are you well? Are you loving well? I am beginning to, like I felt on the day Susanne, my session-crying-partner, began with "I love the feeling of acceptance I feel from you." Her expression surprised me because it came on the heels of me pressing her to lower her anti-depressants, which is scary for her although she is at her lowest amount in many years of medication. I am glad she feels the acceptance as well as the push to improve.

When Susanne leaves my house, we usually kiss and tell each other, "I love you," but on this October day, 2001, she turned back around after exiting the door, and hugged me again, saying, "I love you, I love you, I love you," I lost count how many times. Her love affirms what others cannot or are not ready to feel in acceptance from me. Someday, I especially hope Connie and Erin will know!

As I know the love and acceptance I felt from my father, as I re-read some of his letters where "I love you" was in cursive, filling two-dozen Kleenexes with "pearls of god," that same week. It was as good as a regular crying session, only by my Self. Missing the "I love you" out loud, settling for fear, especially on that traumatic day when I was sixteen. "Oh god" I missed saying those three magic words out loud like I say "Oh god" out loud approaching and during orgasm!

In the past, I took so much for granted when I received dad's letters that forever inscribed, "It's no small wonder that I love you." It took him a great deal of time to write those weekly three-to-four-page letters, my tears inscribe my cheeks and chin even now, writing a heartfelt thank you to him, for loving me even though I was not his biological child.

This is why I will press Erin to respond with "I love you" out loud, because it is an intimacy lacking fear, for "perfect love casts out fear." I was so ignorant, unaware, insensitive in the past, and now I have deep gratitude to take their place. The gratitude of Love.

Love continues to diminish my need for material things, to be okay with making less money. To serve on the Ithaca Health Alliance board, which is a grassroots non-profit organization providing health assurance. It is a model for national health insurance, where everyone has the right to health care, independent of wealth or status. That's Love in action!

Love is the synchronicity of a well-evo-loved world where even time seems to speak of my journey being synchronous with its purpose. I turned off the light and read my clock at 12:12AM. I woke up in the morning at 8:08AM, and another morning at 7:07AM. Could synchronicity be perfection's voice crying out? It is the only sense of perfection I can internalize thus far.

Synchronicity is like me meeting Brian while walking into Taughannock Falls State Park. I did not know him well, but had danced some great synchronous swing steps with him. He was smiling big, happy to see me. It just felt right to run and jump into his arms even though he was not expecting it! We laughed and laughed!

The synchronicity of Love is why I keep in contact with the men with whom I have been a loving lover. When I was at a dance workshop in Rochester, I called up George in a spontaneous moment. I had not seen him for a year and he was available for lunch within an hour. It was good to share sandwiches between us.

Just as I was feeling my relationship with James ending, I drove alone to the Touch of Texas, central New York's newest and largest wooden dance floor, where the cowboys hang out. The Mason-Warrington Orchestra was playing that afternoon, which encouraged me to expand my swing steps into ballroom dancing. On and off for years I had gone to dances by myself, hoping I'd find dance partners. I was especially lucky this day, to meet Robert, who had come with friends, but not a dance partner. I noticed how well he danced, and despite my beginner status in ballroom, I asked him to dance.

Although I have a natural ability to dance, I was surprised to hear him say that I am a <u>divine</u> <u>dancer</u>, who moves so beautifully and glides so effortlessly. I thought: dancing being so graceful, expansive, flowing like tears are. It was the first time I had made the connection of "dancing" "divine" tears. What made Bob's and my connection strong right from the start was his continual talk about emotional therapy work, which he did on a daily basis. He knew what it meant to sob, and rage, and was completing exercises in Dr. Phil's workbooks.

I am very aware of how it is the change in individuals that make it possible for institutions to change. The next day I was attending the Health Alliance Fund meeting, listening to others complain and blame the government, and the corporate control for our country's problems.

Finally, I spoke up and said that we patronize many of these businesses, but more importantly, it is individuals like you and me who make up the government. We should be asking what are we each doing to change the system. Time went quiet. I gave more hugs that night as I left, and felt the group to be closer to one another. If only we could be more sensitive to the individual, the groups would change.

Megan wrote, "Try not to be so sensitive," in an email that same week. This is where love gets tricky: to be able to separate out how one can healthily expect to feel loved in the present, from the unconscious need of not being adequately loved while growing up. I am more and more sensitive and aware not to have my daughters make up the lack of love from childhood, like when I wrote in an email to twenty-seven-year-old Megan:

"I've noticed since my birthday card, signed 'Love you, Megan,' that the usual 'I' was gone, when you used to write, 'I love you' or 'I love you lots' quite often. The last few emails (for 2 months) you sign, 'Love, Megan' which is even less strong or personally involved. Like written to a less important friend. What changed? It hurts to feel less connected or less important to you. You are probably thinking that I'm too sensitive, or too needy…but that's how I feel, and it's a bit scary to tell you these vulnerable feelings of mine. I'm probably more dependent on you because of Erin's lack of love for me, but even so our relationship stands on its own. It is so easy to love you greatly! Mama."

Megan's response: "Hi Mom. Sorry to hear you are questioning my love, only because I leave out a letter sometimes. I don't know if you noticed (I did), but I did say 'I' when we got off the phone last night. Whether I say it long or short, it is all the same, I have to say, I think you read a bit too much into these things. You know that I love you, so don't look for things that you think might counter that. Anyhow, try not to be so sensitive, I LOVE YOU. Megan."

Tears seeped as I typed those three magic words above, again alerting me to my lack of hearing those words during my childhood. I cried out more grief about that loss in my weekly crying session, and felt clear to talk with Megan about the quality and depth of our love, because everything we say and do is a spotlight, reflecting on our true feelings. I sobbed again about having a glass door between Daddy and I that did not allow us to say "I love you" face to face. We were like prisoners who put their hands on the glass when visitors come. It was the prison of religion that kept Daddy and me at a distance, as well as distant from my own bruised and protected heart. I am glad I am so sensitive, and that I know how to heal my hypersensitivity by crying out childhood pain, so that my sensitivity is a healthy balance.

My tears have shed past life grief and light as well. I sobbed as I imaged Erin and me during the Crusades. I killed her with a sword over religion. As I feel sorry for that event even now, and understand why Erin is carefully distant from me, I can more easily accept how Erin is with me. At one time, she agreed to see a past life therapist, but it has not happened as yet. Still, I can accept her feelings as not about me in the present, and I can love her and help her in any way I can. That is a true comfort.

As it was for me to realize that the church religions are not about who you are in the present…but always about working for heaven, to avoid hell, and not to be in your present thoughts or feelings. We had to think and feel as was preached.

Feelings are also reflected in our dreams, and I notice that I have fewer and fewer as I let go of my past emotional pain. One night, I dreamt about being on all fours, pooping all over the place, as well as vomiting a small amount in a bathroom. It was apparent to me that I was letting go of much of my "shit," as many clients say in referring to their childhood hurt or pain.

Having Bob understand these emotional issues as well as literally sweep me off my feet while ballroom dancing ignited my approach to "in love" feelings more quickly than usual. He had taken many hours of ballroom dance lessons, and still said, "I don't want to spoil your style and connection in dancing that formalized lessons do." Wow, I thought, and realized why I do not fit into the expected style of competition dance. Why I stay out of the box of formal dancing in order to be my unique self. Bob said my eye contact was more "genuine" than what he gets from the competitive ballroom dancers. I was surprised to hear that I followed and spun better than some of his dance teachers or partners. It was such a validation of who I am, even through my dance.

During our first date, which was to dance for three hours, we glided over the floor despite our three-inch height difference, me being the one looking downward. We laughed heartily a couple of times when I tripped us up during a tango or samba, with which I had no experience. I was in second heaven. Why second?

We had not made love yet, but I decided to put my fear aside when I emailed him the day after our date, and wrote, "I wonder what it will be like to make love with you." Even though he was three inches shorter than me, and for me a lightweight of 140-145 pounds, I was still attracted to the broad shoulders and muscular arms of this 57-year-old vulnerable man.

Bob had big hands too, which are a major factor in my physical attraction to a man, because they remind me of dads. But on this October morning, while doing my daily yoga, another reason came to me regarding hand attraction. Dad and I had not held hands enough, and the times we did were so important to me, because mom did not love me. Dad and I never had enough physical closeness to support our heart's love for each other. Bob had not picked up that I was interested in a sexual or romantic relationship with him, and I was not sure as yet, but my heart was leading me there.

Just as my healing heart dictates healthier and healthier eating habits as I progress. I used to love to eat homemade cookies, three or four at a time. Now I buy one large mocha chip cookie, and eat half one day, the other half the next day. My body is becoming more in tune with knowing what it presently needs instead of what it wants in order to comfort a past emotional need. It is not new to know that most of us eat more than we need out of a need to comfort ourselves, unaware that past hurts lurk in every mouthful.

I am sad that my overweight sister, Connie, has chosen to take an antidepressant along with a medication to allay the symptoms of ulcerative colitis instead of crying out her pain. She told me that she is aware that she needs to, as she crawled into bed with me on the morning after one of my over night visits to her home. Right off, she began to tell me about her week and the connection she had made to the past. GRRRRRRRRRRRs came out her mouth as she told me how mad she was at her employer of fifteen years, because she did not trust Connie with her car for a week. She did tell her 90-year-old employer that it hurt, but then did not take the car, but instead felt like taking some possession from her home. Once again, I brought up helping her to do grieving work so that she would not feel so vengeful, but she said she does not want to push her process.

Connie was also mad that she gives and gives to her employer and receives so little in return. She is doing the good "born again christian" action and feeling resentful. She related it to our father being very giving, as well as how she felt about us growing up together, sharing her Halloween candies or clothes with me, but I would say that she'd stretch my clothes and that I was saving my candy. I am sure that I had to hang onto stuff because I had so little control over my life, or love from mom. I told Connie how close I felt to have her in bed with me, like we wish we had snuggled as kids, and she agreed. I even noticed the soft touch of her forearm against mine.

Connie is still a born again Christian; I am not. I used to feel hurt and unimportant to her because I was and still am the one who initiates our get-togethers, usually monthly. Now, after years of crying out my connected-grief tears, I can accept that I am the one who needs to keep the connection going because it is important to me! Also I am aware that I am a bit intimidating because I remind her of feelings she doesn't want to face with grief. I will just love her anyway☺

Connie picked me up off my feet as we hugged goodbye, protesting that she was too heavy for me as I picked her up in return. As we stood in her driveway, I told her about a woman that I'd seen in the grocery store dressed up in a black and white cow-design halo, and T-shirt with "Holy Cow" written on it. She'd seen a similar cow-woman in her grocery store an hour from where I live. We laughed hard-heartily, especially Connie, and I knew why.

The "holy cow" of religion had kept me from my "holy child-like self." The thoughts and dictates of religion had denied my child-spirit feelings of innocence and unconditional love. We were trying to laugh the fear of that separation from the god-in-us, away. I borrowed her favorite book, *The Shell Seekers*, partly for pleasure, mostly to know more about my sister. Just now, the title stands out to me as a metaphor for the shell in which religion encapsulates our hearts. If you can find and see the shell for what it is, then you can crack it open to feel the spirit inside, which is what I know I have experienced through my spiritual tears.

Which continue to heighten my sexuality, and created three or four Self-loving orgasms the week after meeting Bob. They varied in their intensity and usually were created for my own pleasure, not originating from being sexually

aroused. When Bob and I danced again, he continued to compliment my dancing, and tell of his frustration with dancers who are so technique-oriented that
they can only follow their own partner. He said that I probably should not take
lessons because I'd lose my "individuality and spontaneity" which he loved so
much.

After the lightness and flow of our dancing, we made love on his waterbed, to
music, dim light, after a full-body massage. It was refreshing for Bob to raise the
conversation about our sexual health, not me for a change. He'd just left a
monogamous relationship of a couple years and had a negative HIV test a year
earlier. My history was a bit riskier, so we decided to use a condom although he
had never used one. It was the first time I ever helped a man put one on,
although I'd seen it done by previous partners. Bob was easily erect and we made
love for more than an hour, orally and with intercourse, neither of us climaxing.
Yet, I felt satisfied from the touching and kissing, he surprised that I was not into
French kissing as I am quite a free spirit.

The next morning he served coffee and grapefruit juice while we sat in bed
talking about many subjects: family, language, making love, national parks. My
tears flowed a couple of times as Bob gave his supportive presence, a hand
clasped with closeness. It was the foreplay to making love again without a
condom, trusting the universe, like I had in a couple of possible risky situations,
where one does not know a lover very well. Marc Rob, James, Bob, I met through
dancing, which is interesting because I became sexual with only one runner
during my twenty-year running career. Dancing has the freedom of self-expres-
sion, creativity and flowing in contrast to the rigid gait of a runner. Bob was a
runner and dancer; aware that I was in his life to teach him freedom, (through
trusting more?) because his two greatest fears were AIDS and drowning.

Bob showed freedom with an incredible full-bodied orgasm where he
screamed loud as a fire engine two times and rocked his body side to side. I had
never been with a man this vocal. It was so opposite of James who barely made
a sound other than a grunt. I didn't climax but felt a long ecstatic wave that gave
into satisfaction and loving to watch his orgasm. And give to him. I knew I had
not been relaxed enough and wished for more touching and neck attention,
which happened the third time we made love later that night.

That afternoon, we ran together for three to four miles, had dinner at the
Skylark diner, then decided on seeing the movie, "Serendipity." I heard myself
laughing heartily several times, hearing mySelf above the audience. No tears for
me at this movie, but some for Bob at the end. How great that the stereotypical
crying roles had reversed. Also, when back at his home, Bob proposed two exercises before being rocked in his waterbed.

The first exercise was to look into each other's eyes for five minutes, facing
each other, close but not touching. Then to tell each other what we saw. I smiled

much of the time, which developed into laughs, but not for Bob. I am sure I was apprehensive with this long intense closeness, true-full-eye contact being new to me. I saw "safety and steadiness" in his eyes; he saw "love me" in mine. Don't we all send the latter message out?

The second exercise was to respond to his statement ten times, "Tell me who you are," with first thoughts. Some that I remember saying: angel, innocence, kindness, love, star, moon, and compassion. He'd done this exercise before and answered in longer phrases like I am the fire of god…I wanted to say "I am truth" when I wrote in my journal. Our hearts were now closer before we retired to snuggle in bed. We made love with drawn out feelings of pleasure and I came by using his penis in my hand rubbing my clitoris, while his fingers rotated my nipples, as he sat astride me. It was a lower key orgasm with "Oh gods" interspersed with "it's so beautiful." He hallowed our intercourse with his screaming orgasm. He noted that I lubricated well despite being well into menopause, which made me think that my tears lubricate all the physical functions. More often, my hands were warmer than Bob's, demonstrating my enhanced circulation. He took vitamins, I don't.

Our orgasms felt loving yet distant, as there was no eye contact, probably protecting our selves from his eventual departure in two weeks to Florida for the winter. We knew it would be a short-lived relationship, but that did not deter us from the loving moments of the present. We continued to hold each other, as our fingers traveled lightly up and down each other's backs, arms, and buttocks, while sharing feelings, which engendered arousal feelings within my body. Then, something spectacular happened.

Although hesitant, I placed Bob's hand over my clitoris, his fingers tickling and lightly rubbing as I touched my right breast. After five or so minutes, I knew I had to help myself, so Bob spooned his body against my rear as I masturbated and he played my nipples. I "oooooohed" and "ahhhhhhhhed" for what seemed like a long time, maybe fifteen minutes, to ride this incredible wave of minor orgasms until I topped off with a goose screaming orgasm. Immediately, I thought of how wonderfully patient and giving Bob was to me, and me to myself, as tears blotted out the guilt and shame for asking for too much pleasure for mySelf. Tears tracked my thoughts, "Thank you for taking care of me." Then, waves of tears as I as thought, "for loving me."

My mouth couldn't help but open and say to Bob, "Thank you for loving me…and I feel a great deal of love for you in this moment." He replied, "That's good and mutual." It really is mutual because as I love myself, by asking for and receiving what I want, I immediately feel love for the other; it is an amazing blend into Oneness. It is like the blending of all the colors of the rainbow into one overpowering arch. (Why our bodies arch at orgasm?) Tears continued to underline my words of missing dad, wishing I'd said, "I love you" to him directly, and not just in letters. That same "directness, openness and honesty on levels that are truly rare, in fact I've never met anyone like you," that Bob valued in me. Because it denotes the loss of fear! And Love casts out fear☺

To pursue the things I love, such as dance, which continued to be an important part of my life, even to barter for dance lessons from Bill, who has taught ballroom and whom I met one day at The Touch of Texas. This married, sixty-eight-year-old man was sure he could improve the technique of this "talented" dancer. I was not motivated to do the needed practice, but I would try.

He taught me the basics of frame and balance during the time I ventured into Cornell University's Performing Arts Center to view some dance films. I surprised myself with tears as I watched Eric Bryn spin across the floor. I already knew that I had been a ballerina from past life regressions, and now I knew why I love to spin and be dipped. I smiled, as I knew that the spirit within is alive from death to death, or life to life.

And I recognize more and more how dancing is like tears: flowing with gracefulness, expanding one's world into playfulness, childlikeness, even innocence with one's body being free to create and express. Our tears touch our cheeks like the gentle kiss of our partner's hand holding ours. We connect, are close, to the heart, especially in tango. I began lessons in Argentine tango soon after Bob left for Florida.

But before he left we had more love to share. One morning when talking in bed together about the book, *The Four Agreements*, Bob told me that one agreement is, "Always do your best." I said that we are always doing our best in any given moment. I told him about a moment I will not forget while a client at the Primal Center. My Primal center therapist, Howard, had asked me to say goodbye to Daddy and to hold my arms out. When I couldn't say goodbye, I said, with strong tears, "I'm doing the best I can." He apologized, realizing that I was where I needed to be in that moment. I truly felt it was okay to be Me in that moment (tears now). The importance of having one's feelings validated is the essence of feeling one's spirit. The true heart, which cannot say, "I love you" unless you are able to <u>feel</u> it! Still, our spirit is always pushing us forward to be better lovers. It is the way the mystery of the universe IS.

I could not respond back to Bob's "I think I love you, no, it's beyond thinking." I did feel love for him, but the intensity was not fulfilled as yet. The next day, we hiked up a huge hill, and I was puffing to keep up with him, a rare moment in my relationships. Usually, the man is striving to keep up with me. And, he was ahead of me dancing, and not far behind in his emotional healing. What a great change; my relationships were becoming more balanced. I was left speechless when we stepped out of his car at the Syracuse ballroom dance when he said, "Do you have any idea how much I love you?"

It is difficult not to return the same feeling, although I said, "I love you too."

I did not feel the "in love" feeling that he had twinges of. We continued to have deep conversations, where Bob cried about his childhood, not knowing his biological dad, and being treated poorly by his adoptive dad. He was surprised that he still had tears about these family losses. Deep losses of love take time to grieve, for these losses have been deeply buried for many years.

Also, tears honor those who we have loved and lost, so I am glad these tears of love do not run dry. A fountain of youthful love has sprung within me. I want to repeat, **"One's ability to grieve is one's capacity to LOVE."** I FEEL it!

The weekend before Bob left for Florida we made love four times, he being boisterous with all four of his orgasms, me not needing to have an orgasm the first night. Twice, I came close to orgasm with intercourse, and it seemed that with practice I could. But, I do not pressure my self to do so, knowing that 80-90% of women do not have orgasms with intercourse alone. I just want to be open to all possibilities. We made love by way of 69, enjoying our rise to my orgasm with his penis caressing my clitoris with our body's own lubricants. There were many "Oh gods", some "Oh goodness," but still no desire to say, "I love you," until after physically lovemaking. He was the first partner I've had who would keep the "serious self-searching" talk going longer than I would.

I reminisced with Bob about my behavior while I was engaged to my first husband. I remembered excusing myself from the dinner table and retreating to the darkness of the upstairs bedroom. I would be hoping that Chuck would search me out, to see how I was feeling, after complaining of stomach symptoms. I had no consciousness of why I was doing this behavior, other than needing a chance to be close to him physically, forbidden or shunned by this born-again-christian family. Shame for sexuality hung like an elevator stuck between the floors of heaven and hell.

And the way to get people to love you was to say you believed in something that in your heart you did not believe. The ultimate giving up of one's spirit. I continued to cry intense tears in my weekly session, triggered by the Afghanistan women being able to take the veils off their faces when freed from the religious Taliban. So, where is god?

I am reminded of religion's prison of fear often, sadly seen in my daughter, when Megan felt she needed to lie to her grandmother, my born-again mother, when asked if she was pregnant. Megan's planned pregnancy was while unmarried to her live-in boyfriend, and she knew my mother would disapprove. After telling me how she hated to lie, (betray her own spirit) she called her grandmother back to tell her the truth. I know my daughters have not grieved their pain of the early years of being taught those same religious beliefs until ages nine and twelve. Unhealthy fear still sadly lives with them.

I am more and more conscious of how I wished I could have cried with Daddy, and how I am healing that need through crying in my weekly sessions and with my lovers. We all hold our pain inside out of fear of non-acceptance. We have imprisoned our spirit's capability to love. It is no wonder I continue to grieve the deepest soul-pain I have survived since that little girl went to Sunday school to hear her innocence being denied. "Jesus loves me this I know" was the song-lie that most hurt me, because I did not FEEL loved. "I can just see my innocent eyes looking at the teacher who took more and more of my innocence away each Sunday," is written in my journal of November 2001.

The reader may think I am redundant about this point of religion imprisoning the spirit. I need to be. It is the core pain of my life.

Still, I know I am healing. I no longer have rage over this injustice to my spirit. My sobs are less intense. Still, there are many many tears. And still, I look to the little white country churches as symbols of the innocence and purity that ought to be held within their walls.

I looked into the eyes of another Bob at a workshop called "Love, Sex and Intimacy," organized by the Human Awareness Institute (HAI). Bob has amazing steady eye contact that I have to work to maintain for long minutes. To be seen IS GOOD. Still, uncomfortable. "One must look within in order not to be without," is HAI's motto. Bob chose me to be his buddy for the weekend and he is married with an "expanded relationship" as he called it. He told me that he is madly in love with his wife of four years, and that they have had an "expanded" relationship for three years. He emphasized that he is emotionally and spiritually connected to his extra partners, as is his wife, and that it adds to the "romance" of his marriage. Could this be a healthy open marriage?

There seems to be much controversy about whether romance is a healthy kind of love. Scott Peck, author of *The Road Less Traveled,* flat out states, "the myth of romantic love is a dreadful lie." His interpretation of the myth as "that for every young man in the world there is a young woman who was 'meant for him,' and vice versa," (page 91) I believe is an exaggeration of what romance is intended to be. According to Webster's dictionary, romance is defined as "responsive to the appeal of what is heroic, idealized, or adventurous; marked by expressions of love or affection; **conducive to or suitable for lovemaking.**" I sense romance is the essential first step into the realm of Real Love. And I love to think of it as a heroic adventure that takes great courage because one will risk vulnerability: be hurt in order to grow into profound love.

Certainly, I was not meant to have the one lifetime marriage. My first husband turned out to be gay. My second husband died. It was difficult to leave my third and fourth husbands, especially my fourth, Gregory, who not only felt like a soul mate, but being with him grew me up big time.

Yet, each marriage began with romance and "falling in love," for which I am deeply grateful! As revealed earlier in this book, I grew like a wildflower throughout each marriage. It is now obvious to me that there is a meant-to-be in all of life. The Design of the Universe. The mystery of the human spirit compelling us to grow into <u>Real Love</u>. What we might call <u>spirituality</u>. <u>EVOL</u>ution.

Connecting lifetimes, as I did with Ben, a thirty-one year old dark chocolate African-American man at this same workshop. I was drawn to choose him for an exercise where we sat face to face naked, first looking into each other's eyes, then taking turns softly touching each other's face and bodies. He amazed me with his words, "Your eyes are a deep love inside me."

My eyes <u>are</u> wider and bigger in their openness as I cry out my fears of becoming close to my Self and others. The inability to touch and to hold was such a vast hole of pain from childhood. As it was to be seen, "You are the most beautiful woman here this weekend," Steve said just before I left the workshop. I had not interacted with Steve all weekend, except now to bend my head down, look at the ground, laugh, showing my fear to be proud of my Self. To be seen with all that beauty was so contrary to my religious upbringing. My beautiful spirit squelched.

Yet, I am gradually finding freedom through each Love relationship, like ballroom dancing Bob said, "You and I are supposed to do some healing work together." Because I have been with several men, Bob said that I have "reckless abandon," which clicked into my automatic thought that he was recklessly abandoned by his father, and so was I by my mother. I heard the message as me being irresponsible in my sexual behavior, also feeling that Bob's fear of AIDS seemed unhealthy. Soon, I was to learn of his greater fear.

At the HAI workshop of sixty participants, we were broken down into groups of four for one afternoon. Two men and two women of our choosing. I was with Ben when the four of us were instructed to be silent, and squeezed together into a very tight shower stall. We kissed, and washed, and I remember Ben leaning to put his mouth on my nipple and how beautiful that image looked. Like mother and child should be…my mother not having breastfed me. It was fun and special being close, and not fully sexual, like kids playing. We learned to appreciate all parts of our bodies with light stroking, not massaging, from head to toe like one needed as a child. We looked at each other like we would look at a baby. No fear, just appreciation. It's sad that I could not hold my father's hand (or my mother's) as much as I needed and wanted to. It was not safe to freely give physical contact in my fear-laden religious home. We did not know that every child is the essence of divinity, like the "Oh goodness, oh god" that spontaneously flies from our mouths.

I noticed that I did not cry all afternoon when receiving individual attention from the other three in my group of: stroking, innocent kisses, looking into my eyes, which I have done in the past during similar workshop exercises. I have less grief about not being seen and/or loved. I was healing into openness to hear that Bob made love with his lover, that morning and how beautiful it was, including some tantric methods.

In my small group of eight that ended the workshop, I said that I carried away more comfort and acceptance, not only for my own body, but also in being with fat people. That was difficult for me to say in front of two fat members, one being a woman who said that she loved her extra 100-pound body. I told her that I was concerned about her health, and her anger, to which she readily admitted. I believe her anger is wound up in her fat, and she appreciated my honesty.

In my crying session that week, I seriously sobbed as I connected with Ben in a past life. I had done a regression years earlier where I learned that I had been a ten-year-old black boy in the 1860s, where I lost my life along with my father, dying in our house that had been torched by the KKK. Ben had been my father. I notice that I have been drawn to people from past lives. I felt the sadness and special love in my solar plexus, which seems to be the spirit's center of feeling.

That divine spirit which makes us feel "all one." Those words made me shiver, as did hearing a woman in the workshop say that she couldn't cry. I sobbed in my weekly crying session as I reiterated her words, and while telling of lost sexuality in front of the workshop. Now my inner child is back, wanting to feel that she can run naked without shame, like children do.

I sob "Oh god, where is god?" I lost that child back in Sunday school, where I learned I was unworthy of god's love. Speaking about that vulnerable child's spirit being broken breaks my heart into tears over and over again so that I can <u>know</u> Love, real love, now.

The Love I use to face my diminishing fear of once again confronting Erin about her inability to tell me "I love you." It is Thanksgiving 2001, when I see my mother give Denali, my granddaughter, some books signed, "I love you, Gram." I feel a pinch in my heart, which leaves quickly.

When I was in the car with Denali, Megan and Ben, Megan's partner, and while we were waiting for my brother, Eric, I mentioned that I wanted to talk to Erin about something. Denali, who was close to nine, asked what about. I told her that it was about Erin's and my relationship, and Denali chimed in, "Let me tell you something, she won't change, she's stubborn and selfish." I was surprised how powerful were her tone and words. I was shocked as if I had jumped away from a live wire fence.

Later, after dinner, a hike and a family variety show, when Denali, Kevin, (Denali's dad), and Niki, Erin's partner, were readying to leave, Erin walked down the stairs into my living room where we were all sitting, and I asked her when could we talk. She looked surprised and Niki looked at Erin as she said that she could not make it happen, that it was up to Erin.

In an annoyed tone, Erin asked, "What do you want?"

"I want to hear you say 'I love you' to me, like you do to everyone else."

"I do love you mom," Erin replies, "so there."

With thoughtfulness, like a mother bird flying to its nest, I said, "I want it to be felt, not said because I want it, like 'so there.'" Tears entered my eyes, as I was stunned to hear Erin say, "Do you want me to tell you 'I love you' every time I see you?"

"Yes, I'd like that!"

My tears and I walked over to Erin, standing as I hugged her, and felt her holding me with the most feeling I had felt in a very long time. It was another Thanksgiving with family witnesses to Love breaking down a barrier: this time a decade of knowing Erin loved me because I was her mother, not heartfelt for Me. Love is not about blood, closed inside arteries where it cannot be seen. Love is full of light, expressed freely, not broken-up by the rules of obligation. Erin's breakthrough has not solved all of her distrusting feelings toward me, but we had made a grand step.

As do I, and chocolate Ben from the HAI workshop, through frequent phone calls where we share our intense feelings of love, as I acquaint him with our past-life connection. We spoke of not wanting the complications of jealousy and avoidance. I am struck by the word "avoidance." It ends in "dance." It begins with "void." Certainly, when one avoids expressing their feelings, there is no dance. There is a void. No freedom to create a beautiful partner connection that dance strongly symbolizes for me. The child-like dance frees the human spirit to love and create.

It is the love that I was capable of showing to my mother as I sat with her in the emergency room, and then cleaned her bathroom and dusted after I took her home. She told me, "You're a sweet lady," before I left. She could recognize my lovingness, although I am not a born again christian like her. I could see the longing in my mother's eyes to be closer to me although there was no "I love you," just a kiss on the lips as I leaned over to give her a kiss. Somehow I felt that mom was longing for the love she could see in my heart. It had been so long that mom has not loved me that tears could not help but make their appearance.

I am reminded of what Megan said on Thanksgiving day, when we each said what we were thankful for: "I thought you'd say you are thankful for tears, mom.☺" YES I AM.

And I am thankful for the reminder that the Design of the Universe gave me as I went outside to run in a light rain that turned into splashing as I approached the top of a hill near where I live. I dashed under the short overhang of a sheep barn, hoping for the rain to lighten. It did within five minutes, and I jogged down the road happily as the clouds lifted. When I turned to return home, I was greeted with the most spectacular sight! A brightly shining double rainbow that claimed my heart. I was sheltered under the arch of a complete rainbow where the inner bow could not have been more brilliant. Its shadow bow cradled me like a baby. I could only smile, feel glee, and run into its beauty, wishing I could share it with someone, and that I had my camera with me. I was amazed by the "high" it gave me with its promise of love and beauty. The double rainbow inspired me to write a poem, talk and email about it for the next few days. Anchored in my backyard, the DoU timed this magnificent "beau" for when I was outside on my run☺

The Perfect Time

It couldn't have been.
Raining lightly as cat paws, I took a chance.
All afternoon, downpours,
Intermissions of gray clouds dancin,
Wondering what's the next move
The sky would make. A chocolate glance?
My Adidas bounce slender frame
Up Gray Road, pounding asphalt hill
To the tune of my breath
Exhaling stale-stance,
Inhaling clean-trance.
My sun-blond hair darkened by droplets from heaven -
Wet as an otter at the top of the hill
So fast ran the rain.
I huddled under red barn's roof,
as heavy drops turned streams, inches from my nose.
Like inches, just minutes found relief –
White-bluish sky pressing toward me
Like a magnet I could not resist.
I ran once more into sky's open arms
Trusting lightness to stalk me.
Still drizzling, I turned back, around,
Jaw dropped, heart pumping, lips open to aaahhhh –
I forgot my step.
The gate of a brilliant rainbow poured over my head –
Perfect arch, earth to sky to earth, all within my vision.
Perfect colors, promise of love as its mission.
Perfect timing, my heart and rainbow without division.
What happened to the imperfect world?

When I spoke to ballroom dancing Bob again, he had revived his relationship with his former girlfriend, Sally, as I had suspected would happen. He said thank you, because my "honesty and directness" was what made the big difference. He also asked me to have an AIDS test, as he and Sally were concerned because I had not used condoms with all the men with whom I had been sexual. I had the AIDS test, being confident that I was fine. I spoke with confidence, non-defensive in tone to the nurse who inserted the needle into my vein. She was warning me about my behavior due to my lack of using condoms. My history with strictly heterosexual men, whose histories were with monogamous partners, and no druggies seemed to allay some of her seriousness. My heart was not pounding, I felt confident in my inner voice.

Like I was becoming with the voice of my orgasm during self-loving two times that week, thinking of Ben, as I said, "Come into me, I want you Ben." Then thought, I wanted the spirit of love to come into me, and I felt it to be growing.

I am still struck by the depth to which my spirit was buried. So unaware of my despair that kept me from becoming closer to my loving father, the despair of believing religion's teachings that I was unworthy of god's love, which encompassed the fear of expressing my innermost vulnerable feelings, especially when I learned he was not my biological father. These two hurt-to-my-core themes, along with my mother not wanting or loving me, are what I continue to grieve.

I am concerned that the reader may be put off by the longevity of this life process. Yet, if we think of it as a practice as important as eating or exercising, it will weave into your life as a form of liberation meditation. The tears will come and go as easily as taking a walk, or incorporating a daily yoga practice. That is what my weekly crying session accomplishes. A time for attention to feelings that need to be expressed in a more deeply connected way than most of us give time for - true attention. It is the healing attention to our feelings that our parents were not able to give. My spirit swims freely in my tears instead of being stuck in the mud of acting out with the reactivity of anger, or fear.

Crying can be like dancing. "The self definition and the trust and the daring, these are the dance. And the dance is the language, the ecstasy connection," as Gina Ogden expresses it in her book, *Women Who Love Sex* (pg.50). And the sexual dance has great possibilities, like that of "Amalie, a violin instructor, telling me of an indelible moment of sexual intimacy with her husband of twelve years: 'the two of us were so close it felt more like a love orgasm than a sex orgasm. I felt it in my heart. My whole chest opened up and I let go in a flood of tears that felt so healing.' Again, re-lease this time moving emotional energy into a cleansing of the physical body" (pg 63). I am happy to see that she is aligning the **love orgasm with tears**.

I would add that it is not just a cleansing of the physical body, but the unbridling of the spirit within, that has been buried and chained for so long by unawareness of its emotional pain. It is about being exquisitely aware and exquisitely sensitive. Why I need the light touch to my genitals and breasts to achieve orgasm, the harder touch deadening my sensitivity. My heart is light and not hardened anymore. Therefore, the light touch mirrors my (en)lightened spirit.

Sex becomes the body-mind-heart-spirit connection. I hesitate to say that such an orgasm is like being literally born again. Yet, it is letting myself trust, be innocent – like an infant who KNOWS how to give unconditional REAL love - the Love that is essential to satisfaction when with a lover.

There has not been much said in this book about the anger that defends us against feeling our hurt or fear, eventually exploding into rage. Most people do not want to admit that they feel such heaps of anger. But, it is inside all of us, dribbling out in daily annoyances or angry verbal fights. I have experienced rage screaming aaaaaaaaaaaaaaaaaaaaahhhhhhhhhhhhs or oooohhhhhhhhhhhhhs to the top of my lungs, or ripping the bible to shreds, or throwing pillows as I voiced, "I hate you mother." Eventually the rage mixes with tears or sobs, beginning to soften our hearts into a tender love that is for Self, then able to be given to another. This process can be read about in my first book, *Tears Are Truth…waiting to be spoken.*

Gina Ogden writes of Rosa's experience, "The weekend I finally burst through to my rage and beat the stuffing out of the sofa, we (she and Roberto) made love after that as if we couldn't stop. There was so much tenderness between us. So much whispering and touching. I remember us waking up and lying side by side in the morning just gazing into each other's eyes. We weren't saying anything. Just observing and accepting. Just being there. It was pure, open connection." (pg. 147)

I made another fascinating connection when I made love with mySelf the day after attending the third level of emotional release workshops with John Lee. The workshop was located on Long Island, and I walked on the beach during the lunch break. I felt the wind blow my hair onto my lips as I thought of Adam, a 6'4" curly-black-haired 40-year-old man that I'd met during the workshop. I picked up several colored stones, looking for one in the shape of a heart that I might give to Adam. I thought of my life as one of those stones, constantly becoming smoother with the tears of the ocean pouring over and through me. I will finally become a grain of sand, soft to the feet, soaking up the sun as a bed for others to lie on, sit on, viewing and knowing the horizon to BE like the endless life of my spirit.

Before our next session, I threw the heart-shaped stone to Adam, who returned my smile, and that evening we talked a long time about our lives before I suggested a walk on the beach under a full moon. It was as easy as the moon shining for us to share our experiences and interests, and for Adam to take me into his arms for a heart-to-heart dance much like the tango. I felt the courage of his openness spring love into my heart for him, as he pushed his large hand as if a glove around mine. Palm to palm. It was a cool, late November evening, the breeze leaning my body into his as he opened his coat for me to feel his warm strong body. When we arrived back at the retreat center, Adam said that he wanted to kiss me, but couldn't because of having a girlfriend with whom he was presently trying to work out his discontents.

In the closing circle, where we looked into each other's eyes, slowly moving person to person, I had only a few tears before I reached Adam. Into his eyes my tears spun as if an unstoppable force that hugged him and made me whisper, "I love you" into his ear. I surprised myself, and probably him. I am now aware of how I am no longer afraid to say the words that name what I am feeling in the moment, unlike when I was growing up, unable to say "I love you" to my father although I felt it, only able to write it on paper.

Adam told me that he falls in love easily and wants to slow that down. When I reflected on whether that was true of me, I realized that I fall in love less and less easily as far as to whom I could be attracted to, but I fall easily when I find the person to BE deeply connected with body-mind-heart-spirit. Real Love is not easy, but draws me like a magnetic rainbow, each of us at either end of the rainbow's arch.

Adam said more than once how attractive my "lightness" is, that I love life and it shows. I talked with Adam a couple of times on the phone, and have not seen him since, yet we truly shared some love, and for that I am grateful. So when I made love with myself the next day, my body felt very alive; touching my nipples intensified my aliveness three-fold. Approaching orgasm, I visualized Ben and Adam making love with me, Adam kissing my lips and touching my nipples while Ben kissed my clitoris, entering me as I climaxed. Kissing, holding, touching, and being entered all at once. It felt intense as a lit-up firefly in the darkest of nights, as my thoughts ushered in my parents giving me all the love that I needed. So that is why a threesome has seemed so appealing to me. Mom, Dad, and Me.

My orgasm came with only an "Oh god." Is that becoming more purely me? "God in me?" A beautiful building cathedral full of orgasmic spiritual ecstasy?

Like me flying over the railroad tie that sits along my driveway, when I arrived home in the dark from the workshop? My hands full of suitcase, backpack, and knitting somehow fell gracefully, most of my impact landed on my right lower thigh; my arms and hands flew outward (like an angel?) sliding onto the grass. All I remember saying was "Oh shit," thinking I'll be bruised when Ben comes to visit, and then glad because I felt the "lightness" of my fall: the beauty of my body being able to fly and not be broken or in pain, feeling joy that my body is flexible, graceful and healing of itself. Again, like a child does many times, falls down and gets right back up. I liked the language of FELL to FEEL to FLYING from pain to joy physically and emotionally.

That same week when I looked in the mirror, my attention was drawn to my crooked right collarbone, which I had never noticed before. When I focused on this new body awareness in my weekly crying session, I broke into tears as an image of my mother shaking me trying to get me to shut up appeared. I did not have enough vocabulary to scream, "Stop, you're hurting me." Sobs roared for minutes, as I understood again why I did not want to take care of my dying mother because I never had a mother who loved me. So, I cry for the loss of not having my mother's love.

And I cry for the loss through death of the father who loved me. Two sides of a picture: the positive and negative within loss. Either way I end up feeling incredibly grateful for my tears. They are the seam that mends all the losses of one's heart, into a flying spirit of LOVE. This mended spirit made it possible for me to say "I love you" to three men within twenty-four hours. Bob, Ben, Adam. And, I do not say those words lightly. It was the difference that Adam felt between "being loving, and being loved." Each man had said, "I love you," to me as well, and Adam and Ben had never made love with my body.

It is the importance of the **heart** connection that causes the body to be more attracted because the feelings are deep within, not just lust under the skin. I want to know more about this HEART of MINE, how it is "softer" after crying about my mother abusing me. Along with an acceptance of her imminent death due to cancer, I also found myself looking into her eyes more closely, as if I was searching for a flicker of love from her to inflame mine. There was no s(n)uffer called resentment.

I was surprised when my mother gave me power of attorney instead of my sister, Connie, to whom she says "I love you." She told me that I had more of a business sense, and that she did not like Connie telling her what is wrong with her, and not trusting her medical choices. I noticed how I wanted to visit my mother, not because I <u>felt</u> obligated. I even brought her a single coral rose because I <u>felt</u> love for her.

Age, distance, and other relationships all contributed to Adam and Ben's exiting from my life, which I understood completely. Pain grows more joy as usual. In one of my last conversations with Ben, I cried, and then as I wrote "home" instead of "him" in my journal. How unconscious are our connections to our true heart…home. My tears came again as I said that my "vulnerability" is the key to my strength of spirit.

These changes provided room for Ted, a sixty-two-year-old man from the HAI workshop to engage in a relationship with me. He also lived in Boston, as did Ben, but had the resources, like a car, to pursue a relationship with me. I wasn't strongly attracted physically, but liked his person: open and willing to grow emotionally, and with initiative.

The next morning when I masturbated-loved myself, I was surprised to engage in a second orgasm about ten to fifteen minutes after my first. I said, "Oh god" and "I want you inside me," with a few thoughts of Ben. Then, the thought "I want you (god) inside me." Shivers traveled down my legs.

The god-divinity enabled me to write an essay called "Cleaning Up," which I read to my mother while visiting her at the hospital while my sister was present. I was a bit apprehensive to read the part about my mother not wanting me, which she disputed by saying she did not want to be pregnant. Then, I was brave to say, "Yes, but I am also the child that you cannot tell "I love you." No response. I read on about my sweet memories that revealed her love for me, even in its limited way. Like the distinction Adam made between loving and BEing loved. Maybe that limited love will have to DO?

"Even the things that hurt are good," swiveled tears from my eyes as I heard those words from the movie, "Tell Me Something You Remember." Then tears as the line, "**You showed me my own heart**" made me remember Daddy, and be glad that I drink tears of the sweet flavor of the love he had for me. Each tear is like watering my love for him; this Love grows and grows.

As Connie and I walked out of the hospital nothing was said about my essay, and I wondered how she felt, but did not ask until a week later on the phone. She had mixed feelings because the first part was painful, and the last part was very positive and loving. She added that mom cannot say "I love you" to me because she cannot forgive herself, making her religion "empty." Because Connie is a "born-again-christian" like my mother, I was surprised by her admittance that my mother's religion was not real, and I told her that religion has brought me great pain. A true barrier to my true spirit.

Once again, I asked Connie how she could believe in an exclusive religion and how can that be spiritual? Connie asked how do I have a relationship with god. Spirituality is inclusive because we are all born with the divine capacity to unconditionally love. My relationship with god is fostered by rescuing the innocent child of god that I was born to BE. My god-given-tears wash away the anger and childhood pain that creates the separation from "god" or divinity, as I would like to call it. (The Design of the Universe) I even quoted a bible verse, "Let the little children come unto me, for of such is the kingdom of god."

I also nurture my relationship to my creator by hiking in nature. Connie had no response. It felt powerful and real and of love as I spoke my truth to her. As did the insight I had while telling her why I was scared to sing a solo with the Mainly Motown group. I was afraid to be seen by the audience, as well as to be heard with my voice, because we had not been allowed to be SEEN or HEARD as a child in the truest sense of those words. The words that express our own feelings.

Like the tears that appeared in telling the above story to Ted, as I said, I didn't have a "voice" of my own, or couldn't be seen for "who I am" and "was scared" to have my own voice. Stronger tears flowed as I said, "Religion has pained me a lot!"

"God damn it" flew out of my mouth as I slipped on my apartment's last two stairs: falling on my coccyx, grabbing Erin's orange tree, breaking off a limb. God damn the pain and suffering? And thank you "god" for the "in love" feeling as Ted asked if it was possible for me to fall "in love" with him. I had to say "no" because I did not possess enough chemistry with him, yet believed I wanted a great friendship. We appreciated the great level of honesty and openness between us.

"As the well of pain becomes shallower, the well of love becomes deeper," I said to Ted with ample tears of truth unknown until this past decade. Ted cried once with me after our appetizer to lovemaking, naked, holding each other. He said, "I haven't been *held* like this since Nancy," his wife of thirty years who had died of cancer nine years earlier. He had been married since for close to three years, now divorced.

My tears continue to hold the key to ushering myself back home to the REAL ME, as sobs underlined those two words in my weekly crying session. I wondered about my need for the comfort of a man in my life, the caring, the love…then thought, this is the way I find and know my Self most profoundly. Through intimate relationships, by following my heart's lead, my tears come up to lay a trail that leads me HOME. "Through my tears I'm bringing myself back home," stimulated a waterfall of tears, bringing home my true spirit of Love.

A Love that would withstand a shocking response from my admirer-dancer-once-lover Bob who had moved to Florida. I told Bob that I had a negative AIDS test result, and he asked me to send a printed copy of the results to give to Sally. I asked, "Don't you believe me?" He said he did, but needed to reassure Sally. I told him that I did not receive any paper proof when told the results, and that Sally should believe and trust him. I related that I felt hurt that he did not believe me because he insisted on paper proof. What a farce that made of all the times he had lauded me for being so open and HONEST. I told him that I felt disrespected and no longer needed to prove to anyone my honesty and trustworthiness. I ended our phone conversation in calm tears without asking for an apology, although I knew I deserved one. But, I also knew that it was his pain of distrust that had been triggered, and that he needed to grieve those feelings for himself. That is a wonderful freedom, to not take his distrust personally.

Still, I was shocked when I received an email from Bob telling me not to email or call him anymore. A year later, I did email him, and received a response that he was open to talking with me☺

Whereas I took the initiative to become involved with Bob, Ted took it with me. One of the exercises he asked of us was to tell about several of our most outstanding orgasms, alternating turns. Before telling of each experience we took one piece of clothing off of the other. It was a very creative mode to develop intimacy over time. I was tickled by what I remembered, some of which I have written in this text. Then, we told of outstanding romantic times, one surprised me. It was a handsome man named Steve who approached me in the P&C grocery store, with his two-year-old son in his arms. He wanted to photograph me, and more.

After I made a tofu stir-fry for dinner, we found ourselves kissing, Ted forgoing the French kisses that do not turn me on. He loved me well with his lips on my clitoris, and enjoyed my lips over and around his penis, and groaned to my light touch over his balls. I ended up having an orgasm my favorite way, with his penis between my labial lips as I move-love over him. He was very patient and caressing of my nipples as I had several waves of pleasure before exclaiming "Oh god." His orgasm came with intercourse and "Oh honey, oh baby." It was sweet but not passionate for me, as I felt it was for him.

Because he snored, I moved into my bed, and left Ted sleeping on the futon where we had made love of some kind. I was glad not to have him in my bed to make love, because I want to feel "in love" or moving toward that if we make love in MY bed. Another symbol of coming closer to intimate real love. Still, I was glad to have this loving experience.

Later, Ted told me how different I am to move up to his face during oral-penis loving, to kiss him, and to look into his eyes before and near orgasm. I want that soul-to-soul, or spirit-to-spirit-connection. That full awareness of Love (desired) between us.

That same week, I noticed a little sign on top of my microwave saying that the clear plastic covering needs to be removed to have the finish truly seen. I had owned this microwave for ten years and not noticed to uncover the veneer. Just like not seeing my true Self for most of my life.

Like not seeing how deeply the need for holding-love exists as my tears spoke while I watched a TV movie called "Angel Eyes," when two people were hugging and saying, "I love you." Just like Ted had remarked about not being held *like this* since his first wife died. It is one reason why I am interested in exploring and reading *Tantra, The Art of Conscious Loving*. And maybe why Ted emailed me that "I have been drawn to you and fascinated by you since I laid eyes on you last month. I sensed your aura, your spirituality. It is about getting to know who you really are…how beautifully and authentically you express yourself in writing and how open you are to true intimacy and love and to new experiences, which we have been denied because of many years and layers of 'shoulds' and 'should nots.' I know that honesty is at the heart of it."

Yes, it is the honest feelings of love and care for my mother that I deeply craved, not just the obligated love. I could genuinely water her plants for her, showing I loved her despite her lack of love for me. It felt like more than caring for my physical needs as my mother did for me as a child, because I could tell her the occasional "I love you" from a small corner of my heart. I wished there was more love for her as I looked steadfastly into her eyes while she laid in her hospital bed, knowing that she'd be gone soon and that I'd cry as hard as a cloudburst.

I noticed the faded stars on my new journal pages and thought about how my father has been the brightest star in my life. How all the other men in my life have faded unless I have been "in love" with them, where a strong love-connection is like a shooting star with a long tale. Unlike the tale I was told by a doctor that I had met through the local paper's personal ads in late December 2001. Hosea had told me that he was a family practitioner, not the psychiatrist that he really was. When I told him that he had set the foundation of distrust, he tried to defend himself, stumbling, finally admitting that he was embarrassed to tell me, and that he did not know why. He said that he had made a mistake and had learned his lesson. In our next phone conversation, I learned that he was married, another lie uncovered. He said he was looking into himself, and knew he was on the "spiritual ride" that I had advertised in my personal ad.

I tell about Hosea to demonstrate that even though one might be in the psychological business, that one can be unaware spiritually of their own feelings of fears and hurts, which made Hosea hide in lies to me. Again, I was glad to be sobbing in my weekly crying session about my mission to disarm religion's wall to being who we really ARE, open and trusting of one's own birthright feelings. "Open up the way to god – look inside — you were born with god's love within you," poured out sobs - sobs of grief for not having that spiritual awareness for most of my life.

That truth became abundantly clear when I said, "I never felt like taking my life but my life was taken from me in a spiritual sense…a spiritual suicide…I had to give up my Self." Sobs ushered those quoted words, "spiritual suicide" that I had never said or thought before, ever.

Oh god, oh god is right! Where were you when I needed you? The answer I guess is that you gave me my dad, and there is no way I can thank you enough, except to show you my tears, to shed the pearls of god." (Notice that the word shed has 'she' and 'he' in it☺)

The next day when I self-loved on my back, I created a beautiful orgasm while saying "Come into me," which did not refer to anyone in particular. Although I briefly thought of Ben, I thought of the spirit of god-love coming into me as I orgasmed! Still, I wanted that experience with a man I love.

Like Christian, my ex-boyfriend from 1983-84, with whom I still keep in contact. At the end of a long phone call near Christmas, I said, "I love you, I always will love you." He did not return those words, but wished me a happy holiday. I was okay with it even though I was a bit disappointed not to hear "I love you" in return. I liked a lot that feelings are more spontaneous, and are markedly more so with love as I clear away my past hurts.

I surprised myself again when I left my friend, Adriana off at the airport, and hugged her good bye that "I love you" flew out of my lips. It was not the kind of close relationship where I generally say, "I love you." I concluded, as I love my Self more, I am more generous with love.

And I liked that Ted had emailed me that he had never had such a sexual, intimate, emotional, spiritual connection before me. He meant all those characteristics at once. And, Ted has had no trouble attracting women with whom to make love.

As the winter equinox passed, the sky was full of radiance, the skies illuminated by coral streaks, which turned the hills indigo. Again, the days began to be longer, the upswing of life which I adore. No longer in the black and white thinking of religion, I am able to ring and sing for the Salvation Army kettles because I know that they give to the needy. I sing, "Deck the Halls with Boughs of Holly" and "Jingle Bells" and "White Christmas." I do not wear the christian label, only the giving spirit of christmas.

My heart is leading me where I need to go. Sometimes, it seems a bit confusing separating the old pain from the new healed parts of Me. Yet, underneath it all, I feel increasing trust of the human spirit to carry me along to where I need to be at any given moment, even in the moments of once or twice weekly sexual-self-loving, where my latest sweet '"Oh god" orgasm melded with images of lover, nature, even my children appeared.

My trust is reinforced by Kiersten's simple comment to her sister Katie, that when she saw me at the weekly swing dance, I was the only one who looked like I was having fun. The others were so serious. Yes, I am smiling now☺

Yes, I will "follow my heart" that floods with tears as I said, with Susanne next to me each week writing down my tear-stained words, "my dad saved my life, I feel that right now in the middle of my chest. My father really loved me, I really felt that," and I continued to cry without words.

I feel the tears appearing even now as I write "the loss of my father is a huge thing, because knowing that my father loved me is partly why I will not settle…I have to carry the torch…the light of Love." The light that showed me the car clock reading 3:33PM, as I spent the last weekend of 2001 alone.

When I awoke that weekend I was not sexually aroused, which had been more and more often the case. I laid in bed many minutes, thinking, enjoying the view of the long green untainted valley, when it eventually felt right to give my Self some loving. The "light" touch all over my labia mixed with vaginal juices that increased as I enjoyed my clitoral arousal. After ten or fifteen minutes I am looking for orgasm, enjoying the long waves of sensuousness that grab me by the hand. After being on my back, I roll onto my stomach where I orgasm more intensely with oooohs and aaaahhhhhs and no "Oh god" this time. I felt my whole body tingle like a smooth hand running all over my body, tightening into an orgasm of ecstasy, not pitched as high as some, yet still beautiful.

My orgasm was mostly with my Self, although a glimpse of oral loving by a man would have been welcomed. I had thoughts of friends, and hills sprinted by, as if I was connected to the whole universe. I was not sleepy afterwards, sometimes I am. Later that day, I called my friend Mike, and he said that he had been thinking of me just as I called. I asked with a laugh what he was thinking. "Of your gracefulness." We had made love once twenty years ago, and were still friends. Is that grace?

"Unmerited divine assistance," says the dictionary.

The same kind of grace given me to be able to help my mother. The grace given me to donate 400 copies of *Everybody Cries* to Head Starts all over the United States. *Everybody Cries* is a children's picture book that I have written and self-published. The grace given me to be able to heal through grace-given tears?

The grace to be able to tell my stepdaughter, Sara "I love you" without hearing it back. The grace to be able to know that grieving is a natural way to live in order to heal loss and hurt. To be able to accept tears whenever they come, like during the video "Falling in Love" when the couple looked into each other's eyes and held each other. The basic needs of being **held** and being **seen** are now known as basic essences of Love. The flowering spiritual journey experience of Real Love.

Sometimes I wonder about grace as this "unmerited divine assistance." Is it the same grace I felt when Richard (with whom I went to the 2001 New Year's Eve dance and we have never been sexual) twirled me a dozen consecutive times, still feeling centered, my whole body tingling as I wrote that in my journal? The same grace defined as "approval, favor, charming and attractive, or a short prayer of thankfulness, or a musical trill, or quality of thoughtfulness and consideration?" I have been most aware of grace when I am dancing, the uninhibited flow of beauty between body and music. It is my spirit exemplifying freedom, which is the closest to divine love as I can express it in words. Fear is no longer in my consciousness. But now, I am most aware of grace when I have tears that connect with my deepest heart pain, because I evolve into truly **feeling** free to be compassionate, not because I am telling myself to be. Tears connected to their painfull source are like spring showers that give roots a chance to grow into blossoms.

Still, is our reincarnation led by our spirit's destiny and drive to be whole, which means becoming divinely loving? Is our journey really "unmerited?" Or is this the religious twist that we have laid on our EVOLution? Grace just might be the "race" to the big "G" that we name "god" or divinity.

I am very grateful that my body is able to dance and dip without feeling aches and pains. And also that my dancing clitoris did an amazing performance as I awoke the morning of New Year's 2002, not feeling aroused. I opened my eyes with the sun rising, and slowly my fingers caressed the top of my vagina, along my labia, up and around my clitoris, creating intense waves of plea-sure. It was one of those orgasms that builds and builds and you *know* it will not diminish. The feelings became more and more intense, like a full moon on a clear night, so big and bright! When I climaxed I was exclaiming, "Oh god, yes, oh god, yes" at least six times. At its peak, I emphatically said, "It's exquisite!" A diamond-like glitter throughout my body. It made me feel like the ocean waves, big and over-whelming, breaking only as they hit the land…of my heart! As I laid in my glow, I found my Self noticing the three 8x10 framed photos on the wall that face me as I lay in my bed. When I had hung them six months earlier, I had only thought of them as pictures of duos, not what I became conscious of while staring at them.

The portrait of my mother and father on their wedding day is the only photo of the three whose eyes I can look into, especially my father's, which watered my eyes, realizing once again his love for me, and the sadness that it had been con-strained. The second photo was of my Grammy Alice holding her firstborn on her lap, and the third photo was of my daughter Megan at age 3, standing above me, holding her hands on my face. All three are the primary loves of my life! How wonderful to notice. Unconsciously I had placed them together, to face me, and I could see the Child in us all. I could not help but recognize the relationship of vulnerability to love, as the same to tears. We cry only when we lose love, or are in physical pain. The loss of our wholeness, either way. My clitoris vibrated as I wrote those last words, and I felt alive as a squirrel jumping from branch to branch, in the openness of my orgasm and tears, which lead me once again to more awareness.

When I picked up my mother from her temporary two-week stay at Oak Hill Nursing Home, she asked me to take her out for pizza, and to pick up some med-ications and groceries. While at Pizza Hut, I asked her if she remembered any-thing about me before I turned one-year-old. With a defensive tone, she said I was probably jealous of Connie, as she was born three days after my first birth-day. She continued by telling me that it was out of fashion to blame parents. I replied that I was not asking questions in order to blame, but to know what's happened to me. I did not want to upset my mother while eating, but she kept the conversation going by saying that Connie and Eric grew up in the same envi-ronment and weren't treated differently than me. I protested by saying that my beginnings were different and "you cannot tell me 'I love you.'"

"I used to like you better before you wrote that I brainwashed you," mom countered with tears.

"I said many good things about you in the book too," I replied gently.

"And you dedicated the book to your father, as if he loved you more."

"He did, mom, he wrote, 'I love you' to me many times and you never did."
No response.

"And you say you are supposed to forgive in your religious belief, if I did do something that hurts you," I added.

We managed to remain in a loving space, enjoying the meal, as I looked into my mother's eyes, fading to life. I reiterated, "I've been able to say 'I love you, mom' genuinely because of all the tears of hurt I've cried out."

I didn't feel tears when I said those words as I do now, but felt good about our sharing, being calm, yet full of feeling the importance of this conversation.

I would <u>press</u> my mother to love me☺

When I left mom off at her apartment, she became very appreciative, saying, "You're a sweet girl." (more tears)

"I know I am, you have borne and raised good kids!"

And why am I crying now? Because there is a huge loss of knowing that I was and am a GOOD kid. My mother's religion saw to it that I believed I was a sinner and unworthy of god's love. I did not feel I was a good kid.

I continued to masturbate once or twice weekly even though I would awaken not aroused. One January morn I turned onto my stomach as I feel the intensity of pleasure build faster than when I am on my back. I let it build without slowing it down and a rich orgasm flowed with "Oh god" said a couple of times quietly. I spontaneously visualized a dolphin on an ocean wave as I had that yummy wave of orgasm. A dolphin is a symbol of psychic awareness, and I have been drawn to these animals for many years, even swimming with them in 1989 and 2000. Interestingly, Megan gave me a small dolphin made of amethyst, to which some authors attribute qualities of healing, lifting depression, and enhancing spirituality.

And spirituality, for me, is listening to the god-voice inside us all that was easy to hear and be seen at our birth. As has been portrayed in this book, our parent's lack of awareness to feelings, brainwashed beliefs and cultural expectations have corrupted and buried that spiritual voice, which I have found to be awakening by tears washing away those denials to our spiritual voice. When I returned from California in 1997, I found myself alone in silence and enjoyed it even though I have always loved music. Without music playing, I was able to hear my spirit's voice more clearly. It has been very recently in 2002 that I began to play music while at home. All along, I have played music in my car and danced to music, but my home time has been stillness, with the quiet to hear spirit. Not only could I hear the birds sing, but also my heart's feelings. They have led me to my true inner spiritual home.

It was in early January 2002 that I not only continued to check the clock at synchronous times such as 4:44pm, 8:08am or 12:12am, but also developed an ankle injury while running. I had been conscious for a few years that I would at sometime put away my running, even though I was running slowly three days per week for 30-40 minutes, usually on soft-earth trails. There is excessive pressure on the joints that feels unhealthy. Walking briskly and dancing are much more beneficial to the muscles of the legs and heart. It has been a constant theme in my life to slow down, and not run away from my Self, my shadow emotional-spiritual pain.

I am no longer running physically or spiritually. For this, I am smiling at this moment.

Nor, am I running from my mother, who was once again in the emergency room for excruciating back pain. I picked her up from the hospital and took her to another supervised living facility, filled her sleeping med prescription, delivered her walker and clean underwear, along with Depends because she was regularly unable to control her elimination.

When I next spoke with my sister, she told me that mom had begged her to let her come live with her. Connie refused, saying, "I just can't." Their "born-again-christian" bond was crumbling before my very eyes, and I understood. Their religion did not carry enough love to dispel Connie's childhood care taking hurt and resentments toward mom. I understood mom's feelings of aloneness, and fear, and found myself explaining them to Connie and Eric.

My brother, Eric, is a successful architect who lives in Washington DC. On the phone he tried to quiet his fears and resentments toward mom by laughing boisterously as he told me that his fantasy was that mom would have to tell dad she's sorry that she treated him so badly before she could come to live with Eric. (Dad being dead 25 years). So, mom had three children who cared about her, but did not love her very much. It was sad to see us siblings bonding in this way. Still, I was glad that I could see the child in my mother, looking me in the eyes and me looking back, wishing there was more love between us. I could only feel this because I have been rescuing the child in me with my child-connected-to-the-past-hurt-tears, which liberate my loving spirit.

Even reliving past life hurts through the present pain in my left ankle, made it possible to remember more of who I really am. My new ankle injury triggered me to cry again about losing my ability to dance in a past life professional performance, where I fell and broke my ankle; I sobbed intensely, and felt more present pain in my ankle for those few minutes. Being in that memory, I was able to grieve about my mother not allowing me to dance while growing up and then confidently say, "Don't ever let anybody take that away from you." As you have read, I had not been permitted to be mySelf in many ways. Therefore, many tears are needed to heal my spirit. Therefore, the importance of remembering!

Pain can truly be a healer. An opportunity to heal. By not running away from your pain through religion, by not letting an outside god take care of it, you are able to find the "god" inside you. It is again why I trust the spirit's "falling in love feeling." "In Love" led me to find Gregory, my fourth husband, who triggered me to regress back to acting like the child-spirit I truly am. It is why I cried when I said to Ted, "one must regress in order to progress." Tears added, "Falling in love has opened my heart for the healing of my pain!"

And now I can hear the little voice inside me becoming louder, because there is less pain from what I have been taught to block out. It is like a dictatorial regime has fallen, and my heart's court is being rebuilt. Like when I talk with my sister about my mother's choice to die. My religious sister told me that it's "playing god" to commit suicide by not eating or drinking. I replied that it's "playing god" to insist on medicines, intravenous or tube feedings, which is not the natural way to die when one is old and can no longer take care of oneself, or contribute to life. I began to cry as I told her that being able to listen to the little voice inside us is what guides us as to what is best for ourselves. To choose to listen to that piece of god within is divine.

As are my orgasms. Ted later told me after we had made love that it is "rare" to see a woman so fully woman, allowing orgasm as I did, and enjoying the longevity of the build up. And I feel especially full of love when I can have my eyes open during orgasm, as vulnerable as a child. It is the same fullness of love that I feel as I gaze longingly and steadfastly into the eyes of my granddaughters with longevity. There is no fear, no need to look away.

A year ago, when I picked up the 8x10 photo of dad, me and my two daughters, and looked only at him, I cried, as I cry now, for our loss of ability to look into each others' eyes to truly see one another. It is sad, and why the eye connection with orgasm is so important.

And why I began connecting more and more with images of dolphins and nature when I masturbated. And why with the **light**est of touch I would reel with electricity into an, "Oh god oh god" orgasm! Incredibly delicious for many seconds, a build up like a rocket off a launching pad. Or a sustained knowing of pleasure that would have to be *exquisite* at its climax! It is hard to think of anything comparable even after several minutes of contemplation. I can't. I look up exquisite in the dictionary. "Deep *sensitivity* or *subtle* understanding." Why sexuality at its best is the vision of our spirituality at its best. Full of loving pleasure. Full of happiness. Bliss. Feeling the orgasm of the divine universe. Making Real Love.

Maybe that's why now I need to eat fewer sweets, am satisfied with a small bowl of "Death by Chocolate" ice cream every evening. When I buy a large chocolate chip cookie at the Ithaca Bakery, most often I can only eat one half of it, the remaining half I eat the next day.

I ask myself why I have certain physical symptoms, like dried yellowish discharge in my nose when I awaken in the morning. It never develops into a cold or any other illness; it is just there. I ask my body "why" when I have my weekly crying session. A memory came up of my mother holding me down in the bathtub when I was very young. My head went under water, as I pushed my elbows down against the bottom (I'd had itchy elbows that week), and water went down my nose. I sobbed loudly as my memory saw her push me down under the water again. Mom was saying, "See, I'll get you back for even existing. You are the one who got me into this predicament."

No wonder I never wanted to be near my mother; I always walked a few steps ahead of her because she had hurt me badly. Now I knew why I enjoyed a conscious memory of wrestling on the front lawn with my mother when I was eleven or twelve, straddling her waist, holding her arms down and reveling in the power I had over her, although it was a "friendly-playful" event.

Many of my crying sessions evolve to tears of missing my father and being grateful for the love and protection he was able to give me. In January 2002, I made a commitment to visit my father's grave every month, because my tears had led me to feeling greater appreciation for him, and therefore a desire to honor him with special time of remembrance, a time to express my deepest feelings for him, my love which has grown deeper for him, and had gone unexpressed for several years of not visiting his grave, or honoring his great importance in my life.

Right on the heels of one of the above sessions, the next day, was remarkable! I was awakened a few minutes after seven by a phone call from the Lakeside Nursing home, telling me that mom had been taken to the hospital because she felt like fainting. I knew my mother had been having panic attacks in the past month, but the emergency room nurse told me that mom was in atrial fibrillation, a fast irregular pulse. She was transferred to the ICU after I spoke with her on the phone in the emergency room. Before I hung up, I spontaneously said, "I love you mom." Even without her false teeth, I heard mom's clear reply: "I love you too!"

Immediately, I began to cry, really sobbing, because I heard what I had never heard before, for fifty years! I wondered if she thought she might die. Still, it felt spontaneous and sincere. Now, all I needed was to hear her say those words to my face, into my eyes.

When I told Connie, she said, good for both of you. When I told Eric, he quickly quipped, "She must be hallucinating." I replied in earnest, "That's not funny!" He was not taking me seriously…that *is*, my feelings. That is, what Me *is*! Feelings are the source of who we really are. Feelings usher in our true spirit of Love, when our hurts are grieved through the washing of tears.

Alas, joy came out of my mother being in pain. And, Love came out of me grieving my pain of lost mother-love. And Love *is* a feeling. The greatest feeling of all because it brings personal peace, then peace to the world. Isn't this the spiritual journey?

That miracle day when my mother spoke those three magic words to me, I talked with my oldest daughter, Erin, and when I said goodbye, she said, "I love you," first. Before I did. Erin's verbal initiative was a first as well☺

That same twenty-four hours provided a third gift when I visited my mother in the ICU, with her teeth and purse in hand. Eventually, I asked her if she remembered what she had said to me on the phone that morning. She readily answered, "that I love you."

Yes! I was surprised that she remembered without hesitation.

"That meant a lot to me," as my tears slid and dropped in front of her pale face.

"That's good you cried." I was astounded again; this is my mother who is usually ashamed of her tears, and I replied, "why?"

"Because it's real." I was so dumbfounded; disbelief caused me to be speechless. I was mute as a pleased smile during sleep. I was a full heart, a full flush, a full daughter.

The next day I ventured into scary territory by calling Gregory at his mother's house in Oxford, New York, where he was visiting from California for a few weeks while his daughter was on college break. I wanted him to know that my mother was in the hospital, as well as how he was. My mother was the only one he had continued to communicate with in my family, telling her not to tell me he called. I knew he was not working and on anti-depressants, and still very distrusting.

Again, the Design of the Universe had timed my call so that Gregory answered, which normally, if his parents had been at home, would not have happened. Gregory was forced to speak with me, and it was indeed good to hear his voice. We had not spoken for about two years although I had called and left messages, or written on certain holidays. He shared a close conversation that he had had with his brother a couple days before, which he felt to be very special. He said he wished that we could be friends, but that he had "too much on his plate" just then.

"I am ready to be friends and understand that you are not," I said in a calm, understanding tone.

"Are you taping this conversation?" Gregory asks.

"I don't have the equipment, nor the interest in doing that," with sadness in my heart to hear his distrust. I went on to tell him about Erin and mom telling me "I love you."

"I wish I could share that more intimately with you. One of my fondest memories is seeing you in the rocking chair at Burlington Flats, seeing us getting old together."

"Yes, I remember that sweet moment too. I still tell my friends and family that I love you and always will."

Silence.

"This is all I can manage at the moment, and a call is coming in that I must answer," said Gregory before our good byes. Even though I am still crying now, it felt good not to be afraid and that I was still loving him. And, of course feeling this meant I was loving mySelf, and that my divine spirit was flying free as water-falls in spring.

If all this newly expressed love was not enough in forty-eight hours; my brother arrived from Washington DC to visit mom in the ICU. When we had dinner that evening, Eric pressed into my eyes, "I give you a lot of credit for taking care of mom, when she has abused you so much!"

"Thanks," I said, as I felt my heart tingle with goodness. "I have to attribute it to all the tears I have shed, and I truly feel no resentment toward her."

The next day while Eric and I visited mom, I asked her about her feelings about dying.

"I want to. I will be better off in heaven, and you know you will go to hell if you don't believe," mom stated despite her being in and out of confusion due to low oxygen levels.

Eric and Connie continued to encourage mom to get better, wanting her to hang onto life. To live in a nursing home? I asked Eric if he had said everything he needed to say to her before she dies. He told me how he'd like her to acknowl-edge how she has caused so many problems for dad, and us kids. He emphasized how her hostility separates him from her.

I noticed how Eric kissed her on the forehead before leaving, and that I kissed her on the mouth, as she held her mouth that way for me. I hugged her and could see she was ready to cry, holding tears back I believe, because Eric had told her not to cry with him. He said that he felt "taken advantage of" when mom cried every time she talked with him. I pointed out again that it is his pain from his childhood that she triggers. I stopped there, aware that Eric needed to take tiny steps into his awareness of his own vulnerability. I could feel Eric's desire to love me for who I really am, by appreciating my lovingness.

When I talked about missing dad, I began to cry, and held some back, because I knew Eric was not ready to be with my tears as yet. I mean hold me and let me cry. Still, love was melting as I spoon-fed him ice cream from my bowl.

Eric did not want to stay and dance with me, and I found myself thinking that I needed to be able to play because I was brought up in such a serious belief system, which dampened my spirit.

I needed to be free to have fun, balance my life, because it was too easy for me to compare my life to full-time givers like Ghandi or Mother Teresa.

Sometimes I've thought that I am too self-absorbed, then immediately feel pleased because I see how all my centering on my Self has resulted in my own healing, which I share with the world in my books, and in my countenance. I may be a dim candle in the light of Martin Luther King Jr., but I know my tears and those of others will shine Love. When I saw a psychic in April 2003, my tears lit up my spirit when she told me that I gave much more love than I receive.

My mission in life is to move the raw anger of grief into its sadness, so we can begin to truly Love. Then, wars will cease. Spell *war* backwards and you will have the *raw* feelings of rage/anger (add one letter to rage and you have anger) that are covering up the vulnerable feelings of h<u>urt</u> (<u>you</u> <u>are</u> hurt) from not being unconditionally loved. The same hurt-sadness that rushed to my eyes as I spoke to the Medicaid worker who would determine the amount of money they would pay for mom's nursing home stay. I was surprised that tears appeared as I told him about my mother being a veteran, serving as an army nurse in England and Germany, and how brave she was. How good it FELT to cry tears of pride in my mother, and simultaneous tears of sadness because it had taken me fifty years to finally love my mother, and simultaneously my Self! Of course! I can feel (sorry) compassion for my mother and my Self all at on(c)e – part of the beauty of my tearful spiritual retrieval of my heart-soul.

The tear rolls down my cheek like I roll from man to man, to find the man who can wholly love me. The mirror of Me loving my Self. Like my continued weekly self-loving on awakening from sleep when not aroused sexually. Yet, I feel the need to love myself with physical pleasure, like a walk in the park. This particular time I rolled from my back to my stomach, the position easiest to create an intense orgasm. The build-ups were continuing to have fuller pleasurable feelings, not insistent on coming, but enjoying the ride I felt the pleasure throughout my body, the muscles tight in my buttocks, back, neck arched, with vibrations throughout my trunk. Near orgasm and at orgasm I was saying, "Oh god, oh god, oh god." The wide-open wilderness was the only image. Forests, hills, mountains. I was one with the universe still not sure I was feeling it completely. More growth to come☺

Still, in January 2002, I am yelling and sobbing in my crying session, "I will never own up to that sin crap…babies born in original sin…such a bunch of crap! That's the damndest message you could give to anyone. Gotta get that song, *Sweet Child of Mine*. I'm so sad that I am still triggered by Gregory's distrust in me. This childhood pain of religious indoctrination (so I cannot trust my own voice) runs so deep!"

"Dianea, you keep feeling…listening to your Self." Yes. Listen to my HEART. I heard my very small voice as a sophomore in college, but was too afraid to believe in my true nature. Like the rusty orange willows, bursting their color amidst dark skeletons of trees. And my sensitive sadness as I stopped to talk with a neighbor girl walking her dog up the same hill that I was walking. As I said goodbye, I recognized the attention that I had given her I had lacked as a child from my mother. My spirit was now freer and freer to feel, let go and reel in self-love.

Bringing my spirit back home became evident again as I teared up while looking at the cover of the book I was reading, *When Life Calls out to Us*. I noticed Victor and Ellie Frankl were holding hands, which I wished I could have done more with my dad and mom. Or, when looking at my pearl ring that Daddy gave me, not able to remember when or why he gave it to me. Most likely a graduation gift from high school, or was it college? I was so sad that I had an important past memory hidden behind emotional pain.

There is an old Indian saying which expresses my sadness well: "All this struggling to learn, when all we have to do is remember."

If only it was that easy.

Like Erin said, "*Just let it be*," after I said tearfully, "I just want to be more connected to you, I miss you. I wish I had spent more time with you last night." I noticed how much better I felt after crying with Erin on the phone, despite my reticence to do so. Yes, just *let our feelings BE* what they really are! The KEY to the door of Love when the varnish of anger is scraped off, and the natural would of hurt tears can be exposed.

Then, the sensitivity of our spirit is exposed, even as I picked up many woodbugs on paper and carried them outside. Also, many ladybugs picked up off the floor, carried to the outdoors. I cannot bear to kill any of them, which I did years ago with a flash of annoyance. Sensitivity to the preciousness of life is a very good thing. Isn't it Love?

While eating dinner at the Moosewood Restaurant, I told Erin and family about how my sister was tired of being nice when she doesn't feel like being nice. My nine-year-old granddaughter, Denali pipes up, "That's scary," surprising me. I asked why? She replied something like she doesn't <u>feel</u> like being nice. Too many people being at the table made me hesitate to pursue what she meant. I wish I had. Maybe, "too scary" to admit her true feelings, or to show her anger?

I was surprised again while reading my sister's favorite book, *The Shell Seekers*, when I cried with the words "Penelope finding a tightly folded blue envelope in a Chanel #5 box, and surreptitiously putting it in her cardigan's pocket." I connected it with my memory of my father giving me that same gift for Christmas, and not remembering if I had received a note with it. I was sad that we had not taken certain feelings seriously enough. Dad had been so good in writing about his love for me, and I still wished that I had told him how much that meant to me.

And the word "surreptitiously" felt like the way I had to *protect my love* for my father. No wonder I cried. No wonder I was sad. No wonder my spirit was not free.

I had turned my heart away from Daddy when I was sixteen, because I had needed him to come to me, I was too scared. My tears turned to sobs as I said, "I didn't know what to do!" I felt helpless. The most difficult feeling to admit to –

you are most vulnerable when feeling helpless.

Like at birth, for mother and baby, I am giving birth to my repressed and hidden spirit through my tears that open up and soften my heart to Love again. For me, this is the REAL born again spiritual experience.

I AM reconnecting to my true Being, then, I am able to FEEL safe with my deepest feelings.

I was not surprised when I cried while listening to a Letterman CD's words, "the way you LOOK tonight." We could not LOOK into each other's eyes without some fear. And so I was delighted while I was LOOKing at the pictures on the wall at the foot of my bed, when my b*rain* rained in a beautiful connection. The names of my children connected to the names of my parents unconsciously! The "E" for Erin was the "E" for Ellen, my mother. The "M" for Megan was the "M" for Michel, my father! I could see and feel the universal connection of names and music Being Oneness.

"It is not our fault" as children that we have lost our oneness with the divine-god. It is no wonder that my client, Sharon, sobbed as she pressed the words from her mouth, having sore lips from holding back her unspoken feelings, "It's not my fault."

Or that people are afraid to express the vulnerability of "I love you." They show their caution in saying, "Love ya." There is no definite "I." Or "you." Interestingly, I have noticed for years that when I have reread my journals or edit my books that "I" is missing in many sentences where the "I" is needed. The same "I love you" I still needed to hear from my mother face-to-face. And, as the Design of the Universe devised, I found myself reading a large print book to my mother on one of my frequent visits to her nursing home. I had randomly picked a story from "Chicken Soup for the Golden Soul," that I had not known would be telling others "I love you." And, my mother appreciated it☺

Like I appreciated my walk into the gorge behind my apartment, following it for a mile, most of the time three to five feet from the water and its falls. I wandered into the light of its icicle chandeliers, humming with various notes of music, which depended on the height and width of the waterfalls. So many varieties my heart sang. Sometimes, I had to climb twenty to thirty feet above, but I kept the water in view…that was important to me. There was a light dusting of snow on the ground, and it was cold enough not to be muddy, yet I could push my sneakers into the earth. The trees and their roots were my special friends that day as I dragged a piece of driftwood up a steep incline. Each step was slow and well planned. I was proud that my body was limber enough to negotiate sharp-angled twists and turns, and that I could trust tree roots to hold me, like I do the roots of my pain exposed by my tears. Tears are what ground me to the truth of my real Being. Why it is important to be close to (one with) the water.

I am smiling the next day, after my tears, while emailing Megan about us being "one" when I gave birth to her. In her email she had written "The Patriots "**one**" the Superbowl" and she had not intended to! How amazing is the universal mind-heart, soul-spirit! When we are finally ONE in spirit, we have WON☺

LOVE and (into) PEACE.

Realizing the GOOD of GRIEF… "good grief," Charlie Brown.

I must repeat, now that the wax and ache is out of my ears,

"The ability to grieve is one's capacity to Love."

Have you ever noticed that water is only white when it *falls*? I was at Lick Brook waterfall in February 2002, and I had never been here in winter. Although there was no snow on the path, the waterfall was frozen, shaded by trees and the enclosed gorge. The water runs behind the ice and snow, a few windows opening the waterfall's face. Cavernous-like stalagmites and finger-laced curtains of ice create see-through skirts of glass-like delicacy. The falls are wide, unlike summer's slim-waist. White-iced waterfalls stand out in white brilliance against the gorge walls of brown and gray, capped by evergreens. It was nearly 40 degrees, and only the water was white that day. The purity of water frozen and *falling*, opening its heart to tears of pearly white.

It is like "*falling* in love." It is the possibility of pure love. Only when you are vulnerable like when you are *falling*.

I was not pure when I made love again with Ted, because I was not all present. I enjoyed the pleasure of the orgasm, but my eyes were closed and I did not feel enough love to be so closely joined. I am no longer willing to be in pieces, separate from mySelf, although I know that I won't have the whole for a while. My true Love that is. I am in EVOLution.

If I am fully IN love with another, then I'll be fully engaged IN the process to Love my Self.

Ted asked me after we made love if it was okay to tell me "I love you."

"Sure. You can say any feelings. I hoped you knew that. Sorry, I cannot say that back."

"I know that you love me (but it is not the "in love" kind), or I wouldn't be here," Ted replies confidently. I am glad that he knows and feels the difference.

And I am glad that while I was musing in bed, I found myself appreciating the diversity of my furniture: chestnut chest, walnut chest, oak desk and filing cabinet, cherry drop leaf table, mahogany bookcase, pine-topped-oak-legged kitchen harvest table. A diversity that creates ONE home like a diversity of Love that creates ONE heart-spirit.

My heart cried again as I shared with my sister how I had cried during interactions regarding mom at the Veteran's Administration, and at Wagner Funeral Home, when I felt pride about mom's bravery in serving in WWII. But, more special was when I shared with mom how I had cried at those places, and that I was proud of her. She reached for my hand, and we squeezed as she, teary-eyed, replied, "You're a sweetheart for appreciating that." It was one of those rare tender moments between my mother and me. Love. It felt like what sweet redemption should feel like, not the church's redemption from sin by accepting Jesus as your savior.

We had shared tears of lost love redeemed! Like the two Hibiscus blossoms close to each other, when the leaves had wilted due to lack of water, and then within an hour of watering (like tears), the leaves are full of life, strongly connected, growing upward, no longer on the path down to death. I knew I had been crying about my own lack of bravery, the sadness of being fearful to leave the religious prison that my heart had been in; where I experienced a false sense of security. Once again, while loving mySelf, I could love my mother. My heart feels so full at this very moment of writing. I wish I could burst off this page and hug you all!

I told Connie that now I felt that god was a part of me, not "out there." I have cried thousands of tears about my inner child hearing and believing that I was responsible for god not loving me, because I am not *worthy*. No wonder we have no self-*worth*.

Connie told me that she likes her Zoloft, an anti-depressant, and that someday she will get off of it, and face her pain, so that she can really heal. Yes, grief brings relief! It honors those we love, because we begin to honor ourselves as worthwhile human Beings. As I have sobbed in my sessions, saying that dad is the "love of my life," I KNOW (k)now that I am crying about the lost <u>love of my</u> (kn)<u>OWN life</u>, way back in Sunday School. "That's getting really CORE I tell you," I said through my sobs. February 2002 was the <u>first</u> time in my process that I had made, because I FELT, that strong connection between "The **LOVE** of MY LIFE" and the lost "LOVE of **MY** LIFE."

So. I am a lucky woman, even though 13 is my lucky number. On February 13th, 2002, my bill at the post office was $3.13. I just so happened to have sent out 13 copies of *Everybody Cries*, on the 13th as well. And can you believe that at Wegman's grocery that same day, the bill was, guess, $3.13! For bananas and milk, when combined, some say can be anti-depressants.

I wonder why I chose 13 to be my lucky number. Immediately, I think that I am trying to dispel the superstition around that number. Dispelling the fears of the unknown, of ignorance.

Hopefully by now, the reader can feel the happy person I am, as well as my capacity to love growing as I cry out my past emotional hurts. Some may be saying to themselves that my crying seems "excessive" as my daughter Megan emailed me. When we next talked on the phone, I asked her why she thinks I cry so often. She wondered why I cry over and over about the same subjects. I explained how they are core pain (1-unworthiness of god's love from religious teachings, 2-my mother not wanting or loving me, and 3-my dad not coming to me when I found out in a traumatic way that he was not my biological father).

I explained how I like my increased sensitivity to tears because they heal me into being more loving, non-judgmental, and compassionate.

I explained how our culture has not allowed grieving like some others (West Africa, Guatemala, etc.) where those who grieve are considered "sacred." Megan repeated "sacred" as if to deeply take in a deep breath. Why not cry as often as the tears come up, a regular exercise like daily yoga, or shower?

I understand it is difficult to be with a woman who does not "behave" as others wish. But as a bumper sticker says, "Those women who behave do not go down in history." I'd like to think I have some Rosa Parks in me☺

Then again, I was shocked and happy to be the object of a man's affections who was very different from my previous experiences with men. On Valentine's Day, I arrived home from work to a clear vase of eleven white and twelve red roses! The Saturday before I had met up with him in the hallway at Ithaca College, where we were both attending a dance. I had barely said hello to this man, maybe danced once with him. I had forgotten his name.

"Dianea, I want to tell you that 'I love you.'"

"You don't know me," is all I could squeak out. I walked on towards the bathroom in disbelief. Surely my face was flushed. Maybe he was a bit tipsy?

Then, I received an articulate expressive letter the day before Valentine's Day, which in part read, "You may be right in saying I don't know you, but I have looked into your eyes and there are three things I do know: you are beautiful, you are kind, and you are modest. Humbly, Howard."

That same week, Andy, at tango practice said, "You have beautiful eyes." I had been told this only in the last year or two. I relate these two incidents because I believe my eyes are more widely open, more in contact with other's eyes, because of all the deeply-connected crying I have regularly done in recent years.

2002 was the first Valentine's Day that I went to my father's grave, using my shoes to scrape a thin layer of ice and snow from dad's bronze marker. Tears fell as I said, "I don't care what happens to these Italian leather shoes as long as I can see some of your face. Your name." I was surprised to add tears as I said out loud, "There are no clouds in the sky, and I can't see or find you, there's no one there." (tears now) After saying "I love you, want to kiss you and hold you," I placed spruce pine cones on his grave marker in the shape of a heart because they are as natural as is my love for Daddy! Always!

Then I drove to Clark's Summit, Pennsylvania to pick up my granddaughter, Denali, where her mother, my daughter Erin would bring her from Baltimore, so that I could drive Denali back to Ithaca to be with her dad for a visit. Two big loves in my life.

Wasn't that plenty for Valentine's Day?

No, **FEBRUARY 15th WOULD BE THE GREATEST DAY** in 2002!!!!

In fact it was one of the best days of my life! I had gone to Lakeside Nursing Home, to take my mother to a test at the hospital, but it had been cancelled. I spoke with the nutritionist and nurse about mom's care. I hadn't planned to stay but mom and I started talking about arranging her room, and emptying her apartment. I said Connie wanted mom's silverware and mom replied that Connie "lusts" after it. I neutralized her dig by saying that Connie is attached to things that have meaning from her childhood, and found out that mom had ordered it from Germany, which is where dad was born. I was fine with Connie having her silverware, but was a bit wishful for the 1976 vase that she had made and was giving to Eric. And what do I get?

I was about to leave and mom once again appreciated me for all I was doing for her. I, spontaneously, looked into her blue-gray eyes as I sat next to her on her side-railed bed, and said, "I love you, Mom." (tears again) For a brief silence, we looked into each other's eyes, and she replied firmly, "**I love you, too.**" (more tears) All I could do was cry and fall into her arms. I could feel her begin to cry, her arms and hands still resting on the bed, but I consciously held onto her. Within thirty seconds she was holding me and I sobbed like a baby. I was.

When I did loosen my hold and looked at her, she said, "Don't cry."

"Why not, mom? This IS the special moment I have been waiting for, for a long time. And if more people cried, we'd have less anger and hate in the world."

"I don't think I ever heard my mother tell me that she loved me, but I knew she did," mom said, now with an open heart.

"Isn't it sad we can't say it though, express how we feel directly, so that we are not so distant? Or afraid?"

"We just didn't do that in our family, not brought up that way," mom retorted.

I went on to tell her how I didn't hear it from dad either although he wrote it often and, how I told my children everyday. After reading their bedtime stories, and tucking them into bed, I would say, "I love you," and Erin and Megan would say back, "I love you too," and I would rally, "I love you more," to their comeback, "I love you more," then I'd say, "I love you the most," and they'd rally, "I love you the mostest," and I'd reply with a louder voice, "I love you the best," and their come back would be, "I love you the bestest," and then I'd up it to, "I love you the bestest of all," and then "the best in the world, the universe," by the time I was on the last step of the stairs.

"That's nice," mom complied.

Our eyes met again as she added, "**I'm glad you're so sensitive.**" I wept again, bending to my mother's ample chest, my tears landing on her breasts. The milk of Love!

"I'm soft-hearted too," mom assured me.

"Yes, that's something I'm glad you were always able to do, is cry – just sorry you've been ashamed of it!" She kissed me on the lips, something I am not used to, as we said goodbye. Another symbol of closeness to love, like a dove with a tender leaf in its beak.

Later, I wondered why mom was proud of my sensitivity. I never did find out why, but I am very glad that she IS, for sensitivity, I've found, is the soul and spirit of Love!

LOVE long sought after was finally granted to me by my mother's "I love you" on that monumental day of Love's appearance, the day after Valentine's. I received an added bonus when Erin said a solid "I love you too" in response to mine! I will never forget!!! They both felt like they meant it!!

And so did I, not only with them, but also with my Self that Valentine night (actually 2am February 15th☺) when I had a whole body orgasm where I felt my big toe tingling. It was of astounding intensity, remarkable with the sense that more intensity was to come, with many "Oh gods" that knew I was just beginning to FEEL my *whole* body. I was more wholly connected with my body's sensations, images fading.

That same day, when I was in the car with Denali, I asked her what love IS. She replied, "Love is happiness."

"What's that mean? Be more specific, like knowing your dad or mom love you," I insist.

"Mom plays games with me, and takes me to school. Dad takes me on hikes and makes good food. You, come and get me in Clarks Summit, Pa., write poems for and with me, come to Grandparent's Day, and take care of me when mom and dad can't." Then she made a wonderful observation.

"Your purpose is to discover the mysteries of the universe," Denali's wisdom reverberates still within Me. Then, she tried to teach me a Madonna song, "Ray of Light."

That's what I felt like after mom's "I love you" flowed from her lips into my eyes. I immediately hunted up my best friend, Susanne, where she worked and took her out to lunch. She hugged and kissed me with loud exclamations of joy! I called Megan and Erin to share my great news! Could I be happier?

That weekend I expressed my joy at the Dance Flurry in Saratoga Springs, New York, where my past boyfriend, James, or J.T. as he liked to be called, lived nearby. I felt very beautiful, walking and dancing tall, all 5'9" of me. James and I had good conversation at dinner, but when we went to bed late that evening after dancing with many great partners, I did not want to be sexual. It surprised me, because James is a cute guy, in great shape, but then again, I was not "in love" with him. We cuddled and he accepted me turning over, not accepting his erect penis. At breakfast the next morning we did not talk about it, it was not in my consciousness to do so. I noticed that I laughed a lot, and commented, "I'm a happy person." I sensed in his eyes that he was wishing for the same kind of happiness. This experience with J.T. showed me how much I wanted ALL of mySELF to BE in lovemaking.

Just now, I sliced a piece of cantaloupe, glanced at the microwave clock, and guess what the time was: 1:11pm, May 12, 2003.

February 2002 ushered in two men with whom I had met and spent little time. Keith I had met once through a personal ad ten years earlier. He had been practicing Taoist sexuality for more than that decade. Although I was not strongly attracted, I was curious about his "spiritual practice." Within a month's time we were at odds over my view of tears being of sadness, not joy. He said, "you're an unhappy person and jealous of others," which hurt. He hardly knew me.

After we watched the movie "The Royal Tennebaums," he called Mr. Tennebaum a "jerk." We talked about the hate the movie portrayed, and how I don't feel hate or rage any more, and therefore do not even feel like calling people names. That victims and perpetrators, both, get compassion from me – no hate.

When I told Susanne that Keith had said I was an unhappy person, she spontaneously offered, "You're one of the happiest people I know!" I knew Keith and I would be short-lived.

But my emotional pain is not, and surprisingly, I dipped into it deeply during my next phone call to Megan. She was happy to share that Ben had bent down on his knees on the Provincetown ocean shore, near where her dad lives, and asked her to marry him. She cried.

I rained on her parade when I asked about the wedding and how would it be for her when her dad was not speaking to me, although I had emailed him twice without a response. My tears were very mixed, as to what hurt I was feeling. Misunderstood, left out, disrespected, all boiling down to not feeling loved. This time, by Chuck. I explained through my tears how I did not want this tension at her wedding, let alone between me and Chuck whom I will always love.

I understood that Megan does not want to be in the middle and believes Chuck will be friendly. Yes, and still would not talk with me? I had a flash of daddy and my sixteen-year-old experience, how painful it was for both of us <u>not</u> to talk with one another after my mother threw "He's not your father" at me. So, I felt and feel that disconnection, pain, with others I love. Also, I was sad that it always had to be me to take the first step to connect, to express my feelings of hurt. I ended our conversation by saying that I will show love to Chuck no matter how he treats me. I knew and know that I am washing my body's cells of pain, like weekly laundry, crying as I hung up the phone. I knew tears are my medication, not just my meditation.☺

Again, I remembered my mother's words, "I'm glad you are so sensitive." They are the best words she could have said to me, because that is my healing work, to be sensitive to Real Love. That is the spiritual quest. To BE the LOVE of MY life. Then, I can Love others better.

I notice more synchronicities, like the license plate on the back of a white station wagon, "CRYBABIE." I thought I saw it park as I drove by, but could not find it after I parked. I wanted to ask why that plate, as I smiled greatly. Now, I proudly wear "CRYBABE" on my red Jeep's license plate. I am a grown up babe who cries☺ I AM aware of what my tears mean, and their purpose. A feeling of synchronicity like that of 2/20/2002 at 20:02? That was a special day in history that I am told had not happened in 700 years, and will not again for another 110.

I, also, noticed at this time that the blotchiness on my neck has essentially disappeared, which although it has not been distracting for years, its leaving added to the pureness of my skin and substantiated even the subtlest healing by god-given natural tears.

And my deepest tears I wish to engrave on my headstone: "Every CHILD is WORTHY of LOVE." It is the ultimate cruelty to tell a child that they are 'unworthy of god's love.' This is the reason Megan cried when Ben proposed marriage, because she heard the same religious message until she was nine years old. Don't let any religion ever tell you that you are not worthy of divine love, my sobs underline.

It is love I feel while holding my sister after I told her about mom telling me "I love you" and "I'm glad you are so sensitive," those words always stringing pearls of god. I had waited a few days to tell her, while we moved mom's furniture out of her apartment. I hadn't needed to call her the day I heard those three magic words from mom. Maybe I needed to tell her face-to-face, like I'd heard them from mom.

The following day Eric arrived from Washington, D.C. and helped me pack up mom's belongings. First, we went for a run after arising from much-needed good sleep. Although I had virtually given up running in January, it was the activity that most connected my brother and me. I smiled inside and out when I heard his words, "Running in the woods with you makes the trip up here all worthwhile." And my happiness grew many-fold that same day when I came across some pictures I had never seen before while packing up mom's apartment. I shouted to Eric who was wrapping dishes in the kitchen, "Guess what I found? A picture of dad holding me!! I've been looking for one for so long!" I was thrilled, like a child finding a frog jumping across its path.

I am a month or two old, cradled in the crook of dad's right arm, he smiling broadly as I sleep. The picture is only 2x3 inches…but not for long…it is now 5x7 in my living room, and 8x10 in my office - like my heart swelling in size. With Love. When we visited mom later that day, she divided up some of her jewelry, me requesting to have her wedding ring that she had not worn since their divorce in 1968. When I read the inscription, I felt elated. "Forever Yours, S.M.C. 6/8/46," meant that now dad's love was "forever mine" as it circles my right hand's fourth finger. The "forever love" I so needed and that he rooted in me.

Which I no longer need from "just sex" with men. My spirit insists on Love being a part of it! I emailed my friend Ted not to visit on his way to New York City because I did not want the pressure to be sexual. He emailed back that there would be none, and I knew that to be true, still, I would rather masturbate-self-love while lying on my back into luscious bodily sensations, saying "oh my god, it's so beautiful,"…me, life, loving myself! Or while lying on my stomach, my whole body feeling the orgasm, flexing a river of lasting pleasure throughout my perineum. It is apparent that I am growing into the whole of Love. And my sexual drive has not lessened as I have grown older, but now my drive is to more Love.

I am saddened as my best friend Tanya told me that she's "crucifying her spirit" every time she is sexual with her husband, Chuck. She knows that she does not love him. He will not go to therapy. She is staying for their three-year-old son, Lucas, because her mother says she should. She knows she needs to cry out more of her childhood pain so she will know what "god's will" IS.

I wish that my daughters knew this truth deeply so they would not want to tattoo their bodies. Gratefully, they have small ones, and I asked Erin why she had an intertwining-lines design on the center of her back near her waist. She liked what it represented, that everything is connected. And yet her tears are not connected to her childhood pain, so she validates her pain with a tattoo needle. Permanent - like childhood pain's effects on our present, unless we drain those infected wounds, hurts, with tears.

Niki, Erin's partner, admits that Denali triggers her childhood hurts because Denali gets to express feelings and do things that Niki's parents would not allow her. During one of our dinners together, Denali made an angry face at Niki because she did not get the artichoke she wanted, and Niki did because it was the last one in my dish. Niki told her not to make that angry face. Denali defended herself, and that made Niki mad because she did not feel listened to or understood (by her parents.) I tried to referee, listen to both, but they kept interrupting each other. Finally, I said to Denali, "How about saying 'I'm disappointed that I did not get the artichoke' instead of being angry." Then, I asked Niki to say "I'm hurt by that angry look. I wish you'd like me to have it."

It was a classic example of how one defends their hurts with anger, and how our unconscious childhood hurt feelings, not being respected by our parents, causes us to shut down. Parents have not been aware that they needed to listen to children's feelings, because their parents did not listen to their feelings. (Remember the old adage, "Children are to be seen and <u>not heard</u>?") Disastrous to our spirits! Consequently, our spirit begins to die, to feel crushed by those we need Love from, the most, our parents. We learn not to feel vulnerable, it is not safe, so we become angry.

Anger becomes the seed of wars…between parents and children, between lovers, spouses, employers and employees, governments, nations, and most of all within ourselves as we then begin to distrust the divine–spirit we are all born with, within.

It is why I continue to cry in my sessions about wishing I could have cried with my Daddy. Why I sob as I say, "Daddy died of a broken heart." Literally, of a sudden heart attack. I felt twinges around my heart as I cried, feeling my stone-like pain breaking up, making space where Love could rush in. "I love you so, Daddy." And, as a result, I am not as hard on myself.

Therefore, I love mySelf more. And loved that I cried while watching "A Beautiful Mind," now one of my most favorite movies of all time. First, I cried when I heard Russell Crowe say to his students, "Hello, eager young minds." It was as if he was speaking to me, and my sadness was that that eager part of me had been dismissed, so that I could not find my own truth as to what the divine may BE.

Second, my tears flowed like a river when I saw his girlfriend put her hands on Russell's face and heart, saying, "This is REAL," and we will try again tomorrow, meaning to go back to the university and fight off his delusions. All my life, I knew and felt that I had been fighting off the delusions or illusions of my religious upbringing. Also, Gregory's delusions that I was having extra-marital affairs, and that he had seen me at his daughter Sara's high school graduation, when I had not been there! Still, I continue to love Gregory despite what he says or believes about me.

Third, tears appeared during the insulin reaction treatments where Russell's eyes rolled back, and I was back seeing Daddy dead in the morgue.

Fourth, a torrent of tears flooded my face at the end of the movie, when at the end of his career Russell was recognized by his colleagues and received the Nobel prize for math. In his acceptance speech, he said something like: there is no logic **in love** like that of his wife (tears now) and that if not for her, he'd not BE there that day! Of course, I was crying for Daddy. It was so much in his hands…the Love he gave me began my journey to who I AM today. Tears stream down my face as I write this day, May 14th, 2003, but not nearly as loudly as that day in the movie theater where my tender sobs could be heard. And I was proud and happy that I was not ashamed of my "pearls of god."

Like Keith, Jim came back into my life a few years after our initial attraction and short "making out" encounter, while out dancing. He called to make a date to go swimming. I knew he wanted to check me out, quite naked. He taught English and Social Studies at George Junior Republic, a youth-at-risk residential facility. He would sing songs to me as we drove along in his red pick up truck. I loved his long, wavy black hair, and sensuous dancing.

When I walked into his place, I felt duly warned not to rescue this man, whose general messiness and accommodation of huge dust bunnies showed lack of care for himself. We began to watch a video called "Cold Fever," which within minutes became hot fever, as Jim's hands touched my skin, candles burning. He said,

"Let's turn it off and hug and kiss for fifteen minutes." I made it clear that was all I wanted. He agreed. Still, he proceeded to try to pull my clothes off, and I said, "We need to talk, we hardly know each other."

We agreed that we would proceed slowly: no intercourse or oral sex. I told him, "I don't want to have sex; I want to make love." As he kissed my breasts, he looked sweet, his long, wavy hair sensually caressing me, as I guided him to be more gentle. " I don't want to frustrate you," I continue as I think to myself, if only he would look into my eyes some times. We enjoyed our nakedness together, but still I wished for more kissing, more eye contact, more touching.

Eventually, he was sitting on top of me masturbating, and came with a large load of semen that spurted onto my chest, face and hair. Yet, he had no vocal sounds with his orgasm, which surprised me. Later, he drove me home without a hassle. Like with Keith, I knew within, I was at a dead end with Jim. They read my book, *TEARS ARE TRUTH*…but as Jim eventually told me, "I am scared of you, you are a beautiful woman and smart, a lethal combination. You know right from wrong, so are not easily manipulated." He also admitted that I made him angry because I set limits. Then, admitted that he's really angry at god.

I asked, "Where's god?"

He placed his hand on his heart, "partly in here." Jim told me that he knew we had been together in a past life because he "feels" it. I asked him what are the three most important things to him in a relationship. He answered, 1) seeing the big picture, and 2) compassion is very important. I began with 1) honesty and 2) vulnerability of feelings. Some distraction prevented hearing our third. I asked him to smell his semen in my hair. He couldn't smell anything, and neither could my mother when I asked her the next day, not having washed my hair. I was proud not to be embarrassed about our sexuality, which I experience as fuel for our spirits to fly.

Flying in the face of society's shame of sexuality and crying, and my expression to Jim that my epitome of making love is to cry at orgasm. He responded, "That's a **good** deal."

As are my continuing masturbatory-self-loving orgasms that arise in the morning, when I awake not feeling sexual. Then, arousal creeps in as I lay on my back enjoying the beginning of a new day, amidst new life-nature outside my window and new life plans for the day. I feel all my muscles flex into my vagina, culminating in an a "rousing" orgasm of "Oh god" and "I want *you* in me." Immediately, I think of "*god* in me" as the-*you* in me. As I evolve I find that the pictures in my mind are more diverse, as if I am incorporating the universal spirit that makes us feel interconnected as One. Like the movie, *A Beautiful Mind,* brought forth tears that validated the beautiful heart of my father without whose seed of love I would not be here, or be who I am today, as I wrote in my journal. The feelings prompted by the movie united my father's love with the growing Love for mySelf, as have all my tears. Again, I felt my clitoris feeling full and sexy at the moment of my Spirit's truth being written down in my journal.

Just the opposite of how my best friend Tanya has felt for over a year: "I am dead," she said to me, "I hate sex with Chuck (her husband)." She has said a number of times that she feels "crucified." Yes, she has shut down her sexuality because her spirit is crushed by her fear of being abandoned by her mother if she leaves the marriage. Her mother tells her that she must stay for the sake of their son Lucas. Her mother has cut her off more than once when Tanya made a decision that goes against her mother's beliefs. Tanya is forty-nine years old, still "crucified" by the fear of her mother cutting off love. The power of parental rejection is truly persistent throughout our lives and rules who we can become. When we part she holds me tightly like a Velcro-magnet, saying she needs to soak in as much love-energy as possible.

As Jim told me, "Relationships are too much work." The work of learning to Love can never be too great, for it is our connection to the divine, where compassion and peace exist. Tanya is learning to cry out her childhood pain, to retrieve her spirit, to no longer live in fear of losing the inadequate love her mother offers. To Love her Self-Spirit.

Then, she will be able to feel the beauty of orgasm and lovemaking again, instead of acting out her pain by hating sex, so much so that she has no desire to masturbate either. Another way to act out one's childhood pain is to not be sexual at all, like Gregory was with me for ten months, or to be promiscuous, or what some might say is an addiction to sex. There is no Love in either extreme.

Nor in Jim saying, "Fuck me, fuck me." I said, "No." Jim then said, "Love me, love me." I looked into his eyes a lot, which he returned, and I caressed his face and hair. He did not touch me much, and wanted me to come. I told him I like to enjoy the pleasure of his penis between my legs, and he learned to touch my nipples, and kiss more, which I enjoyed. I had an incredible orgasm with a huge wave at the end of several smaller ones. The last breaker made me call out, "Oh god" maybe six times, loudly as a town crier☺ I looked into Jim's eyes, as my voice cracked, as if I would cry. I did not feel tears. Jim's orgasm was really quiet with only a few moans as he approached orgasm. He withdrew from me to ejaculate all over my back. As he turned me over I said, "I can't see you." All pictures of his fear to be close, to love. He left my house about 1am.

I couldn't sleep until 3am; even masturbating did not help. I was amazed at how much sexual energy I had buzzing through me, and enjoyed a wonderful second orgasm, saying, "It's beautiful." So, what was all this energy about? In my session that week, I cried about giving into "half-assed" making love with Jim because sexuality should be about making love. I was still grieving not having the Love I needed as a child, because I KNOW in my HEART that I want someone to Love me, not just have sex. That's why I couldn't sleep, because I had accepted some thing less than I deserved and wanted. I was still operating out of childhood need. That pain that runs extremely deep, corrupting the innocence of the child's spirit, because I was taught that I was unworthy of god's love.

That same week, Niki, Erin's partner, emailed me that "Erin says she has lost her innocence. She thinks so much in a way that traps her and bogs her down and that makes her emotionally unavailable. That drives me crazy. It takes me hanging in there while she overcomes her fears. She is a tough one your little Erin! It is like we get really close and have a ball then, she punishes herself for feeling close and distances herself again. I think Erin feels the most alive when she is *really feeling*, either *really* in love or *really* angry, not in the middle, because the middle is not enough of a feeling of being alive!" So true, and I cannot help but think of how Erin really lost her innocence when I taught her those same religious beliefs I was taught, although not to such a rigid degree. It is still inside her. Sad.

That same day, March 11, 2002, my astrological email said to go with the joys of my life…each person stretches me from the inward feelings they bring up. I know that to be true. It is 11:11am as I wrote that in my journal. I visited my mother for an hour, when she told me she'd be too anxious to have back surgery even though she is taking the anti-anxiety-anti-depressant drug, Zoloft. I am aware that many of her childhood fears are near the surface. She is close to her vulnerability, and still I am delightfully surprised as we said goodbye to each other. "I love you, mom" rolls off my tongue easily, and mom replied with a strong tone, "I love you, Diane." (In the nineties, I had changed my name to Dianea) WOW! First time to say my name after those three precious words. Her Love became more real and meaningful…the same thing, right?

Also, I found out I was drawn to Jim because of our past-life connection as Native Americans, as I sobbed during an image of him on a horse galloping away, leaving me. I asked why are you distancing yourself? Why? He told me that he could not be with me because he was from a different tribe. I know that all my experiences are a part of my healing journey. It is why I feel the desire to cry at orgasm, so that it is more love and less sex. And, I am much less hard on mySelf.

My heart was so shut down in 1977 when my father died suddenly of a heart attack that I could not embrace my father's body in the morgue and sob all over him, as I still wish I had. In 2002, I was still grieving my father as well as myself having been "strong" instead of being vulnerable to my soft-hearted-love-spirit. Tears combined with my words, "I'm sorry little Dianea that I shut you down. Sorry I had to. (sad now) When you really Love someone you do not give up on them or mySelf." I will grieve as long as the tears roll; when "the roll is called up yonder," (line from a hymn) then I truly will BE there.

Each visit with mom, I noticed how I liked that she looked at me straight in the eyes. She told me that she likes my visits because she feels less "deserted." As

I do from little Dianea as I continued to wake up in the morning not feeling aroused sexually, yet still with the desire to "make love" to mySelf. Somehow, that was hard to say to my SELF. To give that much Love to my Self?

Once or twice a week I would self-Love in the spring of 2002. One particular morning I went back and forth from my stomach to my back. Near orgasm I had images of big dolphins jumping through the air, with a couple of "Oh gods" over chords of "ahhhhhhhhhhhhha" an orgasm beautifully squeezed from my vagina with intensity. Only a few minutes after, I felt compelled into a second orgasm, which is unusual for me. For ten to fifteen minutes I enjoyed the waves of loving-pleasure before my explosion erupted. No images, only attention to the physical feelings spreading even to my anus. A beautiful ride. I marvel at my sexual energy's role in my life.

I do not dream of sexual subjects, in fact, I rarely have dreams that I remember, and when I do, they are of the present, of routine life. It appears that my unconscious is freer and freer of pressing issues or past pain. I am saddened when I hear Erin tell me, in referring to her self, "I'm bad," on the phone, when relating how great Niki is, and that she her self "is a pain in the ass." I called her on it, and said, "It sounds like you need to be in therapy, even though you jest I hear the old message from your religious upbringing loud and clear." It is so insidious, like the rash of poison ivy, which appears out of nowhere, without a scratch to the skin. Still, at the end of the conversation, Erin surprised me with, "I love you," said first, before I said it, for the first time on the phone. I am so fortunate to be on this healing-into-Love journey, more and more Love coming my way, as I heal little Dianea.

The spirit of Love that we are born with, then crushed with repressed feelings, wants to be reborn, even appearing through novels I read. When I read, "If you sit on the bank of a river, you see only a small part of its surface. And yet, the water before your eyes is proof of the unknowable depths," I cried a river of tears then, added a stream with "My heart brims with thanks for the kindness you have shown me by sitting on the bank of this river, by visiting the echoes of my name." (page 321 from *The Red Tent*)

It is this river of my tears that allowed me to *want* to give my mother back rubs, which she said, "feels very good." I asked her about the 6/8/46 date in her wedding ring. Why had they chosen that date when I was born 8/30/46? She said that she had moved and was living with dad. That was unacceptable in 1946, societally as well as religiously. Denali, nine, asked why mom had not put the real date (January 1947) in the ring. Mom replied with emphasis, "I lied." I thought to myself how that must have been freeing for her to admit her dishonesty, being this "born-again-christian" who was rigid about what the "truth" is. Still, because I was becoming closer to my true loving Being, I no longer felt like criticizing my mother for her hypocrisy, but felt closer and more loving of her, and she followed by opening more of her-heart-self.

And the universal synchronicity continued to show itself to me more <u>fre-quently</u> when I would glance at the clock <u>infrequently</u>. Times like 5:55, 7:07, or 3:33 would pop up everyday. I rarely looked at my odometer, and on the first day of spring, I looked, and it read 100,000 miles! I thought to mySelf that my feel-ing-life must be in closer harmony with my true heart, (LOVE) and the "cosmic circle," a Taoist phrase meaning everything is connected.

How can I say it any more elegantly than our EVOLution is connected to LOVE. It is best felt at weddings, especially at my daughter, Megan's. Ben and Megan were to be married on the anniversary of their first date one year earlier. Originally, they planned to have a ceremony with two best friends present, no family. She was five months pregnant, planned and unexpectedly fertile, as she had been on the pill for most of a decade. They had planned to have a bigger wedding celebration with family a year later.

Two days before the wedding, Megan called me and Erin to say we could come to Martha's Vineyard where they would be married by a woman Unitarian min-ister. Ben and Megan had written their own vows, Ben's in the form of a poem. Megan's tears spread like wildfire so that she had to stop, and wipe them before she could continue to read her vows, which were so expressive of the importance of feelings, and openness. My tears rushed as fast as spring waterfalls, which create sounds like sobs…they could not be quiet. Later, Megan told me that she could hear me crying. I was surprised and pleased like I am when approaching a waterfall heard while unseen in the forest.

There were many wet eyes in this small group of family; even Ben hesitated as he became tearful, holding tears back so he could speak. Megan still wants to believe that these are tears of happiness. My experience, as well as with others who are deeply connected to the source of their tears know differently. (See my first book, *TEARS ARE TRUTH*.)

We cry at weddings because we are briefly connected to the loss of REAL parental LOVE in our lives. In a way, it is like orgasm, a moment in time when our hearts are cracked open, to our vulnerability, so that our spirits can cry freely, making room to love more. It is like the crack of dawn in our awakening to the possibility of REAL LOVE in our lives. I must reiterate,

"One's ability to grieve is one's capacity to Love."

Anne Hillman, author of *The Dancing Animal Woman*, writes, "We need to reclaim who we are. That is why we need the third birth. It is a birth out of tears for the severing of old bonds and for the loss of our selves, our souls and bodies. A birth out of intense grief *into an unbreakable experience of connectedness with all being; a birth into bond with the universe, an immediate care.* (pg. 174)

I would dare to say that this is LOVE, as if I were in love with each expression of creation. This deep integration with all of creation begins to take place during the birth of tears. As Hillman continues, "*For the birth of tears is a birth into care. Care, Kara, is the ancient word for grief.* When I search more deeply among the roots of the word anger, I find it in the Icelandic, *Angr.* That word also mean *grief.* Care brings with it the knife-edge of anger and sorrow. The four are inseparably bonded. Care Anger. Sorrow. Grief.

....*Could we all but weep, our weapons would lie rusting in the deeps.*" (pg. 175)

I agree with Anne Hillman when she says that perhaps your tears are your own greatest teacher. When and wherever my tears pop up they direct me to healing my broken heart. Even with songs, like singing along with "Turn Around Look at Me" on my car radio. "Look at Me" reminds me of how Megan *looked at me* in the eyes, steadfastly, behind Ben's back as I sat on the other side of Ben at their wedding dinner. Her big blue eyes so full of love. I told her, "You are so beautiful and loving." She replied, "It has nothing to do with you, mom?" (tears now) meaning some is because of me. This is the perfect example of why I am on this mission to love more really and fully. *Looking into the eyes* **without fear** reflects the REAL love we need and desire – and I could not look directly into my dad's eyes even knowing that I loved him. The love was too little. The load of fear outweighed the load of love. No wonder my father had lost sight in one eye before he died. We both were operating in the dark – too distant from our true emotions, unspoken fear and hurt, the "dark" sides of our selves.

Even song lines, "Someone who really needs you, someone who really loves you," forced tears to open my heart wider, to find more Love. I know I have not had an open heart because of the anger I used to feel defending my vulnerable heart. When I told my workshop leader, Barry, "I have an open heart," tears came to wash more of my pain away so that it could open wider to Love. Where I could see, then feel the Love from Megan's eyes where no fear dared to linger.

Some define spirituality as the act of waking up, being more conscious. My spiritual practice lies a great deal in my journal writing. Whenever I feel tightness or agitation, it is time to pay attention. There is usually sadness close behind, and many times it is in the act of appreciation, which I conveyed when I left messages for my daughters after Megan's wedding. I need the tears to wash away my hurt of not having been appreciated enough growing up. We all need the expression of the FEELING in order to relieve the pain (agitation, tenseness), in order to take another step into healing. Just THINKING will not heal. It is why many ruminate, acting out their pain by obsessively thinking instead of feeling it. We must take time to focus on our feelings, even the feeling we experience when focusing into another's eyes, where we can feel Love.

In groups where we have done an exercise of gazing into one another's eyes, tears come for many, as they have for me. Now, in emails, writing in my journal, or as you have seen as I write this book, tears flow when I have contacted my **grief,** through being **sensitive,** which ultimately wrap into the oneness, unity of

Love. Perhaps these are the trinity of spirituality. An open heart of Love.

Fascinatingly, I just looked at the clock and it read 10:43am, and I immediately thought of 1,4,3, a short cut for "I love you." (1=I, 4=love, 3=you because of the number of letters in each word). Perhaps this is the trinity of synchronicity?

Anne Hillman expresses this vulnerable journey into love, similarly. "The sensations demanded my attention because they hurt. I experienced them as my body's way of teaching me the truth about who I really am. When I listened to the symptoms, I let go. I began to see my pain as a way of getting honest, of acceptance, and of compassion. Yet when I ultimately dared to feel the honest feelings I was protecting myself from knowing, the pain vanished." (pg. 94)

I also resonate with Anne Hillman in being aware that our spirituality connects us with all of the universe, even the energy of plants and animals, even the stars as I have indicated with astrology. I, too, many times have had deer stop in their galloping tracks, look at me intently, watch me approach them, then walk on their way as if they had honored me as one with them.

My kitty, Maha, is very friendly and affectionate, still, I sense her sensitivity to my loving energy when I do my yoga exercises every morning. When I am in dog position she walks underneath me and sits there while my butt is in the air. When I am on my belly, grabbing my ankles, she walks onto my back and stays put as I slide into child's pose, and then lift my butt up again until she slides off due to gravity.

Somehow it feels similar to the love energy that my mother could not help but respond to, as I continued to visit her several times a week, where on leaving her, I'd say with feeling, not out of obligation, "I love you, mom." And she with sturdiness would reply, "I love you, Diane." Again, my name. That is specific love!

It is like knowing the names of wildflowers, and why I like to teach others their names. When asked why I know their names, I reply with a smile, "Because they are my friends!"

It reminds me of a client session with a therapist, Sue. When she was expressing her childhood pain, she spoke of eye contact, "Look at me!" as important as "Listen to me!" Then you know the person (parent) is listening, that they Love you! Really SEE you for who you ARE. The three L's…Look, Listen, Love united. (Instead of the three R's…Rage, Resent, Resist.)

My brother did visit my mother (a six hour drive from Washington, DC) despite his resentment toward her. He, Connie, and I were becoming closer because of our frequent visits to our dying mother. While having breakfast with Eric one morning, we were discussing the importance of honesty and how it really hurts others less if one is honest from the start. Eric added, "Because it lessens the tension." Yes, the anxiety and fears! I found myself saying "Honesty is always the best policy," one of the few "always." Like I will always love my children. I was surprised to hear Eric tell me that dad had harped on the importance of truthfulness, yet he had not been on some important issues: my biological father, date of their marriage, his affair, and German family of origin. Isn't the spirit of the divine the essence of honesty? Both of my parents being "born again christians," afraid to tell the truth, again illustrates how religion does not bring one to honesty, but to the denial of the truth that we are spiritual beings born worthy of Love. And as must be said often, True Love casts out fear…they cannot co-exist. If one is afraid to tell the truth, our spirits are not free to deeply love.

Eric also talked about mom giving up on getting better, and not wanting to leave the nursing home, and his frustration around mom "manipulating" with her tears. I wondered out loud about Eric's investment in keeping mom alive. I was glad that he asked my opinion of why that might be.

Because my mother would cry easily sometimes while we grew up, Eric, being the youngest and alone the most with mom, probably felt helpless, the truer and deeper feeling behind feeling frustrated. He didn't know what to do, and ended up feeling resentful that her feelings took precedence over his. He said he understood and may need to say this to mom before she dies, and admitted it may be part of his investment in keeping mom alive. To hear face-to-face, "I love you Diane" from my distant brother was another sign we were becoming closer through greater truth telling.

It seems to BE the greatest truth that I keep coming back to, how much we need to be vulnerable with tears in order to be spiritually connected to the divine Love with which we were born. Our birthright. This is the real "born again" process I believe I am experiencing as I cry tears, "the pearls of god." Tears, I began to cry, then wept, then sobbed at the memorial service of Fred, 54, who died of a sudden heart attack while stepping off of the ski lift chair. He was the great friend I wrote of earlier, who shone love close to the unconditional. (tears now) I cry again as I write that I can still feel his arms around me, and what I see most are his eyes, looking so lovingly into mine! That IS why we cry, because we miss that kind of Love! Our tears ARE because we LOVE you!!! (more tears now)

Daddy and Fred were truly magical men, and I thought once that I wished that I'd fallen in love with Fred, but then I would have had another major love *die* on me. My nickname to daddy was *Di*. How apropos. To *die* to my ego, my defended past pain. All of us are nurturing Love for ourselves as we cry away the pain of not being loved adequately, as I explained to Megan on the phone, when talking about our tears at her wedding. She remembered how scared she felt at a Christian camp when she was probably ten or eleven years old. They showed a movie about hell depicted as a lake of fire. How horrendous! To scare a child into Love? Really to death! How outrageous!

And so it is understandable that my sister, like Eric, was annoyed that mom was giving up on getting better and wanting to die, and we discussed why she is so invested in keeping mom alive. Being the "born again christian" still, Connie told me that we shouldn't play god, determining when life is over. I pointed out that in a way she was playing god by not respecting mom's wish to die when she had had a full eighty years of life and could no longer care for herself. And Connie did not want to take care of her either. I also spoke of my belief in reincarnation, which early christianity also embraced, and how our spirits will continue to choose to come back until we have learned to be enlightened, which may well mean learn to BE Love. Tears spoke as I said, "I'll miss mom, but I am okay in letting her go now," like myself into tears. Connie said that she would pray and think about our conversation.

I understand how Connie needs to have control over mom's life, because she has given up so much control to her religion, and lost her way from own spirit's way to live. Although my attractive, overweight, sister is legally separated, and has been in divorce proceedings for five years, she has no interest in dating, or being sexual. I sense that her body is reflecting the lack of spirit aliveness.

In early April 2002, I continued to masturbate-self-love once or twice a week, still not feeling sexually aroused when I awoke, but deciding to touch myself tenderly. All kinds of non-sexual images crossed my mental screen: various men and women in my life, especially Fred. When I orgasmed on my stomach, it was not intense, yet I was aware of feeling sad, and said to myself, "I want someone to love me," as tears gently cried. Then, I said, "Someone I can love." I turned over to my back. Tears gently rolled over the cliff of my cheek into my ears, like dew, as if my ears were the only destination my tears knew. I could not help but think of how tears connect the hearing with the seeing – one must *listen* to one's feelings, before they can *be felt*, then *seen* as important enough to allow the tears to flow into Love. A beautiful picture of spiritual renewal! Within the body☺

After I cry, I feel compassion not only for my spirit, but am urged to call my mother to see how she is feeling, now in the hospital. I told her how sorry I was that she felt so poorly. She thanked me and we exchanged our now regular "I love yous." When I visited later, we talked about her upcoming back surgery. "What if you die during surgery?" I asked with concern. "That'd be good," she replied readily. "It's hard to see you suffering," my tears slide out. Surprisingly my mother didn't cry then. I kept some sobs inside, knowing they were about me, and I held her hand. She squeezed my hand. I knew she was ready to die, and I would miss her, be sad, but also glad that her suffering would end (tears again). Finally, we knew we loved each other. This is why I can say with all sincerity **"I am happy in my sadness."**

Still, how could I say farewell when I'd had my mother for REAL, for only nigh unto two months? I actually enjoyed giving my mother backrubs at each visit, her surgery cancelled due to her deteriorating condition. I sat close to mom's legs, on her hospital bed as the doctor gave her a few weeks to live; this was April 8th, 2002. I stroked her legs, to comfort her, knowing that we both needed the touch that I knew I had been deprived of all of my life.

That same day I said to my mother, "You could be dead in a few weeks, I'll miss you." She replied nonchalantly, "Don't think about it."

"How can I not think about it, you're my mother and I love you!"

It is so important that we do not forget those we love! That's part of truly loving. I'm going to miss her telling me "I love you" and our new ability to look straight into each other's eyes. In my crying session the next day, I sobbed, "I'm not ready not to have a mother. I want to BE there, mom, when you die, I am so sorry we've been so separate for so long." The saddest thing of all is the lesson that I am learning…**you just can't appreciate enough what you have in the moment.**

I want to cry in my mother's arms.

Between Fred's death and mom's condition, I was crying daily, or sobbing, which helped clear out my cold's stuffiness. While writing in my journal about one of my fondest memories of my mother diving off Treman Park's diving board at the age of sixty-five, sobs accompanied my feeling good about being proud of my mother. My new found love for my mother had turned into appreciation and pride with new profoundness because I was giving the same feelings to mySelf. This is the best way I can describe the rescuing of the child's innocent spirit of love, lost soon after birth. It is like the circle without a beginning or ending…intertwining my mother's heart and mine. I was no longer hers because of an umbilical cord, (tears) but because of a circle of tears between our hearts. That is SPIRIT! That is LOVE!

Every tear can be a wake up call, if we allow them to tie us back to our past emotional pain that has bound up our spirit's innate ability to love like a baby. Unconditionally. Like the sobs that came as I watched the movie "Artificial Intelligence," hearing the words from the child to his mommy, "I have always loved you." "I have got to go to my mommy!" "Oh god" leapt from my lips along with the pearls of god.

At 5:10 am, April 10th, I heard a nurse's voice asking me to come to the hospital; my mother was bleeding from her rectum. When I arrived she was pale and breathing heavily. I called my sister to come from an hour away. Mom's speech was garbled; I was glad she recognized me. I helped the nurse change the pads beneath her that were saturated with blood. I knew she would die soon.

I asked, "Mom, do you know who I am?" (sadness now over a year later)

"Yes, Diane." (tears now)

"I love you, mom." (chest heaves now)

"I love you too." (sobs now)

Those were her last words!

She took three sips of water from me, then all she could do was breathe heavily, her hands becoming cooler and cooler. Beads of sweat formed on her forehead; I could not feel her pulse. Connie arrived as I was crying, holding mom's hands, telling her over and over, "I love you, (so many tears) and you can let go." Connie added her hands and voice, echoing each other through a wash of tears. Mom's breathing began to rattle as I continued to look into her gray-blue eyes. Her pupils dilated, three more breaths, and she was gone. I bawled with my head and arms lying on her chest.

Then, I cried in my sister's arms.

As mom was dying, unresponsive, I had told her that I hoped she had forgiven herself for birthing me. That I am glad she gave me life! I thanked her in death as well as in life.

I wished I could have heard her response. Still, I was profoundly grateful to have had this peaceful and loving ending with my mother!

While waiting for my brother to arrive from Washington DC, I found my hands on mom's chest, my fingers in her hair, stroking her hand while talking with Connie. I was surprised that I touched mom so frequently and easily after her death.

When my brother arrived five hours later, Connie and I both fell into Eric's arms. It was the closest we had ever been with each other. We sisters cried; Eric was teary. Although I was saddened that I never saw a tear fall from Eric's brown eyes, he was teary again as he told me that he was glad that he had said, "Stop" when mom would say bad things about me. Also, his eyes glistened when I told him how mom had said "I love you" at all my visits in the past two months. I told my Self how essential those three feeling words are to our spirit's aliveness.

After Eric was able to see mom, we left after I kissed her forehead and one last time touched her hands, which were still slightly soft from lying on her warm, round belly where my life had begun. Connie cried as she said she missed the "warmth" that she never felt from mom.

We went to the Moosewood restaurant for a late lunch, where Connie made a remarkable statement. "Mom **knew** about god's love, but never **felt** it." I made her repeat it to Eric to make sure I had heard it right.

When I called Megan that evening, I felt so close to her spirit as she cried with me, especially as she said, "Sounds like Gram began to forgive herself so that she could tell you she loves you." Erin didn't cry when she heard the news, but was very sweet and supportive.

My best friend Susanne cried a few tears with me on the phone. She knew intimately how much grieving I had done in order to have "I love yous" happen between mom and me. She said, "You are the most loving person I know, and the bravest."

My other best friend Tanya and I had lunch plans the next day, so I found myself crying in her arms tightly wrapped around me for what seemed like minutes on that Ithaca sidewalk. I felt loved like a newborn babe. I also noticed that my cold had left the day after mom's death. I attribute my fast healing to all the crying I had experienced in the past day, washing away the germs because they could not grab hold in the flow.

My friend's affirmations of love were especially supportive as I attended the Radical Honesty workshop two days later, having signed up a month before mom's death. There were nine participants and two women leaders, Raven and Clara. Brad Blanton, who has written excellent books like *Radical Honesty*, trained these workshop leaders to use a specific format of telling others honestly how we feel by saying, "I resent you for ...., then I appreciate you for...."

I cried during an exercise where we looked at a partner and said, "You love me," as well as during another exercise about times that we pretend. It is very difficult to say things that we know will hurt other's feelings, yet know we need to be honest in order to be real, and have deep loving relationships.

Raven, who was about fifty pounds overweight, confronted me by saying that I was defensive because I defend my position with tears, that I was hiding my anger and resentment. I explained that I grew up angry, fought with my mother almost daily, and had voiced my hate for her in therapy sessions. I feel little anger anymore and I am glad for that.

Radical Honesty thinks that society has trouble expressing anger, yes, and even more so their vulnerable hurt through tears, which everyone feels under the defense of anger. They could not accept that I had made this much progress, so I was crying as I said, "I feel misunderstood, and helpless like a child."

I was not defensive, but I did defend myself. There is a difference. I felt alone, as no one came to my defense, and yet, I felt good about being safe in my aloneness as well as defending my truth! I knew in my heart I had made a huge step in **trusting** my SELF.

I felt proud that I no longer had to feel *strong* by defending the beliefs of a "born again christian," but could be on the other side of that (s)word "strong," where I can trust my own Being, my truth through "orgasm(s) of grief." Tears have brought me divine Love.

It is the kind of Love that does not need to be returned, like when I called Chuck, my first husband, father of my two daughters, to wish him a happy birthday. We had talked rarely because of Chuck's resentment toward me, but he responded to my friendliness, and appreciation for him initiating our love affair with the National Parks. He was now applying to be a park ranger after retiring as a high school music teacher. At the end of our conversation, I spontaneously said, "I love you Chuck, and always will." It was easy to say, unlike the silence that followed, then, "Thanks."

I am happy to love, and not expect it back, although I would like it to be returned. It has taken much grieving to be able to come to this giving of Love without expectation of return. My childhood "born again christian" friend Mary who lives in Michigan told me on the phone that I gave such Love to (my "born again christian") mom so that she could eventually return it to me.

When I spoke with mom's primary doctor after she died, I asked why they had not confirmed the original multiple myeloma diagnosis, a type of bone cancer. He pleaded his infallibility, along with other doctor's assessments. I told him that it would have been easier for my brother and sister to let mom die, and not push her to get better, if they had known. I was the only child who sensed that she was dying, and needed to be present with mom's process of dying. Doctor Law replied, "You're wise." I answered, "It's the **feeling**," so wise feelings can BE, when uncovered from their defenses.

Mom's death brought more family connectedness, including phone calls to my step-daughter, Sara, and her dad, Gregory. Although I received the reply, "I love you too," from Sara, I did not from Gregory when I said, "I love you and always will." And I was glad once again to be able to feel and give fuller Love.

Ten days after mom died, I was awakened at 7am by an earthquake, the lamp shaking, as I laid in my double bed, and thought, 'maybe mom was coming back to be present with me.' But actually she was more present the day before when I had gone to her nursing home room to retrieve some of her belongings. I sobbed in that room, and tears ran fast during my walk out to the car. Maybe because it was in that room that we exchanged love that had been held back for fifty years.

The day before, I had masturbated with the images of Gregory, Alain, Reid, and even Chuck. All four ex-husbands giving me oral loving, orgasming with "Oh god, I want you to come into me," from my satisfied lips. Love is *com*ing into my heart more and more, staying, be*com*ing more a part of Me, than being dependant on men to give love to me. Love is in the inside, not from the outside, like the egg from the ovary, not dependant on sperm from the penis to feel good about its eggness☺

As I walked along the glen behind my apartment, I noticed the steadiness of the waterfalls, each unique and beautiful in a different way. I love their steady flowing, not shaken by the bumps of rocks, or turns of the banks. Just go with the flow! My heart's <u>aim</u>. (see the I am in the word aim☺) The water falls into whiteness, amidst the blackness of the stones, and I just thought of how my eyes have white as the outer color, black as the center color, the pupil, and blue in between. It is a great metaphor for the color of love. For Love is not found in the black and white thinking, where religion classifies what is the right and wrong way to god, ending in exclusivity as to who has access to god. But love is the color of life, in the middle, where moderation includes all ways of being. Blue, brown, hazel, green eyes are the windows to the soul-heart's desire to deeply Love.

I am also aware that my memory is improving with age, as I become less scared, for perfect Love casts out fear. I am also more creative in the moment when I am dancing!

When I was reading mom's journal from 1989, amidst her usual recounts of the day's activities, she wrote, "Very depressed and tired." She never shared that with any of her children, and I wondered what she was depressed about, and how she dealt with it. As she was 200 pounds, I knew she ate to comfort herself, while she put on the front of being just fine and happy in her religious faith. She had left the "I" out of the sentence "I am very depressed," and I have noted for years that I have left out "I" in my sentences as well. In religious doctrine, I was taught that "I was to deny myself." "I" did not exist. Other rare feeling journal entries said, "Diane annoys me to death." And, "Connie gave me the business today for not telling Diane I love her."

How could she? She hadn't forgiven her self-spirit for conceiving me. And her tears were not accepted either, especially by my brother, who stated that even my tears felt manipulative when I had one or two tears in response to being disappointed that he did not attend a Radical Honesty meeting with me, when he had said he would. According to Eric, my response was "exaggerated," that I reacted as if it was a tragedy, "like he'd chopped my arm off." One or two tears? WOW. Looks like the projection of him exaggerating what a couple of tears might mean. I had been calm, and kind, and just showed my disappointment, how important he is to me.

I smiled explaining to Eric how our society is not comfortable with tears, and how his response is a conditioned one. He affirmed it felt the same as when mom cried with him, manipulated into a space of feeling sorry or blamed. Or helplessness, which most of us are not aware of feeling under the resentment, nor know how to be or deal with. We are back into being the little hurt girl or boy, whose feelings had not been taken seriously. Our spirit has been hurt, and we don't know how to BE with our hurt, or express it so others will understand. This is the work I do as a psychotherapist, to heal broken heart-spirits through listening, accepting, connecting feelings so they can be constructively expressed, and grieved into Love making. Therefore, healing emotions, I believe, is closely aligned with healing the spirit, whose purpose is to Love profoundly.

When one lets go with orgasm, we have a taste of that possibility. As David says in Deborah Anapol's book *Polyamory: The New Love Without Limits*, "We'd be exploring the nature of emotions and all of a sudden we'd find ourselves back at sex. We'd be having a lofty discussion of what truly is unconditional love and bam! Straight up against sex…what's happened in the last 4,000 years has been that we have unduly devalued the potency of sex as a positive spiritual energy. And what it came down to for us is that sex is spirit. Are we not talking about a fundamental life energy that connects us all? Is not the moment of orgasm the moment of enlightenment – an outrageous idea to us at the time…it was our commitment to Truth that kept us going." (pgs. 119-120)

I know that it is not just sex that brings spirit home. We all know that sex does not have to join with love, although I am more and more convinced that it is meant to be.

It IS our EVOLution!

I am reminded of a dream I had the same month mom died. The man was unrecognizable, although I thought it was some form of dad that seemed to be in the role of Freud. He was trying to make me his lover and I wasn't attracted, but I was friendly. Another man was leading me into a fog, and I was reticent to go. I was a little afraid at the end, yet had a sense of confidence to go my own way. That is what feels true; that I can be more confident in my Self. I don't need Freud, or sex, just Love.

And my heart needs to be broken, fall apart, as it did with mom, so that Love could flow. Synchronously, just like the journal I wrote in during her dying, which I bought on sale for nine dollars, and had been $30. The cover is of Italian bonded leather, and yet the pages within eventually fell totally apart! What about the binding? Sex is worth only what the binding of Love costs to retrieve our spirits.

Despite the pain in our life, the child within continues to come out and play. I was surprised as I watched my sister pick out clothes from huge boxes at an Angel Heart barn sale. We tried on clothes together in a big dressing area where twenty or thirty women were in different stages of undress, and gave each other our opinions on how we looked. At some point Connie exclaimed, "I'm having the time of my life!" It was so childlike, so beautiful, and loving as we marched across the parking lot with our arms around each other. So different we are, yet not when the love-child comes out!

It is difficult for me to be materialistic when others have so little. DO I still need too much attention? My Hibiscus was flowering two buds daily again, and again, the same rosy red with a glint of pink. I wear the same clothes two or three days in a row, but still like to change from dresses to pants, to frills, to plain, so can I be the same? As a flower?

I do not want to be a nun where I need to hide my true feelings, like the priests who act out their need for love by sexually abusing their congregation's children. In the new millennium, more and more reports of priests abusing children continue to be reported in the media. On NBC news in 2002, 87 priests in the Boston diocese alone were reported as guilty, and 70 others in other cities. All due to the fear of vulnerable exposure of one's needs and feelings. There is no safe place in heaven or hell. We need to make it safe here on earth.

When Connie and I met with the minister of the Bethel Grove Bible church, where mom's memorial service was to be held, he listened well to my story of "redeeming" mom's love through my tears. Still, he affirmed his teachings of the bible, John 14:6 says, "I am the way, the truth, and the life, no man cometh unto the father but by me." Therefore, being "born again" by accepting Jesus as your savior is the ONLY way you can have eternal life with god. Sad. Still, I felt good because it seemed like spiritual grace that this religious man could see the Love I am able to BE without the religious hiding place where mom, Connie and he live. Also, it was wonderful to hear my sister affirm that it was my love for mom that allowed her to love me. Connie cried a few tears before we left saying that she missed ever having the close warmth of mother, so she was wearing mom's *black and white*☺ T-shirt in order to feel it. The same for me, as I wore the brown sweater mom had knitted for me in high school.

Afterwards, I thought of the above bible verse as: "I am the way OF LOVE, the truth OF LOVE, and the life OF LOVE." That is the Real message: Love is for all, not just the followers of Jesus, who is an example of what Love can be, just like Buddha, Krishna or Allah. LOVE is inclusive, not exclusive.

The fear I have lived with has become clearer and clearer to me, and my stomach was tight when thinking of saying my truth in that bible church. I would be brave in my Love. As I listened to James Taylor sing "Secret of Life" tears formed circles as I imagined mom as a child, running across a field in play. I know she was once that adorable girl! "So long ol' gal."

Can you believe there were snow flurries on April 29th 2002, and fog, and rain, and a smile and tears on my face all at once? Isn't that the circle of love and life?

The circle that comes with orgasm, the mouth forming the "O" of "Oh god," masturbating into that self-lovin' feeling. Tingling feelings more frequent, and images less frequent…more present with my Self?

It certainly seems so, and the Design of the Universe confirms my growth as synchronous to its plan to evolve into deeper Love. Taking into consideration everyone's schedules, we decided to have mom's memorial on May 5th 2002, three weeks after her dying. May 4th is my father's birthday, and May 6th is Megan's. May 5th is my mother's father's birthday. Why so many significant births during the celebration of death? And why did I sob and so many others tell me that their tears could not be held back as I ended my memorial piece to mom with my favorite memory of her: at 65, diving off a diving board next to Treman Park's huge waterfall?

Tears were strongest as I said the word, "awe" in the sentence, "I am in awe of her." I was clearly aware, as I have come to realize after years of crying, that it is about me, to have not felt the awe, or respect for mySelf. Most of us have not felt that deep respect during our growing up, and later, I sobbed most about this memory, when I read my memorial to mom over again. Why is that?

Awe is the <u>image</u> of who I am…and every other soul-spirit. It is the courage to be freely ourselves, which has been lost for so long. Finally feeling the AWE for self as I let go of my tears of loss of mom and her love. I love you mom!

And then, I think of the sound of "AHHHHHHHHHHHH" as the same sound as "awe." The "AAAHHHHHHHHHH" of orgasm, as we approach that moment of letting go into "Oh god." Our life's journey is to find the divine in us daily, not just at orgasm.

To let go of more and more fear, like that of Erin, who decided not to say anything at her grandmother's memorial because she felt "self-conscious, and shy." You mean "scared?" "Yes," Erin replied. Later, Megan told me that Erin told her that she was afraid that she'd break down too much. Megan did read her memories of mom, and cried, in fact, sobbing at one point, when she said, "I knew Gram <u>loved</u> me."

Again, KNOWing that your family loves you is not sufficient to FEEL loved. My daughters' tears and fears are an affirmation to me that they have not felt enough love growing up, in great part due to their first nine and twelve years being under the fear and guilt of the "you must be born again, or else you will go to hell" religion.

I felt very good about how I stated with sadness my disagreement with the exclusivity of "Jesus love" during the memorial. I also appreciated the minister, and church members preparing goodies for the reception afterwards. They were helpful and kind. I just wish for god's Love to be founded in worthiness. Two of my friends, Adriana, and Susanne, who attended the memorial told me that my words were wonderful and that my honesty was what more people needed to hear.

I was surprised how generous I became in promoting my mother's memory, by giving several family members 8x10 photos of mom taken when she entered nursing school. What a loving-spiritual change came about between mom and me as we felt love together in our last two months together. It was a deeper love because we finally FELT Love. Our minds finally joined hands with our hearts.

A couple of days after the memorial, as I was eating dinner, I burst into tears while thinking of mom eating her dinner alone at Lakeside Nursing Home. I knew what it felt like to be alone while a child, when mom left me alone in the crib, or alone with my feelings when sixteen. This is the spiritual connection with another, when we can feel, be sensitive to what others might feel, and then accept them. To be spiritual is to be connected to Love. What a wonderful circle where tears are about the loss of Love, and then open our hearts to love again☺

Megan validated my feelings by telling me that her favorite part of my eulogy was the deep feelings of love that changed between mom and me because of my tears, more than my appreciations of mom, or the funny entries from her journal that I read. This kind of deep love made it possible for renewed connections with the father of my children who came to my home for Megan's baby shower, and with a therapist friend, who has not been able to tell me why we are no longer in contact.

The spiritual-synchronous connection filled out the big picture even more when Erin signed a lease to rent 410 Marshall Street here in Ithaca. She was returning primarily for her daughter, Denali, to live in the same city as her father. And get this! Denali's dad, Kevin, was renting a house at 410 Madison Street! Not only were the numbers the same, but both streets begin with Ma! Ma, who is me☺ Since then, both of them have bought their rented homes! Doesn't the spirit connect us in synchronistic ways?!

As do the eyes most vulnerably, which I noticed at mom's memorial especially. When I looked steadily into other's eyes, tears appeared like streams that flowed into hugs. Like Love wants to flow, and fear wants to hide.

Bradford Keeney, an internationally acclaimed scholar and teacher whose academic books are deemed classics in the field of psychotherapy, quotes a Kalahari bushman doctor: "There is a kind of light that connects you to another person. When you see and feel it, you become a brother and sister to that other person. From that point on, you will completely understand the other person. This experience can take place during the dance. *You must look into their eyes in a strong way.* If you are lucky you will feel and see the line of light that connects you and the two of you will come together in your heart and mind." (italics mine, pg. 51, *Spirituality and Health* magazine June 2003)

This is the kind of Love we find in a baby's steadfast eye gaze, and wish to continue to nurture in our children. That same May, I spoke at the local public library for Children's Mental Health Day, where mostly professionals working with children attended. Although I used Aletha Solter's book *Tears and Tantrums* as the basis of my discussion, spontaneously, I was asked to read my children's book, *Everybody Cries.* My message is to preserve the Love all children are born to give and BE.

Like me, when I was smiling cheekbone-to-cheekbone after I ran into my long time friend, Ken, who immediately said, "You look like a child, a five-year-old." In the midst of giggles I asked, "How so?"

"That **child**like **spirit** shines through!" Ken beamed to me. It was the greatest compliment I could hear. I hope all of you readers find it too! Tears will lead you home to open-hearted Love, as I have described in my mother, through my process of grieving lost parts of myself. Just days before mom died, Eric had asked her if she prayed. She said she couldn't, which surprised us sibs. Connie concluded that mom was not as strong in her religious beliefs at the end. I concluded that she did not need them as much because she felt more true Love in her heart.

"My tear is a kiss of love for you," I emailed back to Christian, a 1980s boyfriend, when he wrote how my mother's death brought up great pain for his six losses, including two brothers, one a twin! All of whom he loved dearly. It is much easier to feel genuine compassion when the tears flow. And I can smile as I planted the two flowering trees that Connie and I picked out: a crabapple tree over mom's grave and a weeping cherry over dad's☺

Also, in May 2002, I met Johnny at a tango workshop, but had to leave before I could talk with him. I did wave him over, and gave him my business card with the message, "If you'd like to dance, call me." He seemed very interested and appreciative, so it was hard not to hear from him for a couple of weeks. When I next masturbated, I envisioned him, and Gregory, into a very strong orgasm while lying on my back. My vagina pulsated as it did the tango with my clitoris. The music was six counts of "Oh god," to the drumbeat of "IN ME" It seemed too long since I had made love with a man where there was no guardedness. Like…

"No holes barred," was the phrase I used with my friend Sue, how I wanted our friendship. Right away I thought what a great metaphor. No emotional holes from unmet childhood needs will be barred; they will be exposed through tears and rage, so that we are free to express all our true feelings, which innately are of love and compassion. Sue, being a therapist, understood when I told her that going to therapy once a week can be similar to going to church every Sunday your whole life, to find your lost spirit of Love.

The difference is that religion covers up the emotional pain, which covers up our true spirit, which is born to love inclusively, wholeheartedly. However, feeling psychotherapy can be seen as a spiritual practice, because it frees our Spirit, by letting go through feeling our past pained-feelings that had not been respected, but shamed by our parents and society. There is a CD called *Love Is Pain* by Ja Rule; I disagree because it makes sense that Hate is Pain, because the hurt-fear-pain has not been felt, let go of. It is the releasing of emotional pain through vulnerable tears that unleashes Love. We no longer have to protect ourselves from: "Don't be a crybaby." Love is revealed like a glorious sunset streaked with clouds of tears! Love sets in!

Someone has said, "**Grief is not a problem to be cured, it is only a statement that you have loved someone.**" That *someone* is usually understood to be a beloved parent, family member, or friend. But most of all, it is the Love we lost as a child for one's Self.

This process is validated again when I continually notice how I have better eye contact with others as I continue to cry out my grief-pain. At the memorial, I even checked out the <u>eye</u> colors of Bill and Lucille, who have been like my second parents. I have a new deeper noticing through the <u>eyes</u>, because of less fear being inside me. "I" is more prevalent, more noticed, the "<u>I</u>" that lets go of the ego, which is our guardedness, another word for fear.

Spirit feels like: eye contact of lovers, the Beloved, connection, passion, unspoken love. I felt it with Eric, a young tango dancer who kept long eye contact with me while dancing. I can still remember his deep breathing, the in and out, like a time-lapse photo of a blooming lotus.

If only we would pay attention like children do, like Tanya's three-year-old Lucas, who wanted to read *Everybody Cries* three or four times a week for a month or so. He would ask Tanya about the photo of three-year-old Megan on the cover, crying. "Why is she crying? Where is her Mommy? Why doesn't her Mommy pick her up?" As I wrote earlier, I sense that, unconsciously, I needed to pay attention to my own tears and was trying to by photographing my daughter's tears. Surprisingly, one of my clients brought in pictures of her childhood, and one was of her crying as she stands in her crib. Why do parents take such pictures?

And why is it that now I am drawn to the thundering brown waterfalls of spring? I have rarely worn the color brown because I have seen it as a dull color. It is the substantial color of the earth, although supremely covered by lush green grasses and leaves of tress, whose trunks are brown. Yet, I love brown eyes! You guessed it, my father's eyes are brown☺ Now, I have gained more appreciation for the color brown, as I have for the color gray. As my heart expands its ability to Love, so does the loving of all the colors.

And the theme that expands my heart is when I am saying through tears, "I have to be more sensitive to my feelings!" Then, I am sensitive to others, like when I witnessed a mother yelling at her three-year-old daughter for running because she had fallen down. Here she was physically hurt and her mother was yelling at her. Tearful as I was, I almost stepped in to comfort the little girl. My heart was broken open to sensitivity to another. I like what my client Cherise said to me, "If I wasn't so sensitive, I wouldn't have a heart at all."

I love the way I feel as a tear travels down my cheek: its steady flow, its importance, its comfort, its flavor – salt of the earth, watering the thirst of my heart to Love. It is why I love to look into the eyes of children; they are my most treasured attraction. They are wide open to the power of the sensitivity that is Love.

The sensitivity that I am continuing to bring to my orgasms. One May morning, as I touched myself into a wider feeling of impending orgasm throughout my genital area, and into my vagina, I imaged a shiny penis, and wanted to kiss a man, undress Johnny, and feel the fullness of our loving union. It was an "Ohhhhhhhhhhhhh" orgasm with one "Oh god" fully said. Immediately after I thought, "I want someone to love me," tears flowed into small sobs, until I was interrupted by a phone call. Isn't "I want someone to love me" the universal CRY?

And when you love, one wants to forgive, right? So why was I astounded when my sister said to me, "I can't possibly ask Heather to forgive me?" Heather is her oldest daughter, now in her thirties. Connie said that she had not protected Heather enough from her father who had tried to strangle her, although Connie had jumped onto him. I responded, "Of course you can ask for forgiveness!"

"And where does that come from that you don't think you can?" I asked.

Of course, her religion – that we are not worthy of forgiveness; we deserve to go to hell. Her facial expression told me that she saw the connection. She was speechless. Earlier she had said that she sees "sinner, as devoid of god."

But, LOOK at a newborn child!

And, LOOK, how I have added two more mirrors to my home in the past year, finding them at a huge warehouse-type building with so much stuff you could barely walk down the cramped aisles. They were inexpensive oak-framed mirrors, not cheap flimsy department store wall mirrors. I was reflecting a greater feeling of quality in my Self. I could LOOK at Me. My home is becoming complete, beautifully simple, cared for, with life-giving plants nourishing each *chamber* of my heart-home.

I was blessedly surprised again when I self-loved a week later. Varying mundane thoughts mixed with the day's activities ahead, Erin and Megan, Johnny, until I was centering on my physical sensations, the tightening and loosening of my vagina and anus, contracting and feeling intense pleasure building especially in my vagina. I was saying,

"Oh god, come in me," but I did not cry until my second orgasm about twenty minutes later, which was clitoral as well as vaginal. I was saying, "Oh god, come into me, come into me!" Although I also asked Johnny to come into me, my tears made it feel it to be "god"…both together. My thoughts added, "I don't want to be alone." As I was crying, I felt pleased to be so present with loving my Self.

Then, I thought about writing a poem about how my tears run down my face, joining my eyes (seeing), to my ears (hearing), while lying down. And, as I sat up, running to my nose (smelling), and into my mouth (tasting.) All the senses being joined in order to be Me.

It is like the mixture or combination of feelings of love and sadness, how they run together. One of my clients said that joy and sadness are two sides of the same coin. I would rather say that love and sadness are the two sides of the same coin because we cry when we lose Love – the essence of our Being. Human Being. Joy is the outcome of having someone love you!

Love is why I fell apart when I wrote the word "honor" in my journal in telling about the memorial bench I designed for my mother and father. I'll actually have my hands on the bench and sit in the laps of their memory. I sobbed as I spoke of the moon and shooting star carved into the back of the bench, because Diana is the goddess of the Moon and the Hunt. I will become a FULL moon as I continue to learn to Love, and my father is the Shooting Star that brought that possibility down to my earth-life. Now, every time I cry I am aware "there is more of god inside me." When I cry at orgasm, I feel vulnerable, OPEN. I've become aware of how Orgasm and Open both begin with "O." Said "Oh" with "Oh god." Then, open can be separated into O-pen. I write with my pen so that I can be more connected to the openness of my mouth with "O god." I love the inter-connectedness of language and tears and the synchronicity of the Design of the Universe. It feels enlightening. Opening to Love everyone and thing.

Therefore, I cannot "shut up" as my sister tells me to do when I gently confront her decision to treat her ulcerative colitis with another pill. "I am not going to shut up because I care about you, Connie!" I am going to continue to tell the truth of my heart's love for you. The truth hurts but it also sets you free☺

And develops patience, like emailing Johnny for one month before finally meeting for a date in early June. He lived two hours away and had recently ended another relationship, as well his semester teaching. He also is an active father with his two teenage daughters who live with their mother one hour away.

Johnny arrived at my home, expecting to spend the day with me. After I made French toast topped with fresh fruit, we hiked into Treman Park, where he earnestly folded his hand into mine. It felt particularly good because I had not wanted to hold other men's hands for over a year, except for one short walk with Jim. I was very attracted to Johnny's big artistic hands and earthy brown eyes that reflected his great openness about his past three marriages and recent relationship. When we came to Lucifer Falls, marshmallowy white, Johnny suggested that we swim to the other side so we could view the falls fully. That meant nudeness! I hesitated, wondering if I wanted to show my body to him for the first time in this setting. But why not?

As we sat a foot apart, surrounded by a weeping wall of plants and a roaring-splashing waterfall, we looked into each other's eyes for what seemed hours. I couldn't hold the tension any longer and leaned into him for our first kiss, long and luscious as the deep green enfolding us. I couldn't have imagined a more beautiful setting for our intimate beginnings.

After spending the afternoon at the Ithaca Festival, where I performed in the "Mostly Motown" singing group of twenty, we continued to share ourselves on the red sofa in my open view-of-the-valley-living room. Johnny had brought some of his poems to share, and read them to me while his tears watered words of emotion spoken. He also played a torch song on his laptop, to which our bodies sweetly danced.

In light darkness, on the flowered sofa outside on my front porch, we "made out." Johnny appreciated the dark sky that shone stars, because he lived in a city. He wondered out loud why he liked the darkness so much. I suggested that it makes one feel close to oneself, and he added, maybe it is because you can hide. Was that to be telling?

The darkness represents the shadow side of one's self.

We kissed and fondled for an hour before we touched each other's genitals through our clothes, although I had felt Johnny's strong erection long before. He had planned to return home that night, but suggested that we sleep together without being sexual, "holding my head to his heart." I liked the metaphor for his journey with me. He slept easily; it took me more than twenty minutes to fall asleep, sleeping lightly next to this very in-shape, attractive man.

Johnny had told me that he wanted to progress slowly and not be in a committed relationship because his pattern was to jump in too quickly, and he found it difficult to be himself because he would be too responsible for hurting the woman's feelings, negating his own.

So, I was surprised when we awoke, that Johnny wanted to make love with me. When we were about to have intercourse I put on the brakes, because I want to be falling in love before I become one (with Love?) Johnny was a very good lover, and with his soft erect penis gliding over my genitals, I came easily, screaming "Oh my god" several times along with Johnny's name. It was a very full orgasm, which felt full of tears. I did not cry. I could tell that Johnny felt torn about coming so far into our sexuality because his penis showed it by fluctuating from firm to less firm. He said, "I feel very vulnerable." I felt great that he said that so openly! "I'm disappointed in myself" for going farther sexually than my mind wanted to. And to my surprise added, "You're the most beautiful body I've been with." (He's 48, I'm 55.) I'm embarrassed and proud all at once, like a surprise birthday party just for me.

After breakfast, another surprise, when Johnny told me that he wanted to have an orgasm and cry with it! I hadn't said anything about how that was my ideal either!

I thought, "Wow, we are meant to be." I asked why he wanted that experience.

"It would be a relief," Johnny offhandedly replied.

He told me about making love with Lisa, (third wife,) and Ellen, (recent girlfriend,) and that it would be good except that he would orgasm about every seventh time, and that he'd like to more often. He said that he was aware that it was emotional, and didn't know why he held back, maybe because he was so concerned about his partner's pleasure. As he'd said earlier, "I don't know that I deserve all this pleasure."

Can I write that I was surprised again that same morning, when we made love again on the living room sofa, still without intercourse? During my "Oh god" orgasm, I looked into Johnny's eyes, and tears trickled when I said, "Here's looking at you." Silence took hold of a couple tears coming out of my nose, then I said, "I'm crying because I wasn't really looked at as a child, for who I AM – my opinions and feelings." He took it in, wiped a tear away, and I felt calm in loving as I shared my whole heart.

And body, as Johnny carried me over to my new mirror, stood us side by side, admiring our bodies singly and together for several minutes. I was not used to such appreciation of my body, even though I had learned to like it by then. Even though we had moved further sexually than both of us had planned on, I still held the line of no intercourse, which Johnny felt was mute since I had crossed the stated line into Orgasmville, so why not go for "penetration?"

I answered that it made a difference to me because I call intercourse "union," a special difference on more than one level. I see union as one with Self, therefore, "making Love." Whereas, penetration seems like a one-way view, and not a joining: more mechanical than loving. I wanted to be able to tell each other "I love you," and say that we are making love, not having sex, as he had described his sexual relations with Lisa and Ellen.

When Johnny stepped into his Miata to leave, he said, "Thank you for giving me 100%, no, 200% in being with me."

"What's the greatest percent?" I retorted.

"It's already over the top," Johnny smiled. I knew he felt fully supported, understood and accepted. As did I. I wondered how we would evolve.

The next day, when Johnny answered the phone, I asked, "Is this Sean Connery or Tom Hanks?" Johnny laughed loudly and I appreciated his cool laugh. He appreciated me more than once for how tender and gently I had touched him. He said that it felt like "mother" when I touched him, even licking his buttocks felt like mother wiping his bottom as a child. Certainly, it was not my image, but I was glad he could admit to his. He told me that he wanted to back up physically. "Put the car in reverse?" I replied with a laugh, joining with his.

I liked that we would slow down sexually, enjoy more kissing, more lovingness instead of appeasing old-unmet-emotional-physical need. I did not feel rejected. I felt more loved as he read a beginning email to me expressing that he had never had such an enjoyable long conversation with anyone before. And, that my emotional consciousness was what he needed in his life. He'd been in several years of psychotherapy in the past.

I asked Johnny what he had meant by "relief" as his response to my earlier question as to why he wanted to cry at orgasm. He easily responded that it was a relief to not have to make himself lovable to someone and that it connected to his father. Yes, it is about the loss of his father's love, letting go of that pain is what heals us with source-connected –tears.

One morning, on waking, I thought of splitting up my middle name, Alice.

Al…I…C(E), or "All I see" sounded out. Because Alice means "the truthful one," I tell all I see, the truth☺

When I self-loved the next time, I briefly envisioned Johnny's eyes and penis with Robert's shoulders, then orgasmed saying "Oh god" and "Enter me," three or four times. That was a change from "Come into me." 'Enter me' was more direct, meaning to take me over more fully, inside all of Me? I was aware that I was a little scared that I'd move away from needing men, maybe because I'd want them instead of needing them. I liked that! Cool! What a paradox, as fear is the barrier to finding much better. Love.

It reminded me of one of my male clients saying, in the midst of his sobbing, "I don't even know if I know how to grieve." I believe I am learning how to grieve in my weekly crying sessions, my journal writing, and other writings such as the article I was writing for the Ithaca Journal, "Thankful for Persisting Family Love." I cried several times as I wrote, while **remember**ing what I appreciated about my father and mother, and how long I had not **remember**ed! My pain had blocked much appreciation of them, because I had blocked my own pain of appreciation for mySelf for so long. We need to **remember** our tears in order to Love.

And, greater Love seems to be coming my way more and more as I become older…yet younger in spirit! The next weekend in June when I am with Johnny, he surprises me again with "I want to say 'I love you.'"

I was quiet, then said "I have love for you as I wrote in my emails, and I say 'I love you,' when I feel deeply for someone." On that June Sunday he also said that he felt "bliss" with me at certain moments. I had never heard "bliss" spoken of in regard to me. Although Johnny and I were compatible on many levels, he was unusually so in his ability to see the value of making love versus having sex. He has wanted this in his life all along and we carried it out our second weekend together, where we kissed a lot and necked, *making eyes*, but did not touch each other's genitals. I believe he is the first man I've been with to dislike the word "fuck" in everyway that it is used.

When he said that I am "unusual," I believed him despite feeling slightly embarrassed when he added, "the women I have known are either "thoughtful," or "uninhibited," not both, like you."

My tears made their appearance in my next email to him, which said how much I loved his **child**-like **vulnerability**. He seemed to say what he felt at any given moment, and I love that my tears validate how much that vulnerability is Real Love. I was surprised again when I burst into tears while listening to the BeeGee's *Too Much Heaven*, even as the instrumental introduction began on my car radio. It was as if I was a wave that knew it would crash on the words, "Love is such a beautiful thing!" I couldn't help but sing the song to the top of my vocal chords and heart!

The next day, I sobbed deeply as I heard the BeeGees sing *How Deep is Your Love?* The day before, while in bed with Johnny, I had wept while telling him of a childhood dream, after he had shared his present dreams. I was surprised how strong my tears felt, although I did not allow myself to bawl. He laid his head on my heart after he had wiped away a tear. I had been crying about how my dad had saved me, wiped the long nose off of me with a washcloth after I'd lifted my head out of a bag of fertilizer. Dad had revealed the truth that he loved me; (not the church religion) that I was and am lovable. I wondered if I was falling in love with Johnny.

In my next crying session, I began to cry as I said, I can't settle for less than I need or want when I say to myself maybe I should be satisfied. "My spirit says no that I cannot settle, that I want so much to be there fully loving somebody," with tears of truth and wisdom. And that somebody is ME! Sobs say, "I keep looking for *you* Daddy." And now it connects that *you* is LOVE, what Daddy began in Me. Doesn't this sound like spiritual work, when we connect with Real Love?

I seemed to be at a crucial landmark in my growth. I was crying more about the loss of the good loving (by my father) now, instead of the loss felt by not being loved (by my mother and the church) This process of crying is the gift that replaces the denial of emotional pain by religious abuse. Grieving (pearls of god) is why religion no longer matters.

Johnny's and my third weekend together cemented our mutual understanding of wanting to keep an "open, non-committed-meaningful" relationship. We had arrived at giving each other what we really needed, a gratifying balance for a change. We felt love for each other although I was not ready to say, "I love you." I felt it coming, or becoming. Becoming is another fascinating word, as it is used in saying, "that dress is becoming to you." It is a beautiful thing to **become** Love! As it is a beautiful thing to **be coming** at orgasm.

Well, it happened. On Father's Day 2002. The night before, Johnny talked about how he was not sure that he was ready to be naked with me, and what it would mean to make love all the way with intercourse. I was accepting and supportive, and soon we evolved into each other's arms and bodies with fine oral loving, and finally union. I nearly came when I was on top with Jack (his penis) inside of me. But, it felt "exquisite" when Jack kissed my clitoris along with smooth caresses throughout my genitals, so that "Oh god" escaped as I looked into Johnny's chocolate eyes. I closed my eyes right at orgasm, which showed me that my full feeling of "inloveness" was not there. We both said our first "I love yous" to each other while making love, not at the moment of heated orgasm.

Later, when we climbed into his convertible Miata, I said, "I love you." He replied, "You do?" I replied, "I just said it, and not in the heat of passion." We had great conversations, where I even said apprehensively, "I'd have to get used to so much body hair." Johnny said, after our talk about fearing to hurt each other's feelings, "Tell me the truth even if it hurts my feelings." It was great to hear him say that!! (Not me.) And he is not a psychotherapist☺ This is the kind of intimacy that breeds deep Love.

He had cried in my arms that same morning while saying, "It hurts that I hold back from you. I have given up too much of myself before." He was making the connection of why his erections were not as full as he'd like them to be. After his tears about being afraid to reveal his true being, he became erect.

So Love grows with the experience of tears. And flows.

Like when Susanne's card arrived the same day my mother's ashes did. A swan diver graced the front, while the inside read "Nothing is Real until it is…experienced!" In her swooping handwriting: "I've learned this and so much more…especially about Love and courage from you – I love you, Susanne."

When I next self-loved, my orgasm alone said, "Oh god" and "In Me," as my vagina contracted with thoughts of wanting Johnny inside me as well. It seemed clear that I felt "god (love) in me" as the central point of lovemaking. Seeing 'god' in each of us. Especially, easily seen in the face of a child, then in their profound words.

Three-year-old Lucas told his mother, Tanya, "Daddy hasn't forgiven you Mommy," and "I forgive you Mommy." When Tanya asked Lucas, "Forgive me for what?" Lucas replied, "You know, Mommy." In her session with me she realized as she cried that he was saying "I forgive you for aborting me." She had had more than one abortion.

Before Tanya's session, we had eaten breakfast together, and she told me about a Caroline Myss tape she had listened to and how it tells about what needs to change but does not tell you how. She reminded me of how she'll always remember her "profound" change by tears in order to become pregnant with Lucas. She was forty-six when she gave birth to him, and had given up hope of having a child. She is still in the process of re-birthing little Tanya (herself), as are Susanne and I, and my clients, and others who cry primally.

The fourth weekend that I saw Johnny, we shared about our time spent with others, like me dancing with Bill, and him going to a party with his friend, Nickie. The difference being that he kissed Nickie for minutes, and I did not with Bill. Johnny said that they have an understanding that "kissing is as far as it goes." We both felt a bit funny about this different way of being in our relationship, yet wanted it to be open in every way, which means that we would tell each other about what happens with others and our feelings about it all. We concurred that we were a primary relationship and would check it out with the other before becoming sexual with another.

I was very aware of my feelings as I questioned whether this was a healthy openness, unlike my acting out of fear of vulnerability in my second marriage. I knew I was not "in love" with Johnny although I loved him. I enjoyed being affectionate and making love with him even if I did not always have an orgasm. I was happy that he had had an orgasm with me, showing his progress of letting go of his fears that he might not be pleasing me. We loved our foreplay: our walk in the moonlight into the gorge of waterfalls, kissing and touching all over, my nipples setting off fireworks. This particular evening, Johnny just wanted to be affectionate, and, remarkably, I was able to fall asleep with a very erect clitoris.

After lovemaking in the morning, Johnny stood at the side of my white iron double bed, staring at my naked body for seconds, then into my eyes for minutes.

Tears formed and one ran down my cheek as I said, "No one has looked at me like you do – you SEE Me." Johnny then held me and said, "I am here; I'm present."

I loved in return, "Yes, you are a present!"

The theme of the eyes ('I' s) being the opening to our heart-soul cannot be overstated! And the tears that want to flow from our eyes, like at breakfast when Johnny picked up the 8x10 photograph of my father holding Megan, me with Erin. I was sad that I had not been held more by my father, or had pictures of him holding me as he did my children. And I became excited as I realized that the two large pictures of dad and my children are of <u>holding</u> them! How unconscious is that, my need, once again shown in the photographs I took years ago.

And now I was in relationship with a photographer and filmmaker, who in one of our discussions said that emotions are really what direct our lives, not rationality. Yes, feelings are a deeper source to truth than reason; we must dig into the **mine.**

We talked about his spiritual life, which had evolved out of a Bahai background that he chose as a teenager. He believed that we are all interconnected but never concluded as to what gave his life meaning. He did not accept astrology or psychics as I do, but we accepted our differences as edges of a page in the book of our evolving story-lives.

The world of America was living with more "terror" alerts in June 2002, as well as hearing of suicide bombers in the Israeli-Palestinian conflict. All over whose religion is the best or "right:" the muslims, or the christians. How sad is the present plight of humankind – not feeling loved enough, so must compete to be superior: to feel safe, and secure.

As Johnny and I became closer, I asked Johnny if he'd be interested in exploring Tantra with me. Tantra is a spiritual system in which sexual love is a sacrament. It has come to us from ancient Indian books over two thousand years old. Charles and Caroline Muir refer to it as the Art of Conscious Loving. He was open to it, but it did not happen because it did not become a priority.

Just like Connie does not make it a priority to work through her emotional pain. When she went to the doctor who was treating her ulcerative colitis, she told him that I'd said that if she cried more, she wouldn't have to take the medications. Surprise, surprise! He agreed! I was not surprised when Connie told me that she did not miss mom, dead then for two months. She said that mom would not listen to other opinions and would only vent and that she did not miss. I understood her emotional pain, and wished she would grieve it.

Johnny continued to email loving expressions and to tell me how he liked intimacy in small doses all day. That he wanted me to be affectionate and not aim to turn him on…just what most women want! When I self-loved again, I imaged many different couples like: Erin and Niki, Chuck and Kimber, Megan and Ben, and then a bit with Johnny, wanting his penis barely penetrating me at orgasm of "Oh god, oh god, so GOOD!" Now my GOODness was being validated!

"Traditional religious teaching has blinded us to the fact that flesh and spirit are two poles that belong together. Romantic love is undeniably sexual, yet it contains the potential for great spiritual experiences…The word kama (made famous by the book of erotic lore called Kama Sutra) is used to describe not just sexual desire but the desire to unite with god. By implication this is the same kama that makes you want to be united with your Self." (pg. 133, *The Path to Love*, by Deepak Chopra) I was happy to see my Self appearing more and more as "god in me" through the joining of sexuality and spirituality - as "Go(o)d!"

The joining paralleled my increasing awareness of nature's detail, as I gazed at my Hibiscus, opening a new blossom everyday. I finally trimmed it back as two branches covered too much of my view out of my living room picture window. Another branch needed to be trimmed back soon but I found it too hard to cut off those small buds "coming." The Hibiscus is becoming wider and deeper: more central green branches grow because of the pruning; like cutting back my pain, I blossom more and more.

And I wondered if I was blossoming into a healthy open relationship with Johnny. He became mad at himself for being in a "confused" state, being used to knowing for certain what he wants to do. He wanted to think of himself as making love to only one woman, yet now was considering otherwise, as his ex-girlfriend was calling to entice him. Confusion is just a feeling when one is in transition or change. Therefore, I was flowing with the process, and not being "pissed off at myself."

Johnny and I continued to discuss the words "having sex vs. making love" as descriptions of what we do. He said that others see them as the same. That could be, but I was imagining the evolution of our language in sync with <u>evol</u>ution's goal to make Real Love as the prominent description and motivation for the sexual act.

Doesn't it make sense that the more we have real Love in our lives, the more we will describe it as that instead of the physical act? We will become more vulnerable with the EMOTION – motion toward making Love in the world. The process of becoming more intimate with our emotions and their roots seems to be the function of monogamy at this time in history. Monogamy functions as a structure where it is not as easy to run away from our emotional pain and encourages growth into Love.

"One thing I like about you is that you make me uncomfortable," Johnny said as we walked into the Bistro Q restaurant. At the table he continued, "You're everything I want, I must be an idiot not to want you." (Exclusively, he meant.) But, we were in sync in our growth process because I wanted the same freedom to explore, and told him that I was going to Italy for two weeks to allow myself to be more open to meeting an Italian man, whom I had ignored during my last trip. Now, I would be operating out of less fear, or need to control.

WE both appreciated the beauty of our physical being, and more so the important way we could talk to each other about less revealed parts of ourselves. Johnny said that he felt really safe with me, more so than with his previous girl-friend because I was more understanding, less reactive, and accepted him as he is right now.

I was glad to cry with Johnny as I spoke of how evolutionarily I had to give up the community I was raised in, in order to BE Me – that religion has to go – in order for us to evolve to a love that includes, not excludes. Where I can listen to my own truth, where my tears of truth lead me. I feel so lucky, even as I cried with my client, Sharon, as she looked at a picture of herself at age four. Sharon said, "She wants me to *know* her." I made sure my tears did not distract Sharon, and at the end of the session told her why I had cried, about not looking at or knowing little Dianea for most of my life. She wondered if she or I would get over that pain. I replied, "I welcome my tears; they make me a more loving-compas-sionate human being. It is a process and I do feel lighter and lighter, crying less and less intensely."

Now it is easy for me to be with others' emotional pain because I have been with my own. One night, just after we had crawled into bed, Johnny's oldest teenage daughter called him and they talked for a half hour or more. When he returned to our bed, he curled up into my arms and sobbed for five to ten min-utes, saying "I'm not enough," for Meira. He meant that he couldn't love her enough (himself of course); she has nobody but him. We fell asleep holding hands.

The next morning, Johnny began to touch me, look at me, and soon we were kissing, morning mouth and all. This time he was much slower, touching many parts of our bodies, more kissing and looking, more tenderness and affection. His penis was very hard. We masturbated each other, orally loved, and eventually he was inside of me. We enjoyed the waves of pleasure, touching, looking into each other's eyes with intention of love. Neither of us had an orgasm. It was the best yet – really "making Love." I called him later and told him so.

We both told each other "I love you." Before he left that Monday morning, he looked intently at me and my naked body, like he was mesmerized, looking into a mirror, and said, "You're so beautiful." I walked gracefully toward him like a confident gazelle and said, "I feel beautiful and innocent," with a smile on my lips and a tear in the corner of my eye. It was the first time I could say that out loud to anybody. That's why tears hugged my words.

My eyes and mouth seemed to grow stronger and stronger in their connec-tion. As I held my newborn granddaughter Riley Shea the day after she was born, and her eyes opened to mine, I said, "Grandma is **look**ing at you," a glistening tear in attendance. Later that afternoon, I thought, "Riley's **look**ing at me," and tears settled on the top of my cheekbone, settling there as if invited to dinner, and then they fell down my cheeks, two or three of them. I had to choke back my tears; all of us were trying to take naps.

I love remembering the touch of Megan's skin as she pushed Riley Shea into this world, (July 3, 2002) her left leg against my abdomen, my fingers on her soft creamy legs…I was a mother "in the flesh" again. I loved that our blue eyes met frequently, as they did with her husband Ben's who held her right leg as she pushed. And when Megan nursed Riley she was at ease with me touching her breasts to help Riley latch onto her. We were all one "<u>in</u> Love.'"

That evening I read until 1:30am, and still was not sleepy, so I self-loved with images of various people other than past boyfriends, some unusual to appear, and then Johnny, until I finally climaxed in a haze of calm "Oh god oh god, I love you, I love you," feeling that I was saying it to Me! When I returned to the hospital the next day, Megan told me that she had cried when she asked the nurse to take Riley for a couple of hours so that she could sleep. I was so happy that she felt it easy to share her vulnerability, her heart, with me.

Later, I initiated a game of sorts with Megan and Ben. I had been thinking lately of what my best characteristic or quality IS. So we told each other what we each thought the other's best quality was. For a long time, I had heard others say in conversations how persistent I am. Persistence to **grow**, to **love**, to **know**…all four-letter words. It dawned on me how four-letter words truly ground us to who we really are and can be…to **LOOK** being a big one during those days. Ben admitted spontaneously that he had cried when *look*ing at Riley. Even **hate** and **soul** and **hear**, to **kiss**, to **bear**, to **fear**, to **hurt**, to be **seen**. To **mean**, **lean**, **help** and be **born**! (And hell, damn, kill, rage, shit, evil, live, safe, good, home, all like the <u>four</u> seasons.)

When I returned to Megan and Ben's apartment, I vacuumed and as I dusted, I came across a postcard I'd sent Megan fitted into the frame of her mirror, then, just a pretty picture of me in that same mirror. I am also in a photo on the refrigerator where Megan is holding me…I sobbed as I realized how important I am to her, and have not been to my Self, and how much love I have now and had lost because I wasn't that important to my mother. I had snot running into my mouth as I sighed and felt my chest filling up with love for <u>Me</u> and <u>Me</u>gan right then☺

Megan told me that my best characteristic is my honesty; that I am the most honest person she knows. Ben said that my best quality is that I can take criticism. It was a fun and revealing game to all of us! I felt so loved and close to my precious family who wanted me to participate in the birth of their first baby.

When I returned home from Boston, I met Johnny at a swing dance held in a pavilion on the shore of Cayuga Lake. Later, we had a slow lovemaking shower and then climbed into bed before he entered me. Within ten minutes he was so hot that he came full blast with loud vocal sounds that lasted more than a minute. He ejaculated a puddle, afterwards saying, "I feel so safe with you, I don't think I have ever felt so safe. Thank you for letting me get close to you." It felt like he was all there with me. Being there. I was very hot after his orgasm, but fell asleep easily, surprisingly. He was very caring, and I said I was okay, and if I had to wake him, I would. In the morning, he began making love with me, and it seemed that I had an internal orgasm instead of an external one where I am very vocal. We had our eyes open for much of the orgasm, a subtle beautiful wave where I did feel satisfied. As Chopra states, "Love is not about orgasm; it's about surrender to the other person." (pg. 264, *The Path to Love.*)

During a conversation that we had the next day about whether we could still be sexual with our exs, whom we have loved and do love differently at this time, I said that I could if they continued to take care of themselves physically. I need to be attracted on all levels including the physical where lovers keep their bodies attractive. Johnny was elated that I felt this way because for twenty years he had heard others say that the physical should not matter. Why not? It is part of the whole person, and reflects how they feel about themselves. As I have written earlier, religion tries to deny parts of ourselves that threaten its view of the world: it needs to control so that we all can (falsely) feel secure. Their message being, if tempted by our physical beauty, which god created in us, we will fall out of Love.

Before I flew to Italy for two weeks, Johnny and I made love deliciously, in various positions, ending in sixty-nine, on our sides, where I screamed an orgasm that the neighbors could hear. Immediately, I wanted my lover inside me. WE enjoyed intercourse for a long time; Johnny came close to climax, but didn't come, and was fine because our lovemaking was really good. And again at dawn, when we held each other in various ways, and Johnny remarked how wonderful that part of the morning was. He was truly a full-course lover, not just aiming for dessert.

After he read his newest poem, *Good Boyfriend*, which he felt he had to be with his recent girlfriend, he cried, as he said, "It's not fair," to have all that pressure in order to be loved. I just sat with him, like a dark coral lavender sun sets stretching. Like a cat stretching out long as possible. Like the mother who needed to stretch herself to accept all his little boy feelings.

The morning I left for Italy, I called Megan, and sensed that she really needed me, although she had no new-mother questions for me. She told me how hard it was to have Riley nurse more at night than in the daytime. She told me that she loved me, the second time, "I love you, Ma" which I had not heard with "Ma" for years, if ever. She had this desperate childlike voice, and I immediately felt sad, and cried when off the phone, Johnny holding me as I said, "I really love that girl!" I tell you this because I am becoming-feeling clearer that as I cry, it truly is for my Self. I am really saying those words to 'little Dianea,' as I say them about

Megan! My tears are bringing the loving spirit of Dianea back home.

As I drove out of my driveway, listening to Rachmaninoff on NPR, I was moved to stop the car at Treman Park's entrance; Johnny's car followed suit.

I said with tears revealing, "I'll miss you!" His holding understood, and we just looked intently into one another. Like Riley's eyes do at me.

How powerful is the child's LOOK – who truly sees us and gives love totally. Completely OPEN, as I kept wondering why I was taking this second trip to Italy. All I could come up with was to BE OPEN to the universe, what it wanted to give me. Johnny said that if some Mario stopped his motorcycle, jump on.

Yes, I would miss Johnny, but not terribly. It would be a good missing, an open missing – the mix of stability with flexibility: another view of openness?

Like the experience I had the first night in Italy? I was traveling with my Lindy-dance partner, Brian and his painter friend, Bill. They had arrived a week earlier, and I met them at the Todi bus terminal. The first morning I slept in while Brian and Bill went to paint the landscape. I had awakened briefly to be disappointed by the price-included continental breakfast and knew I needed more rest. I masturbated because I felt that I might fall to sleep quickly if I touched myself warmly. But instead, I orgasmed in silence. Amazingly, after another thirty minutes I climaxed again, coming in tune with the lyrics "Oh my god" sung ten or twelve times, adding "Oh Johnny" as the last note. It enlivened my whole body like a candle melting down its sides. I slept until 2:30pm when Brian returned.

I had dreamt a very amazing feeling, like I was astral-projecting into a delusional state. It is very difficult to describe. I wondered in the dream whether I would return to a "sane" state. I felt afraid and excited all at once. This happened exactly a year ago today, and had never happened before or since. I wondered if it was a direct reflection of my subconscious knowing that I was in process of becoming more "enlightened" (more sane?) in the realm of Love, as the image in the dream also had huge flashes of light, smoother and fuller than fireworks could be.

When we visited an old church that same day, I felt an un-at-home distant feeling: a bit repulsed by the confessionals and gold-lined art work reminding me of how religion covers up unhealthy behaviors with ornamentation and tradition. Money, I believe, that could be more aptly used to help the poor.

The next day we traveled in our rented station wagon to Florence, where something very special happened. The rain was a welcome relief to the heat of the previous day. We stopped at the Piazza d'Michelangelo, where I had turned away from the "possible love of my life" two years earlier. Despite the rain and fog, I decided to step out of the car, and LOOK at the statute of David.

A deep sadness grew over me like the enfolding fog. Tears, like raindrops, I could not stop! As I viewed the city of Florence, a sense of lost love overwhelmed me. Maybe a past-life love as well? I thought of Johnny as a soul I have known before. I would do a regression to find out later. Brian gave me a hug, and Bill gave me a pat on the back, both not sure what to do.

Throughout the two weeks, we visited many museums and churches full of art that was impressive in detail and ability to show life as it was. Still, I was continually distressed and saddened by all the emphasis on religion, such as Madonna and child and the crucifixion of Jesus. So ornate, in some of the churches I felt overwhelmed, a power play by the church to keep people under their control. I was aware of being open to learning about art, but my biggest lesson was seeing the ignorance and torture by the church.

One painting showed two men with sharp tools placed on the nipples of a woman, ready to cut them off. It was obvious to me that a few rich families and the church ran the people, and did not care about them.

To top my grief off, listen to my experience at the Basilica of San Lorenzo, a church in Florence. While exploring, we saw that a concert was to begin inside, so we sat and waited for the music to begin. When it did, a few tears crept in to say, "You are sad to have been taken in by the church, partly through its music." Church music had caused me to be emotional, cry, and feel badly about myself, so I would be walking to the front of the church, feeling pressured like being with a herd of animals. "Just as I Am" was the usual hymn played as the invitation to accept Jesus as your (only) savior was given at the end of the preacher's sermon. I could not trust my own heart of doubt that knew their words were not true. True, my heart IS!

Unlike the shame I felt as I entered another church where I was closed out because my back showed, wearing my daisy sundress. Shame, shame, shame of the body. At first I was disgusted, then I became sad, then glad that I was out of that prison enclosing heart!

The body is beautiful when cared for...loved.

Brian and I showed this as we danced at three different outdoor plazas, to live music in Florence, Venice and Rome. I felt as light as the clouds that continually caught my eye. And, when resting, reading *Women Who Love Sex*, I remembered and appreciated how Johnny had looked at my vulva, describing it with love and tenderness, how it is delicate with smaller petals than others he has seen.

In Cortona, Brian drew me nude, outside, on a hillside next to a church, overlooking another church. One would have to strain to see us, therefore, I felt comfortable modeling for two hours while holding still for fifteen to twenty minute stints. While I was standing in front of his paintbrush, he asked me what I was thinking about. Surprisingly, I had been thinking about the torture by the Nazis, how Jews had to stand for hours, with no sleep, seeing others shot. I was glad to be looking away from the church, looking higher for real Love.

Brian wanted to know some of my "aha" experiences, many being while crying, making connections with past lives, and present truths like I had had with Brian the day before. While he was driving, I told him that I liked his hands, his large palms reminding me of my father's, handing me tears to wash away more grief of losing his love through death, while filling up my heart-well with Love. So profound is my love for my father that it runs deep enough to lift a tear over my eyelid to slide down my cheek as I said to Brian, "the tear is the **kiss of god**." I love that image! On a bare cheek (which one!) and body!

How Would I Like to be Kissed?

By the light of a crescent moon circling my buttocks –
A ray of touch felt like a distant lightning known as Giovanni's lips.

By the breeze of our breath brushing untouched lips
Close as angel wings.

Dark and light eyes are open – wide – begging
"Look into Me" –
see the shine that presses a tear

to caress my wide cheekbone-
it is the kiss of god.

Roman Italian's molten mouth delicately wisps
The saltiness into our lips,
Flavoring the desire of love.
It is the divine-god in us.

German father's lips are far away as the moon –
A fear pressed by the stamp of church control –
Love flows like the shot of an arrow.
Only my wedding day gave a permit
To know dad's lips to dance on my cheek –
A second of time I must keep.

It is the treasure of god.

The breeze flutters a kiss to my nipples
As I stand on Cortona's grassy hill,
My nakedness covering the church below,

As my eyes look away,
Stayed by the royal sky's rolling clouds,
Strippers of shame –
It is the angel of god.

Our chins lean in slow,
so slow, time stops.
Steady, a hair's width distance held.
Then, sinking like two white butterflies
Together, fluttering, circling for minutes –
It is the tender kiss of love
I find to BE on my lips.

Love is the contrast to the "outrageous" (Bill's word) religiosity I experienced at the Vatican, where, again, I was not allowed in because I had shorts on and my back was exposed. It was no great loss, as I was overloaded with the pompous, superficial, ornamental, gaudy (not goddy:), overindulgent way of these churches. One of the last churches I visited had two fat priests hearing confession, one using a rosary, and I made a strong statement to Brian about the repression by the church, and its arrogance to say that one has to go through a priest to talk to god! Or use rote prayers because we cannot communicate what is personally on our hearts?

Brian reacted by saying that I act like a priest, because my clients confess to me. No, I said, they are not confessing their sins to me; they are "confessing" their hurts, fears, and other feelings to me. Not their wrongdoings! Besides, I am not saying I am needed to find god, or the only way to god. I am helping others to find their own way to the divine within themselves as well as without.

I liked the architecture of many of the old ruins, buildings as well as churches. The power of their simplicity and the human-form statues heartened me like the reality of the bare truth of our feelings. Why I am glad to no longer be ashamed of my bare-naked body, simple on the outside, complex on the inside?

Brian and I had spirited arguments, or disagreements, which later got termed wrangles which he did not like. Bill said that he did, because it expands who we are to be open to different points of view. By the end of our two weeks together in Italy, I knew that my purpose there was just to be OPEN, the word kept ringing in my ears and eyes and cells of my body. I could share a room with two men-friends, walk around naked and be perfectly safe. As Brian and I slept on the cold floor of the Rome airport, waiting for our 6am flight home, it was cold in air temperature, but warm in heart-spirit as Brian held me in the spoon position.

We had shared much beauty together: the fields of sunflowers, the art and architecture, the food, the swimming, the canals of Venice, the marble statutes, the dances, the exploring of new people and places, as well as the old, and sweet laughter. I remember noticing my ready and boisterous laughter, louder than the guys while watching performers at the Piazza Novana in Rome. I was coming *home*.

When I woke up at 6:30am in my bed, I knew I needed more sleep, but my feelings took over. I thought of the Italian man I had left behind two years earlier, and my eyes could not help but cry and sob about my lack of openness, acknowledging my coldness to ignore the man who had made an honorable attempt to talk with me. The connection came clearly as to why I had to return to Italy… "I have to come back to remember." To remember my feelings, lost inside a closed-up heart. "To make a place in my heart for you," meaning my Self, then, others can come in. I cried for a half hour, a self-session. I cried again as I related these same feelings to Johnny.

When we began kissing and hugging, I reminded Johnny how he had told me his desire not to be as sexual, just to be inside of me, still. He stopped touching me and began to cry, with a few sobs accenting, "I don't know what to do." I held him and asked if he wanted to talk about it. We eventually began kissing again, and he asked me if I wanted him. I did; I was easily turned on by Johnny. After much face-to-face intercourse, he barely had the head of his penis inside my entrance, my G-spot feeling very lovely. He said, "I love you," after two days of not saying so. We had had a long talk during the weekend, where I learned that he had been sexual with his recent ex-girlfriend, and he knew that he didn't want an emotional relationship with her. He could even admit that it felt like a sexual addiction.

It came out that we both knew that we would not be together for the long term, but still would be primary to each other for the present. We talked more specifically about how I cry at orgasm with masturbation-self loving as well with a lover, and how that experience connects with the real Me, or what "**I am meant to BE**." My tears became heavier and heavier as I told him about finding more and more of "god" coming into me, by grieving the loss of feeling loved for who I really am, not what others want me to Be.

The truth of being able to really Love being the lifeline to our true Self-Spirit validated big time by my "pearls of god."

And again, when Johnny and I made love before leaving my apartment that last weekend in July. We were slow in progression, tender kissing and touching all over our bodies. I thought and then said, "Please be inside me and be still." He chose not to be still, but did move more slowly, which became really arousing on a very subtle touching level, as if feeling the softness of a rose petal. We looked into each other's eyes steadily, Johnny saying, "I like making love with your eyes." We could not help but say, "I love you." Plain, pure and simple. Johnny had been on top of me for maybe thirty minutes, then, I went topside, and rode his penis outside my vagina, sliding through my vulva, which I had not done since our first lovemaking. This time, he seemed to really like this position, and said so later. I was very wet. I came saying strongly, "Oh god, oh god, oh Johnny," flowing into a scream as rich as ice cream. My eyes were open to Johnny's, and my heart could not help but cry out with sobs. I thought, then said, "You stayed with me." I meant that he cared enough to love me, stay with me trying for an orgasm the way I wanted it – not entirely new, but, Johnny looking at me with intent love was more (k)new.

After I told Johnny these connections, he told me, "You're beautiful," me with tears that IS. His words caused more tears. His body joined mine again, and felt that he did not need an orgasm; he was fine. I was surprised that I had met that spiritual place in my body because I had not intended to. Must be, I was open. There was an overflowing **feeling** of Love; I could not resist orgasm.

Clear as the water in my eyes, I was <u>staying</u> with my feelings, to Love my Self.

Tears continued to fill my heart with Love, where inadequate love growing up could not. I had experienced the widest freedom to cry at orgasm with Johnny. He was smiling; he seemed so pleased to be a part of the whole experience, and said that to be true, later.

I wondered about my new openness in regard to an interaction in a movie that felt very real to Johnny. It happened in *Vanilla Sky*, when Cameron Diaz said to Tom Cruise that having intercourse was your body making a promise to be together. To Love. But does that mean one needs to be monogamous?

It makes sense to me that for the majority of us, in this time of our evolution, that monogamy functions to help us not easily flee intimacy, the expression of vulnerable feelings, the key to Love. My own exploration into a healthy non-monogamy will have to be left to my next book.

It is clear to me that Johnny being able to communicate his feelings safely for two days after my return from Italy, is what led him to say again, more than once, "I love you." As was my openness with many tears in acknowledging my rejection of the Italian man two years earlier as due to the coldness of my heart…due to fear of being wholly OPEN. Open-hearted!

It had been a monumental weekend, where Johnny had experienced a very vocal orgasm, and I had a body-wracking orgasm from oral loving, when after shouting "Oh gods" I rolled off of Johnny and laughed and laughed, saying, "I can't do anything!" I was so out of control; Johnny laughed and smiled widely.

Also, I had had my first real intercourse orgasm without clitoral stimulation and him fully inside of me. (I had had a rare intercourse orgasm predicated on clitoral feeling when the penis was not totally inside.) The intercourse orgasm was full, but not as intense as my clitoral orgasms.

Maybe clitoral orgasms are the wave of the evolving individual who can be secure in their own sense of self, and grow into interdependence, not foster the co-dependence of being as one, where we want others to be the reflection of ourselves. Our lack of Self-Love has promoted our disconnect from reality (realness) by eliciting vows of security ('til death do us part) in the traditional marriage vows, instead of growing to KNOW and FEEL that we are lovable and can bear the loss of a love partner.

The fears of being abandoned by my parents are the reasons I cried at orgasm with Johnny and during my session that week when I said, "You stayed with me." In my session I cried loudly, and kicked my feet when I said, "Why couldn't we talk about it?" Daddy had left me at sixteen, alone, to feel the pain of learning in anger that he was not my biological father. I was hurting badly and needed my father to come and stay with me and my feelings…talk about it…be reassured of his love.

Sixteen was a huge turning point in my life, unconsciously, realizing I had to handle my hurt-grief-sadness on my own. My heart had turned cold, and contributed to me turning my back on the Italian man who just wanted to talk with me.

My dad and I were so close, and yet so far, because of feelings being oppressed by our religious beliefs, and learned defenses, which protected our selves from feeling our vulnerable feelings. This is true for all of us to some degree depending on how well-loved we have been in childhood. And, hopefully the reader is recognizing how crying, especially at orgasm, has drawn me into the integration of spirit and sex, having what I would like to call "spiritual orgasms."

Johnny and I continued to see each other on the weekends and to make love both days, usually twice each day because we were sharing deep feelings that caused us to feel very close and loved. Our lovemaking joined with creativity. After dancing one August evening, it was still very warm in my apartment, so Johnny wanted to go for a walk under the stars, and we ended up under an arbor where the neighbor's relatives were married the previous weekend. We began "making out" which led Johnny to remove my underpants, and me to unbuckle his belt so that his pants fell to his ankles. Soon he was inside me, with me hanging from the arbor, becoming my favorite flower, the Morning Glory.

I saw a short shooting star as Johnny had a long loud orgasm of "aaaaahhhh-hhhhhhhs" after saying, "I love you," "You're mine" and "You're the best." I enjoyed watching his ecstasy. I knew he was becoming freer with his orgasms as he was being more open about his true feelings. We climbed into bed at 1:11am.

When Johnny woke me the next morning with his erection between my legs, my buttocks began to gently pulsate, squeezing and hugging him. We had slow foreplay with his tongue titillating my clitoris, before he entered me. When we slowed intercourse, really slowed, I felt increasingly excited, like stepping onto a plane for a visit to a new country. After thirty minutes or so, Johnny said he was ready to stop. As I laid next to him, I felt like touching my self and so lightly feathered my clitoris, while Johnny fingered my electric nipples. With in five minutes I commenced a beautiful orgasm of "Oh gods, and oh Johnny," looking at him as I came. Once again, I began to cry for several minutes as I said, "I love you so much." Immediately, I thought: I am loving my Self by proceeding with what I needed. And Johnny gave so readily.

I had allowed my Self to Love Me! And, that is the loss: the grief of me having not been able to give Love to mySelf. Just like Johnny's pain. Mirrors.

When he finally left the bed, we just gazed at each other's nakedness, he saying how beautiful I am. As he stood at the bedroom door, me leaning back on the bed, I said, "I love your dark eyes and how you use them," with tears to accent how I AM really SEEN. He kissed my tears with smiles of Love. We were so free with each other. Freer to come closer to Real Love!

"Art is the culture of the beautiful, but the greater art is to live well," a quote I read at an art opening. Johnny being an artist, I shared it with him on the phone. Then added, "The greater art is to Love well."

Isn't it fascinating that "art" is an integral part of the word, "he_art_?"

The next time Johnny and I made love, we began in the evening outside on the porch sofa and continued in my double bed that looks out across a long green valley of trees, with only sky above. Neither of us orgasmed, yet we created several sweaty "I love yous." When Johnny woke up the next morning, it was raining. He asked, "Can I get inside you?" before I was awake or warmed up. I said yes and we made sweet pleasurable love for close to an hour. Later he told me that he wanted to be connected with the rain.

What a metaphor for connecting with tears!

After doing yoga together, and while eating bagels with sips of Ovaltine, we became engrossed in a long conversation about my book and we disagreed on my use of EVOL=LOVE as a reflection of how everything in the universe is connected, even language. Johnny said they are "coincidences," and that it is "superstitious" to put so much meaning into these coincidences. I continued on about synchronicity, by asking what words he could see in the word HEART. He replied firstly with "*art*," then, "*he, hear* and *ear*."

I knew in my heart that he could not know or feel this truth about synchronicity (connectedness he had just sought by wishing to be "inside of me" while it rained) until he experienced more letting go of his emotional pain. That is why I can also see the word "tear" in the word "heart." Just switch the "h" and "t."

Johnny did admit that reason does not run our lives, that emotion does, and that my therapy-type would help his oldest daughter. He is glad I can be my own person. Be naked not only with feelings, but also with my body as I walked around the kitchen naked as he watched. Again, as I watched his eyes looking into mine during my next intercourse orgasm, I was on the brink of tears and laughter. Was I expanding my orgasm capabilities as I moved forward in my growth toward Love?

I was the one who pushed Johnny to be more open in what we shared in an intimately loving relationship. I don't want to hide anything, whereas he believed that it was considerate to not burden one another with having to consider what the other might say…like how one spent their extra money after the bills were paid. I want to be able to hear the approval/disapproval, and still accept one another's differences as well as have the opportunity to learn another way of being that might be helpful to me.

Johnny admitted that he could not have shared his opinion about me being "superstitious" with his recent psychotherapist girlfriend, because it would have caused too much conflict. Whereas, he felt safe with me because I am non-reactive while being strong in my opinions. As well known psychotherapist Fritz Perls stated, "Contact is the appreciation of differences." It is refreshing as rain to notice how I am growing to accept my Self without other's approval.

As refreshing as one of my client's statements, "I thought what I was thinking was a FEELING." Katie had been treated for depression for ten years before reaching me, mostly with cognitive (thinking) psychotherapies. She'd been on and off antidepressants as well. She cried easily and a lot, and had recently reached her rage which scared her. As I supported her to connect these feelings to her childhood pain, she realized, "I'm so much more aware of how I don't want to feel my feelings – being with them versus surviving them. I got so lost from feeling my feelings like children do. Oh my god." The "Oh my god" came spontaneously, I believe, as recognition of a huge change in being able to connect with her true Self.

One August morning I had close to a full body orgasm after debating whether to masturbate. A cool breeze swept over my clitoris, urging me to touch myself while lying on my back, then while on my stomach, where within minutes I was exploding "Oh god, oh god, oh god, oh god," waves of pleasure. Up from my feet, into my trunk, not quite reaching my head. I was reminded of a spontaneous statement I had made to a client, "I listen to god at orgasm."

Now, because I am connected to little Dianea, I feel the divine (god) whenever I cry. Both instances, crying and orgasm, are at the moments of losing control, being totally vulnerable to our spirit's true Being. Human Being at its best. "There is no such thing as crying too much – we simply cry until we are through, and we are through when the underlying energy of hurt is spent. Likewise there is no such thing as laughing too hard or getting too angry or grieving beyond measure." (pg. 265, *The Path to Love*, by Deepak Chopra) And, all those feelings NEED to BE connected to their source or else you will not be freed of them, but caught in the unending patterns or cycles of resentment underlying depression and anxiety.

When Johnny and I next made love in the morning, I had initiated by rubbing my clitoris on his thigh, eventually moving my hand up and down his penis, undulating together for maybe ten minutes. It was very erotic for both of us, and it seemed that every time we made love, something different happened. We were inside and outside of each other as I climbed a high wave of pleasure for a long time. Eventually, I had a vaginal orgasm accompanying many "Oh gods" and "Oh Johnny I love you," our eyes reaching for each others', his fingers on my high-volt nipples. I cried as I thought to myself, "I want you to tell me I love you," and he didn't at this time. I thought of Daddy and how I wanted to look into his eyes and have him <u>tell</u> me "I love you." It was so clear to me how my tears were connected to parental loss of love, and that I was loving Johnny for supporting me into that connection to my vulnerable true Self.

The next day while writing the above in my journal I was aroused to masturbate, and had a bombastic, legs elevated off the sofa, head arched way back, orgasm, where I said, "I know you love Me the best!" several times. I knew I was talking to my Self. I remembered how a stranger had come to our table at brunch that weekend and said to me,

"You are so gorgeous, if I had a figure like yours, I'd flaunt it too." I took her hand and thanked her, as for one of the first times in my life I was not embarrassed to have my physicality appreciated, yet it is still a bit difficult to write it down here. I had on a beige tango skirt that covered my knees and exposed my navel; Johnny said my hips and waist are very sensual. It is still not easy to appreciate my outer beauty, yet it reflects the inner.

When we returned to Johnny's apartment, he opened his mailbox, and there laid my postcard to him from Venice sent three weeks earlier! All I could say was, "Isn't this synchronicity?" He just smiled.

After Johnny and I discussed which of us was more innocent or naïve, I read some of my journal to him, which unleashed tears. It related how dad had proposed to mom in Tarrytown, NY, where mom was considering giving me up for adoption. Johnny looked at my tears and said, "You can't love him enough, can you?" (tearful now) No, I can't, because he is the doorway to loving my Self, and I had written, "I hope to love him more and more."

After our powerful conversation, Johnny cried briefly while saying he's confused and doesn't know how to make decisions for himself. I knew we were becoming more intimate, as he also confessed that weekend that he had made love once with his ex-girlfriend while I was in Italy, and had been dishonest with me. I was hurt but had little bodily reaction. He tried to defend himself by saying that we had not agreed to tell each other about our sexual encounters. I knew that I had specifically said we needed to when there was more than kissing or hugging. That hurt me most that he had not respected me enough to clearly remember. I'd asked him if he had been sexual when I returned from Italy and he had said no. That hurt the trust between us, although he had chosen to tell me now. He didn't like himself for not being honest, good! He agreed that having sex or making love with someone is significant and should not be hidden because we were learning and wanting to be whole. In Love. He still feared the rejection, ultimately to be unloved and alone. He told me that he believes that pain and hurt are here to help us grow yet, he is still afraid to practice facing his fear because he has not grieved enough of his own childhood pain. He took a step and I loved him for it, feeling he loved me the best to be able to take that vulnerable step with me. I noticed what I predominantly wanted my life goal to be: to be the 'best' in the ability to give Real Love.

I wrote in my journal, "I have the freedom to move into other relationships that will bring me more real well love. The 'well' was not intentionally written, my pen just wrote from my unconscious 'well.'☺ "So I can see that my pain and joy are one."

Or is it Love that IS ONE…the One connecter to everything? Why I told Johnny that I do not want any hate in my heart. He tried to argue that there are good sides to hate because it makes you change things. I would call that anger that motivates change and the true motivator underneath anger is our ability to Love that promotes the most change. For we know that being angry alienates people, whereas kindness and non-violence bring lasting change. Martin Luther King, Rosa Parks, and Ghandi are just a few who have given worth to my words.

I am trekking toward an ideal world where real love can exist, and hate cannot abide there, like oil and vinegar do not mix. I know this world is far off, but I am a stepping-stone into it, as was my father, who was born in Germany.

Now, my link to my German family is through my twenty-four-year-old cousin Damien, who emails me bimonthly from France and when he visits my Aunt Resi in Dreis, Germany, where she and dad were born. Resi is my father's only living sibling, his youngest sister who cannot speak English. Yet, when I called while Damien was visiting, Resi said hello, and "Ich liebe dich," as we said goodbye. It means "I love you" in German, and astoundingly, my first husband, Chuck had chosen that titled song to sing to me at our wedding! Are we not all connected?!

When Johnny and I went to bed the night of his admitted lie to me, I read out loud a Reader's Write article about "Falling In Love" from the SUN magazine, which made us laugh and relate to these personal journeys. Johnny was sleepy so we did not make love which we were both fine with, sinking into our acceptance and love of his "Glad I told you." It was good to notice that we did not have to reinforce our Love physically. We felt more within our spirits, coming alive in honesty and openness.

We made very special love the next morning without bombastic orgasms, but I felt two or three internal ones with oral loving. What was so special was how we looked at each other, and me saying "I love you" without him returning those words, when Johnny was inside of me. Because I felt so much love for me from the way Johnny was kissing and looking at me, I said, "I love you too," once more. And I was fine not hearing it back. I knew I would hear it when he *wanted* to say it. When we walked to his car he said, "I love you" twice. All I responded with was, "You know my love for you?" "Yes."

We had given each other much pleasure in our lovemaking with much touching, kissing, looking, slow-talking, telling him what physical qualities I appreciated about him: his muscles, his dark eyes. A wonderful lover. He picked me up in his arms, carried me out of my bed, over to the large mirror, where we gazed at each other's aging bodies for several minutes – really LOOKed with eyes and arms around each other.

After the mirror gazing, I asked Johnny to get inside me and for us to be still with each other for a few minutes. Although he was not totally erect, we were connected with love. I felt it like how a turtle might feel its shell without seeing or hearing its presence.

The day before when I had asked Johnny what he liked about sex with Ellen that was different from me, he became embarrassed and didn't want to say. I understood and knew that he would eventually tell me, one exposure at a time. I had told him how sometimes, I saw images of friends, family, and recently flowers instead of mountains when I self-loved. And, on that weekend I had thought of a respected friend, Paul, who I am not attracted to, while orally loving Johnny. It was rare that I would think of others while making love with Johnny, and it felt strange to do so, although good to be able to tell him. It was interesting to notice how my images were changing, and how they happened less and less often. It was my growing openness to be able to share everything I wished to without being afraid.

I would whether he did or not. Johnny admitted that maybe he didn't want to hear of a sexual-making love encounter I might have had with another man, as he was doing with Ellen. It appears all connected; all of us are afraid of losing love, as we did as young children. And, as Johnny and I shared vulnerable questions and experiences, we helped each other become less fearful. Feel safe. Feel loved.

Even though we loved each other more deeply as we spent more time together, I wondered if I could be "in love" with him. I wondered how I had not picked up on Johnny's lying to me. It was good to realize how trusting I am; being very grateful for having that childlike quality still in me. Paradoxically, triggered by Gregory's distrust; trust deepened in my Self through grieving, resulting in a stronger belief in core human goodness.

Johnny validated that human desire to be good with truthfulness when he emailed me the next day that he had told Ellen that "we (Johnny and I) have no secrets!" I continue to sense that it is the purpose of life, to evolve to the best real love that can be known. And synchronicities continue to happen frequently to underpin my confidence in our human journey.

I was looking for a piece of paper on which I had written notes for a poem about Johnny. I didn't see it in my journal at first, so searched in my recycle bin, and found two pieces of unopened mail. One was a check from a client. What a great way to turn a mistake into a whole lot of gratitude!

It took only a couple of days for Johnny to tell me that he remained in an ambivalent relationship with Ellen because of the sex. When I pointed out that he did not feel the need to make love with me the night that he revealed his dishonesty to me, he admitted that he used "sex" to patch things up, to feel connected. (Really, to feel loved, I thought to myself.) He had not noticed the connection of not needing sex after I had been accepting of his vulnerable disclosure. It was good to hear him say that he grows with me in his life in ways he has not before…that he is in a deeper honesty.

He was realizing how he softened the truth because of fear of Ellen's reactions, feeling helpless to get her to understand him, to accept him, and so he had also protected himself from facing his fears. The growing understanding of our true selves grew more "I love yous" between us. That same week, when Johnny saw Ellen, she invited him to sleep with her and he refused. She became "pissed off" and he reacted in anger, repeating their pattern of not sharing their hurts, and therefore not feeling understood. Johnny told me later that he loved his new way of being: without secrets, and being more independent. Initially, Johnny had been annoyed with me "pushing" him to this point of greater intimacy, but now he was happy for it. As a plant pushes up through rocks and dirt, so must we as human beings…it is painful and oh so rewarding.

A poem for Johnny:

> Making love with Johnny is like a mathematical theorem,
> Making infinity only a fraction of what love can be.
> It needs no proof -
> He scales the roof of my mouth, my vagina,
> The roof of my soul.
> The urgency to add, subtract, or divide
> Succumbs to the equalizing of finite fingertips flirting with my nipples,
> Resulting in real numbers of ooooooooooooohhs and ahhhhhhhhhhhhhhhhs,
> "Oh gods" one more time,
> Be inside me, without movement,
> Eyes open, filling me with Love.

This same month of August, I began to respond to my interest in a dancer named Bill, whom I had met a year earlier and danced with a few times at ballroom dances. He taught ballroom steps to me, and I felt attracted to his broad shoulders and long, wavy silver hair, as well as to his smooth graceful dancing. We felt the music the same.

At an Argentine tango dance, Jerry had literally swept me off my feet during a move I had never done before. He thanked me for asking him to dance. I began pursuing information as to how to get hold of him, as he lived an hour away from me. And I told Johnny.

Ellen continued to ask Johnny to have sex with her until she found another man in her life. I had mixed feelings about it. He said he was afraid to have sex with her, fearing I'd leave him. Yet, he didn't want to be controlled by that fear.

I knew I was loved most, but still did not like having her that close to him physically. Why not, I asked myself. Maybe because he tells her that he loves her? So what? Why not share the love? I wanted to be *special* on all levels of intimacy: physically, emotionally and spiritually. I concluded that I needed to talk about the sexual differences between Ellen and me. That deep intimacy level is what I really wanted.

When Johnny called late one night after being with Ellen, but choosing not to be sexual with her, I was relieved to hear that he wanted to know what he was getting out of being sexual with her, and didn't know as yet. I responded, "That's great!" Johnny began to cry. He said, "I feel understood, what I don't get from Ellen." He said that he felt interrogated by her, and although I asked similar questions, he didn't feel that way with me. "I trust you!" came pouring from his quivering lips. That was the best statement I could have heard. Trust being the foundation of Love.

I knew that I did not press him with expectations to always please me. I gave him space, time, to process and feel his feelings as I pushed for change, insight into deeper intimacy. Johnny also told me that he sees that I am not hurt as easily as Ellen, yet I am vulnerable around feelings that connect to my past. I take responsibility for my emotional pain, feel it, grieve it, therefore, I am less reactive and needy. And, able to find a deeper love within.

When Johnny emailed me later, he told me that Ellen's love for him, being desired (she wanted to marry him), and being pleasured contributed to his vulnerability with her. A few days later, he added that it was her devotion to him. His surety of her love, which he admitted he was not sure of from me…on a long term committed basis that is.

When I cried in my session that week, I made the connection of needing to feel special with my fear that I would not have anyone to love me if Daddy left, because my mother didn't love me. I grieved more loss of mother's love, as I continue to do, knowing it was my childhood "unloved" feelings that made me feel if I lost Johnny, I wouldn't have someone to love me. I feel whole when I know and FEEL the distinction between past and present feelings.

I reiterated to Johnny how we were not willing to settle. I am growing sure that I will not settle for anything other than Real Love where I feel I want to commit to someone I am "in love" with. This was why we were in an open relationship where we could be really truthful, loving each other because we would go deeper and deeper by sharing our vulnerable feelings.

We were in similar feeling places, as both of us said, "I love you" as we said good night.

The next morning when I self-loved, I found myself saying, "Come with Me," meaning not just with orgasm, but with me on this deeply loving journey. I confirmed in my heart that I want the whole thing *in love* – the body reflecting the Love within my heart-spirit. Like when my body has a bombastic orgasm with several "Oh gods" and I feel more like god is in Me.

As I do when I look up at the clouds - a full feeling comes over me, like clouds are, full of fluffiness, creative in their shapes, dancing lightly, warm and wise, like Johnny said of my face.

After a few more days went by, having not spent the weekend with Johnny because he was with his daughter and friend on a camping trip, I awoke slowly, enjoying the new day as I have done for the past few years, not knowing what creates in my body a desire to self-love. I had not awakened aroused. I began touching my clitoris while lying on my back, then turned over onto my tummy where I sprinted to an orgasm. It was a very tender light touch on my clitoris, like fluttering hummingbird wings. It was a very steady intense climb to an orgasm of "Oh god, oh god, oh god," being very aware that there were no images; I was purely with my body's sensations – a divine feeling – pure love of some sort! No mind. A universe of Love?

My wardrobe seems to reflect a whole diversity of feelings as well. I have clothes, many from second hand shops, that are elegant, or feminine with lace, or casual as blue jeans and slacks, or sexy clingy tops, or childlike 360 degree circumference skirts with polka dots. When my friend Ken saw me with Erin and nine-year-old Denali, he said Erin and I looked like Denali, not that Denali looked like us. "You all look childlike," Ken laughed. Childlike at fifty, what could be better?

Johnny's huge orgasm? He arrived early Monday morning because he missed me, not being with me over the weekend. He crawled his naked body into bed against my naked sleeping one, saying, "I love you." My body was not aroused although we hugged and kissed, so I licked his penis and then he used it to rub my clitoris and vagina only an inch inside. It was too much pressure to turn me on and he wanted inside me. He "Oooohed" and "Ahhhhhed" intensely like an excited animal and then thrusted with loud "Ooooohs" and "Ahhhhhhhhs," and within a minute or two said, "Can I come?" I said sure and was happy that he was so excited and free to pleasure himself, as his pattern had been to always focus on the woman's pleasure. He had a huge long intense orgasm with ejaculation, as he tried to look at me in the eyes. He was exquisite in his delight and I delighted in him. I was glad I was not turned on myself so I could focus on him, and told him so. Still, there were no "Oh gods." He snoozed as his arms held me in togetherness.

I loved how Johnny looked into himself and expressed his feelings and motivations, as well as took responsibility for them. He also had some awareness of how he was feeling-behaving due to his parental upbringing. We both felt great safety and he told me that he had had the most orgasms with me, greatly due to that trust.

Once again, I am grateful for Daddy who was the foundation for me to build trust so that I could feel that he was the *Love* of my Life, so that I could find Love of *my* Life within Me, through grieving Daddy. Full circle. Whole.

Therefore, I want to honor my father's memory more and more. On a whim, I had sent to SUN magazine a picture of my father holding my sister standing on his right hand, arm extended. Connie was close to one year old, her broad smile reflecting the epitome of trust. I write to this magazine every month on a topic they choose for a Reader's Write column, and I thought this picture would fit their topic of "safety."

I had written SUN every month for three years, and never been published, so I was surprised to receive a letter saying they wished to publish the photo! The only photo I had ever submitted. I was elated until they called to say that the photo did not have sufficient contrast to be published. I was disappointed, but then asked my sister for her copy of the photo, which I had given her. She refused to part with it, even though I said she could have mine if hers was lost somehow. Her fear and lack of trust was amazing to me, although I connected it with her "born again" beliefs, which instill fear big-time!

I began to cry as I told her I wanted it printed to honor dad, and I wished that it had been me he was holding in that picture. I began to feel frustrated: a defensive feeling-word that covers the true feeling of helplessness, because nothing I could say would change her mind.

I even pointed out how unhealthy it is to be so untrusting, while she pointed out that she's healthier because she is saying her feelings, whereas before she would please people. I agreed that was a good step. Then, I gently pulled out the hurt-focused argument. "That's why I am not in your religion anymore because you say you believe god will give you what you need, yet you don't TRUST god to get that photo back to you." I was crying as I said those words, because I had had so little trust in my Self for all those years that I believed in that religious dogma. Spell dogma backwards and you have "am god" and going backwards from that religion, I feel in my spirit that I "am god." We all are. We all have the god-divine born in us. And I am smiling now that I can still Be full of truth about not trusting religion.

"Spirit isn't a phenomenon; it is the whispered truth within a phenomenon. As such, spirit is gentle, it persuades by the softest touch. The messages never get louder, but clearer." (pg. 97, *The Path to Love*, Deepak Chopra) I sobbed in my session that week about how religion sucked away that basic trust in my spirit, and then, as I felt sorry for my Self, I also did for my sister, still under that oppression of the spirit.

It is why I need to honor my father's spirit, to remember what true Love is through feeling my tears, which make my spirit feel more REAL, the word on which I cried loudest.

Sometimes, I wonder if others think I am too serious, when talking about crying like I am throughout this book, thoughts I said out loud when Ben and Megan visited in August 2002. Ben spontaneously said, "You're a good balance of serious and fun," and he is a twenty-nine-year old guy who owns an auto detail shop, jokes much more than me, yet can pursue a serious conversation. His perception of me was a good surprise to hear.

While having dinner with Megan, Ben, Erin, Niki and Denali at the Lost Dog restaurant, we had a discussion about using the word "hate." Erin and Megan decided to pay for the dinner as a birthday present for me. I said, "I strongly dislike that for my birthday present," making us all laugh.

Denali had said, "I hate you," to Erin that week and Erin wanted her to say, "I hate what you do," instead of "I hate <u>you</u>." I ventured my opinion that it was okay to say the feeling hate as she had, as that is what she felt in the moment. Focusing on "what you do," which is the behavior, does not address the feeling of hurt underneath Denali's anger; most likely disappointment, not heard, or misunderstood. It would help everyone if we learned to express our hurts, which then enhances understanding, connection and comfort. Really Love.

What I had become opposed to is the use of the word "kill" in "I want to kill you," when one is hurt-angry. That phrase used to be said by my kids while growing up, and as I became more aware of healthier ways to express feelings I would not permit Erin and Megan to say "kill" because it addresses a behavior and continues the avoidance of saying our true feelings. Also, killing is an act of violence, the language of which does not have a place in a loving household. I was glad that I was becoming sensitive in the 1980s, but I had a long way to go in learning to truly let go of my hurt-pain.

A few days before my birthday in August 2002, I was to experience a healing orgasm that would be unforgettable. The reader is aware that when Johnny visited on the weekends, that we have made love usually morning and night, with growing vulnerability and expression of pleasured Love, although we were still not "in love," as we both wished to be.

After kissing lips, then penis, then penis and clitoris simultaneously, I was satisfied to stop. Yet, somehow, Johnny, who was very respectful of my feelings, began kissing my clitoris lightly, driving me into ecstasy. I had to stop kissing his penis, to be totally with my self, enjoying the waves of intense "please" (pleasure) as I wrote it in my journal. For another ten minutes I knew I was going to orgasm; I knew I was taking care of my Self while Johnny was taking care to love me tenderly. Only a slight hesitation to hear myself think: I'll take too long. I kept enjoying the wonder of it all! "Oh god, oh Johnny, oh god," loudly several times until I spilled into orgasm with shrieks and squeals of Love without "I love yous." Immediately I began to cry before the orgasm could end. I brought Johnny up to my face, not pulling his penis into me as I usually do. A first. I only needed to look into his dark eyes, with tears thinking, "Do you love me?" Then I said my question.

Johnny replied tenderly, "I love you." Kissed me softly. Another "I love you."

He hadn't said those life-based words all weekend while making love, although he had said it once on Saturday after an affectionate kiss. I had said those three love-filled words more than once while we made love without the feeling that I needed to hear it back, which was new in my EVOLution.

But when I was crying I felt like the child again, who wasn't sure of the love of its parents, especially from my mother. It was so CL<u>EA</u>R to Me. In my crying session that week, I added sobs as I said, "Johnny gave to me because he wanted to - can you just love me? I don't have to do anything to get Love…that was such a gift, and made me love him more." And, my Self, of course☺

I am not sure that I can say this too often or too **well**…that these moments of connected childlike tears of grieving lost love are what foster Self-Love. The **well** of pain becomes shallower, as the **well** of Love becomes deeper.

When I asked Johnny how he felt about what happened in this last spectacular orgasm with tears for fears, he replied that he felt "my vulnerability." I answered clearly, "Yes, it's the mirror of you," because he'd been the one to ask me more than once in recent conversations, "Do you love me?" It was one of the most outstanding orgasms of healing, that I will not forget.

I knew that I was becoming stronger in my self worth as I felt less apprehensive in hearing that Johnny made love with Ellen and that he had two Match.com dates in the coming week. He told me that it took too much of his energy to take care of Ellen emotionally, and was glad he didn't feel that way with me. Isn't it the wonderful paradox that being with someone like me who cries easily, no longer angry, yet stands up for herself, is seen as not needing to be taken care of! Because I am now able to take responsibility for my own feelings and not project my insecurities onto someone else, expecting them to make me feel whole. Loved.

As one of my clients said recently, "The easy road is not the happy one."

Johnny said it felt "right" to be with me primarily. As it feels right to me to realize that we talk about raising one's self-esteem, or self-worth, but not self-love. Why is it that most self-help books promote self-esteem or self-worth in their titles, and not self-love?

They all mean the same thing according to the dictionary, with the exception that it does not list self-respect as self-love (amazingly), but as "regard for one's own happiness or advantage."

I find those distinctions as sad, when Love makes: a human being able to be peaceful with one another, a child able to thrive in this world in a constructive way, engenders kindness and tenderness toward all of creation, ultimately to have compassion for all…then why is it that we are not promoting the source-feeling of self-LOVE? Is it still seen as selfish in an unhealthy way? As I said before, as does the bible, "god is love;" it is the divine in us and the best we can Be.

We have much to learn as we EVOLve toward Love, therefore our goal can be said to be to Self-Love, to "raise our self-love" so we can become divine in the way of our BEing. Notice how we have learned to avoid feelings (love) by saying "esteem" or "worth" instead. Our language again mirrors our difficulty developing intimacy with our feelings.

As well, self-love can be reflected in the clothing we wear. Although Johnny was becoming more intimate with his own feelings and their connections back to his family, he did not spend time in a practice that would encourage this spiritual healing. He was not interested enough to finish reading my book, *TEARS ARE TRUTH*. Although Johnny liked me to dress me in colors, he had very little color in his own wardrobe, mostly black, white, or dark shades of blue. I am a child of the rainbow.

I could be more open, tolerate more uncertainty than Johnny. It would be why I would begin to entertain the possibility of a healthy polyamorous relationship. "If you wish to use your relationships in order to become more conscious of your own dysfunctional patterns and buried feelings so that you can release them and increase your capacity for intimacy, polyamory offers you an unparalleled opportunity to do so… Learn to forgive yourself, accept yourself, love yourself. (Doesn't love include forgiveness and acceptance? Parentheses mine) …For many people this will involve parenting yourself and working with your inner child." (*Polyamory: The New Love Without Limits*, pgs. 27, 37) Read about my evolving and exploring in this regard in my next book.

As I let go of my inner child's pain, I find myself becoming more generous. Erin had asked if she could have one of my antiques for an end table in her new home. I thought about it over the weekend and ended up giving her the one that said "Family Soap Company" on it. She was very appreciative and I was proud of my Self for *letting it go*, not being as attached to things. I was practicing my "Family Soap Box" and I even liked the way my room looked better once it was gone. It had more space, as did my heart.

That same week of my birthday, I received two wonderful firsts! Erin telling me "I love you" before I said it, as well as giving me a birthday gift after several years of receiving no card or gift. Still, no card. And my brother sent me a birthday card with, "I love you" written by him. He had said it before, but not written it.

My intuition was improving too. And what does intuition mean? "The power or faculty of attaining to direct knowledge or cognition without evident rational thought and inference," says the dictionary. (Sounds like a feeling defined as "appreciative or responsive awareness or recognition.") I wanted to find an autograph that my mother had written to my father while on the ship where they had met at the end of WWII. I looked in my filing cabinet for a few minutes then paused, and asked where; it is in one of my twenty-plus journals. I scanned through four, paused again, asked where, and the brown one came to mind. I opened it up and there was the autograph in my mother's hand. A surprise of joy!

When I pause and ask, my intuition, or feelings of remembrance have a chance to bubble up, guide me. Next, I thought of my father guiding the autograph to me; I began to cry. He is my guardian angel, who wakes up my intuition, or unconscious, because he has been and is the seed-source of the Love that I AM growing in this lifetime, who guides me to what I need to feel in order to Love my Self again. This is the true "born again" I am genuinely feeling when I said, "Thank you" out loud. Isn't this the spiritual journey of Love we are here to experience?

Isn't this the gui-dance of the spirit within us all? The Great Spirit that the Native Americans speak of? No wonder I love to dance with my guide, my heart of feelings. It is why I ended my essay to SUN magazine's Reader's Write topic, "Falling in Love" with, "I keep falling *in love* with my dad, Michel, every time I remember his great gift of love for me!" I can only think of grief as a lathering-body-wash of love. A spirit wash. For ever so slowly **as I have grieved for the love I miss from my father, the process has melded me to a conscious loving of my Self.** It is very difficult to describe until you experience it through your own source-past-pain tears. Maybe I am like the embroidery thread sewn into a design on cloth. Like the design I created in the seventies on the back of a denim jacket. I drew a copy of a couple dancing, skirt flared, arms holding each other's shoulders. Then I embroidered the design with various colors of thread. The embroidery thread and denim become one, yet are separate. I am like the child in the womb again! That perfect unconditionally loving spirit! Unconsciously, I was falling *in love* with the real Me.

My journal entry September 1, 2002: "I am so glad that I cry about my dad's love for Me. It makes it even more true, if that's possible."

Which became more evident when I made love with Johnny on the weekend of my birthday. After making love for a spell, Johnny wanted to quit and I said,

"What if I masturbate?" "Can I watch?" was his curious reply. I said, "Sure, help me." Johnny played my nipples and soon plunged two fingers inside my vagina, as I feathered my clitoris. It was more difficult than usual to orgasm because I felt some pressure to finish because of Johnny's plans for the day to meet with his children. Still, several "Oh gods" came along with my orgasm, experienced as being the most integrated with my tears, then small sobs like a baby feeling safe in the arms of its parents. I looked into Johnny's eyes, his body over me, without intercourse. Nor did I need him inside of me. The last two times we made love with tears I did not need to be joined with Johnny. I did not need a man inside of me to feel loved…this progression IS so amazing to ME! I love it! Johnny looked into my eyes so lovingly as I cried, looking and hugging so connected with Love. I said, "I love you" into his eyes. Immediately, he replied, twice, "I love you." I said those three world needed words again at the finishing of my tears.

When I asked how it was going with Ellen, Johnny shed tears as he said, "I am not like this; I am a one-woman-man." He told me that he had made love with Ellen the morning of my birthday, and felt badly about it because it felt as if I had been present. I told him that I understood, took his hand and comforted him. We both wanted, ultimately, to be with the one person we are totally in love with. I wasn't quite fully conscious that that one person was my Self or he, himself. Now, I aaaaaaaaaaaaammmmmmmmmmmmm. And, it is fun to see that it is more **ME** that I need to Love than the **ME**N I need for love.

Johnny was not used to being this open, where he would tell each woman about the other. I have expected this kind of openness and honesty, and made it safe, possible for him to say, "I'm glad I told you about this." He didn't want to because he thought it would hurt me too much, when it would really hurt him to see me hurt. SEEing me hurt would trigger his own pain. I reiterated that it shows respect for someone when you tell the truth despite the hurt. It means that the person is capable of bearing the hurt, grief, which ultimately brings us into deeper intimacy, a capability to Really Love. I replied, "I'm hurt and I'm resilient." I liked that a lot!

As I do our spirits' continual push to EVOLve into profound Love, where violence of any kind does not exist. Like the conversation Johnny and I had over his use of the word "kick" when he said he'd like to kick Maha, my cat, out from between us. I noted that it was a violent way to deal with Maha, and that I wished that he'd used a gentler word. He responded that I was too precise in my use of words, and that he wished to be able to talk in a way that allowed levels of meanings of words, and that he missed that in our relationship. I did not pursue the discussion, just remarked that I am trying to encourage a gentler, kinder, more loving world where harsh words are not necessary. Like: kill, bitch, stupid, mother-fucker, asshole, etc. To see more of the gentler side, like Johnny and me picking up garbage along Cascadilla Gorge.

Or me not having to worry whether Johnny replies in kind to my "I love you," knowing it is more real if said when he feels it, not said for the purpose to soothe my insecurity. My fear. How wonderful it was to laugh with Johnny in the shower, when I told him about my son-in-law's idea to put duct tape on Johnny while he was sleeping, to pull off the hair on his back. I was proud to be with him.

And, to be more with Me as I told about my growing vulnerable orgasms to my friend, Sue. I cried as I spoke, "How I knew that when I said, 'I love you' to Johnny, that I was saying those three immense and intense words to little Dianea. How I didn't need a man inside me to feel loved. How excited I am to have the immediate integration of orgasm and crying, which I sensed as truly being 'in love' with one's own spirit."

That's the whole "IN LOVE" purpose! To integrate sexuality with spirituality!

That was the main purpose of Johnny in my life at that time, and I felt very lucky. It was my first Labor Day weekend alone where I felt I was metaphorically in labor, the birthing of a major part of my true Self. I was at a place where I was accepting things as they come and go easily. I was learning to "go with the flow." Like my Morning Glories, big, blue and beautiful, as they wound around the trellis, growing with the flow of the (di)vine.

I understood how Johnny would feel more warmth from Ellen, who was in love with him, and I was not quite. I was more detached; yet very connected through our long conversations, our heart-to-heart tear-present *interchanges*. I felt more of being a "separate" person. I cried big tears during that week's crying session as I said the word <u>separate</u>, when I said, "I'm more of a *separate* person, more attached to my Self, my inner Self, understanding that I am a separate human being." Meaning: I am who I am, and not what others want Me to Be. Johnny told me again how he valued the honesty and growth that I pushed him into although it is "uncomfortable." This is what I can call "good hurt."

Then, Johnny noted how he loves me more when he sees me being playful, like when we hiked with Erin, Niki and Denali in Treman State Park. The child-likeness: one minute able to cry and hug, the next to laugh and snug☺

That childlike ability to show all of ourselves comes from a foundation of trust. The lack of being trusted is what broke Gregory and me apart, and triggered me again when I received his poem in September 2002. Many sweet loving words, but so little Love, because he once again asked me to admit that I had been at his daughter Sara's high school graduation when I had not. In his delusional state, he thought he had seen me just three feet away, yet he could not speak to me. Love cannot lie! He does not trust that I don't lie. Therefore, there is little love. I was sad and hurt that I was not known for who I am. Just as Gregory believed a lie about me, I was triggered into my old pain of living a lie as a "born-again christian." I grieved more of this core pain of abandoning myself to religious beliefs, and was able to let go of the hurt Gregory triggered in me. This is the beauty of this spirit-retrieval process, where anger and resentment do not abide. And TRUST does. (My next book, *TEARS ARE TRUST…waiting to be felt,* is expected to be published in 2006.)

At this time I was impressed in a deeper way by the importance of remembering, not only the present, but the past, the necessity to feel it, then you become more present. The fascinating paradoxical circle of life.

My remembering of the past happened often and again as I looked into Johnny's eyes once more and began to cry, as I said, "It's the way you *look* and *see* me as I am!" He replies, "I love you," which speeds up my tears. We hold each other for maybe thirty seconds before I feel like saying, "I love you back." Later, I asked how he felt when I had cried that morning coming off an orgasm with intercourse where I looked into Johnny's eyes as I vocalized "Ohhs, ahhhs" and "Oh gods." He was so present with me that my tears appeared as if a curtain was lifting from the stage of life, where there is only real love. Not love, buried by fear of what others think or disapprove of. Tears of freedom to Love! I remembered saying "I love you" in a whisper, into his eyes, well before my orgasm, on my way, to more love. And after my orgasm, I said a poem so naturally:

It's when I look and feel,

That our love becomes real!

My spirit appeared totally free in those moments. Thank you Johnny.

He said that he felt "normal" as he witnessed my tears, and "sympathy." He did not say loving, but agreed that one needs to love the Self before one can truly love another. That is why he was primarily with me, and not Ellen, because he was listening to what he needed more than pleasing another out of fear of not being loved by her.

And my Self was more aware of receiving Love from my Self than from men, or sex with men, as I had in the past. A complete wonderful circle where I would feel growing love for Johnny after vulnerable moments of tear-filled sharing, exposing our true Being. The child who had hidden for so long.

Still, Johnny would ask me, referring to Gregory, "How can you love someone so emotionally disturbed? Abusive to you?"

"By feeling my childhood pain (and sometimes past life pain); a 'letting go' yes changes how one's heart feels, that's how!"

Johnny was beginning to understand, but still couldn't feel it inside himself, until he released more of his childhood pain. Because he was becoming more real with his feelings with Ellen, they had better lovemaking, was less about sex. He was loving himSelf by saying his real feelings. He appreciated how freely he could express his feelings with me, and recognized he could express more with Ellen because of safety with me.

Still, he told me that he was thinking about breaking up with me because I was not "in love" with him and not a part of his artistic community, and lived too far away. I was surprised that I did not feel more rejection, even though I had no illusions about us being "the one" for each other. I was really okay with Johnny loving us both, and I knew he appreciated me and valued me for the growth in his heart. And I, for mine.

The process is like seeing, from our canoe, the huge one hundred-year-old tree stump root system that had drifted onto the Adirondack Stillwater Lake's shore. The intricacies of the root system were/are (w)holy beautiful: smooth, curvaceous, interweaving like a tapestry of ropes that connected to the heart of the earth. Roots so full of Love! A life metaphor for the work I do, deep into the ROOT of Love.

As does the other side of the earth, the sky full of stars at night. We saw the Aurora Borealis show up, flashing lights over and on us as the stars reflected in the lake's smooth surface like fireflies of the sky swimming at night. When we saw a short shooting star, Johnny told me that he imagined that my father would be looking into the stars and **know**ing the universe. Is Love? My tears appeared like the short shooting star, out of nowhere. The sadness of not **know**ing Daddy or my Self deeply. The Oneness of it all equals Love, which constantly dashes and flashes to us the universe's glory. If we can more than notice. Slow down. Be still. Take time to <u>feel</u> as Johnny did after a scary fire while making dinner on his camping stove.

He had made some navigating mistakes in the car, and on the lake, which were small and easily corrected, and had not screwed the camp stove valve on tight enough. He laid nude on the bear blanket, and said that he felt like crying. I rubbed his back and head, and hurt arm, then his tears flowed as I heard him say, "I feel lost, I've lost my self-confidence." He sobbed, and cried for fifteen or twenty minutes, then sat up and leaned into my arms, saying, "I miss my wife; I feel alone."

All I could say was, "Yes," and BE with him. I felt happy that he felt safe with me. Later, he asked again what I get from him.

"You are open to my pain, patient, give support, look, do not run away."

"Is our relationship equal?" he queried.

I could not answer.

When I asked Johnny what was the soul purpose of life, I was surprised by his answers. "Fulfillment," then "Happiness," then I asked what made those possible?

"By accomplishing something," Johnny retorted.

"And how does that happen?"

"Through Love," Johnny said slightly exasperated.

"Yes!" How difficult it is to reveal the source, deep Truth. None of us want to face pain, although it is our greatest teacher. I am beginning to embrace, HOLD, this awesome teacher☺ because my tears are becoming gentler in their flow.

I embraced my Beloved, then flowed through Johnny as we began to make love under the twinkling stars on the sandy beach. Although, at first, I was not into "it" I knew I would change as we slowly touched, although I thought and felt that he wanted intercourse too soon. I let the stars above us bury me with awe, as Johnny had a full- blown orgasm with "Ahaaahhhhhhhhhhhhhhhhs" and one "Oh god." It was the first time that I heard him say "Oh god" and it came as he was coming down off his orgasm. I loved enjoying his orgasm, making jokes and laughter. Joyful! As the trees clapped their hands for us.

During our three-day camping, canoeing trip we had deep conversations where our differences became more reasons to leave each other. Johnny said that I was not showing my "intuitive" side enough. Also, he thought that it was "ridiculous" that I thought that more positive experiences and opportunities *come to me* as I emotionally heal. Also my experiences of feeling past lives or life while in my mother's womb were not "rational."

"Yes, it's not rational. It's intuitive!" I replied spontaneously.

On our drive home, Johnny apologized for "abusing" me. I told him that he hadn't abused me, but had been judgmental for saying my experiences are "ridiculous." I felt steady with my Self as I answered with calmness.

Like I felt steadily satisfied with the caressing waves of orgasm rising with the sunrise meeting us on the beach of our last day at Stillwater. Johnny had held me in his arms at night, and then his penis held my vagina in the dawn. We both had many intense "Ooooohs" and "Aaaaaaaaahs." We whispered, "I love you" more than once as if melding our Love more simultaneously. It was fine that that neither of us had an orgasm. Later, Johnny told me that we had just the right amount of lovemaking over that weekend.

When I gave one of the three pieces of driftwood I had brought back from Stillwater Lake to Erin, she asked how had I thought to bring her one. It was easy to reply, "Because I love you." She did not reply or look at me, but I saw the reflection of my pleasure on her face. Love is in the air!

Like when I called up Jerry and began to learn about another man whom I was attracted to through dancing an Argentine tango or two. This Czech man and I talked for two hours, feeling a depth of ease that I shouldn't have been surprised about, but I was. It was the one-year anniversary of 9/11, and I would be vulnerable once again, the important lesson of 9/11.

As is the lesson of crying tears at orgasm, underscored in my weekly session while recounting how I cried at orgasm with Johnny as we looked into each other's eyes, because when you *look* and *feel*, you know the **love** is *real*. Tears flowed as I said, "When somebody really sees you, and stays with you, you know you're loved."

Sobs intensified this truth as I spoke, "**Another one of those beautiful sexual and spiritual moments**: my spirit totally free in that moment." Thank you Johnny; thank you Design of the Universe.

When I self-loved again, thinking about Jerry and Johnny, neither were in my thoughts as I orgasmed. I felt a streak of pleasurable energy travel down the back of my legs and then up my back as I said, "Oh god" at least seven times – that's all there was! An intense being with god.

I was also excited about Johnny's ability to touch up the photo of my dad holding my baby sister with his one outstretched arm. He was able to send the picture digitally to SUN. I have shed many tears for not being able to give dad (and Me) honorable Love, Real Love. Daddy was the seed that would eventually grow the flower of Love for my own life. Let's face it! It's all about LOVE-TEARS, which enable ears to hear tears of healing spirit wisdom.

It was Friday the 13th (my lucky number) of September 2002 when I received the call from Rachel at the SUN that they would use the photo! When I asked when the photo would be printed, she did not know. I told her how I had intended it for the issue on "safety," and she said that the November issue layout was finished. But, later that day she called back, and they had decided to use my photo instead of another that had been in place! I felt elated, like a hot air balloon rising and rising. Again, the lesson of how the Design of the Universe works all things together for go(o)d. Even my sister's resistance to using her photo turned into a good thing for me, as Johnny used his expertise to enhance the photo so it could be printed. Her photo was in very much the same condition as mine, most likely would not have passed the criteria to be printed anyway, and we would have lost more time so that the photo would not have made the November issue about safety. As both of my daughters said, "Awesome!"

Another Friday the 13th gift was hearing that I would receive an $800 car rental refund incurred during an accident that had not been my fault. The other person's insurance company had been fighting me in arbitration, and I won due to my persistence over a year's time: finding the witness to the accident, and the correct police report of the accident. I would not give up. I screamed with happiness.

And when Johnny called just after midnight, I spontaneously said, "Hi, Midnight Cowboy" (he grew up in Dallas). He laughed and laughed, then asked, "Did you plan that?"

"No, it just came to me as I picked up the phone." Sometimes, I am a funny crybabe.☺

Johnny told Ellen that he was just coasting with her, and growing with me. I noticed how I needed to be loved the best, what we all want, but I knew I needed it to be in a healthier way.

I was wide awake after talking with Johnny and felt the subtle impulse to touch myself for twenty to thirty minutes as I climbed to a fine orgasm, on my back, resisting the pull to roll onto my stomach where it is easier to attain orgasm. I thought of Jerry and Johnny until I was in the zone of orgasm, then I was with my Self only, saying, "Oh god, oh god, get in me." That was all, as a float-ing tingle spread throughout the top of my body. Then, I thought of "god get in me, more and more," as I do this emotional release work; I have back more of my Self. Back to how I was born – god in Me - Love.

And it is Real, like the sycamore tree I discovered on my new walking route to the bank. It has three huge trunks with a common base, so tall, so wide; I just stare. What a star! What you are! With an "e" eeeeeeeeeeeeee. This magnificent syc*amore* felt like "amore" as the Spanish say for love. Love, that protects me with strength and safety unbounded; no fear, as you can *see* in the centerfold of this book.

And *hear*, like I did when I returned to Tallmadge Tire, after a hike into Buttermilk Falls State Park, where I picked up a huge fallen brown sycamore leaf that was perfectly whole in its 12 by 11 inch dimensions. As I walked into the business to pay for my tune-up, one of the mechanics said, "Is that real?" He had never seen such a big leaf before.

I placed the sycamore leaf on my kitchen table, and again I heard, "Is that real?" when my friend Susanne came for dinner and our weekly session. Can we believe that our hearts can become so big? That it is our nature to be big-hearted?

As I expect my self and Johnny to be when we disagree about me being pres-ent at a tango milonga in his city where Ellen usually dances. It was four months into our relationship and he still wanted to protect her from feeling "humiliated" if I came to the milonga with him. She had requested that I not come; it was her safe place.

I told him how I felt helpless to have him understand, because he had not felt his childhood pain enough to understand how it is beneficial for him and Ellen to face and feel their fears. I explained that it is not respectful to either of them as avoiding their fears says that they can't handle this new growth.

Before I arrived at Johnny's, Ellen had just left with her couple belongings because he had told her that he did not want to take care of her emotional bag-gage. Still, he was mad at me for pressuring him (he'd been up all night) even though he agreed with my viewpoint.

"You don't want me to challenge you? Yet you say that you value the personal growth I en*courage*." We did go together from 9-10pm, and he called Ellen to let her know of our decision, which gave her 10-12pm to dance if she chose to come. It was a loving gesture, and Johnny actually enjoyed himself.

When we made love that night, it was good without the need for orgasm. I noticed that I kept my eyes open more than Johnny during lovemaking. I told him "I love you" twice without hearing it in return and felt fine about it. I felt proud of my growing ability to genuinely give without expecting return. We fell asleep close to one another for a few hours before driving to the airport for my 6am flight. When Johnny let me off at US Air, he was the first to say, "I love you."

I remembered with fondness how Johnny had crawled on top of me when we first got into bed, looked into my eyes and said with a smile, "I was mad at you and going to sleep in the living room; now I feel grateful."

Johnny also thanked me for not getting hurt by our argument. I told him that I was hurt although he said that it didn't seem that I had been. I had expressed it in "my helplessness to have him understand." I didn't have big reactions because I can express my hurt constructively and I know the hurt that I am feeling and can express it constructively because much of it has been grieved.

I flew to Phoenix, Arizona, where I met my brother, Eric, who drove us to the Grand Canyon National Park for a five-day and night backpacking trip down into the canyon. Eric reminded me of the summer he spent with me while working with my first husband, Chuck, landscaping. He remembered Louie, a teenager we had taken in temporarily to help him let go of his drug addiction, finding his drug paraphernalia in our bathroom. I realized how our memory is clearest when experiencing extreme moments or happenings in our lives: most scary or most beautifully loving. It's like the extremes are the hard cover of a book, whose pages are the everyday living that makes life meaningful.

The "hardness" of life, or pain, is what needs to be felt so we can become flexible like a paperback book, which I would much rather hold in my hands. It's lighter, easily opened. Maybe pain is the front hard cover that needs to be melted through everyday tears, leading us to find a sturdy loving back cover at the end of our lives. The pages in between then become what I am most grateful for: my healthy body, my family and friends who love me, a job I like, growth through writing about my everyday triggers that cause tears of healing into Love. The dance of **life,** which I **love** and literally partner.

With a 30-pound pack on my back, I joined my brother and ten others, and our leader Rich, being an accomplished guide to the many wonders of the Grand Canyon. Hiking from the 38 degree North Rim down to the 100-degree bottom and back up to the 70 degree South room engaged all my awe some senses. It was the best way to connect with my emotionally-distant brother, who tries hard to care about his two sisters.

On our drive back to Phoenix to catch the plane, I asked Eric, owner of a flourishing architecture firm, how he felt about Connie asking for money to have her teeth repaired, estimated by her dentist to be $13,000. Quickly, his tone was annoyed as he told me that he was not responsible for how she or I might need money from him, because we have chosen to live our lives as we do, and he's worked his butt off, 80 hours a week in order to have a decent retirement. It was true that I could work more hours, as my psychotherapy practice is three days a week so that I can use the other days to write. Connie could find a nursing job where she is paid more per hour. Neither of us have health insurance.

Eric told me that he designed ten years for low-income housing and thinks that it is a crime to enable people to stay on welfare and not work. In short order, I asked, "What makes these people unmotivated?" They have been very disrespected, blacks oppressed by our white predecessors, and many Americans are still prejudiced against minorities. Eric replied, "I didn't do that."

"Sure, but what about compassion for their oppression and ongoing lesser degrees of racism? We need people in social services who care enough to turn this cycle around. Where are they? We have not been loved enough, so we go after money for beautiful homes, cars, material things to help us feel better about ourselves," I replied.

We discussed the reasons that I am writing books: to help guide our evolutionary journey into becoming more loving human beings. I gingerly said, "It's not about responsibility or obligation – I understand that from our religious oppression we have learned 'me last,' and too much obligatory 'care-taking of others' when we as children have not been emotionally taken care of as needed."

I could understand Eric's resentment, which covers up his own hurt of not being loved enough, as is true of everyone in varying degrees. We talked about our values, reflected in where we place our money, and when we choose to help. He had offered Connie a plan where he would match whatever loan offered by Joshua, her twenty-four-year-old son, who had a good-paying job enabling him to build a new house. She was afraid to ask Joshua for money.

It took courage for me to point out Eric's paying $5,000 for one piece of art, a large painting, of which he had several, as an example of how we choose to spend our money. I have never paid, nor could I, over $100 for a piece of art. I agreed that Connie needed to work on her abilities to take care of herself. Eric asked why I didn't help her financially. I replied that she has more assets than I do, owning her home without a mortgage, and that I have much of what I have because I am careful with money: buying the cheapest gas, many second-hand clothes, owning a second-hand ten-year-old car. The opposite of Eric's buying habits. He learned that I have some savings, and a small retirement, so he knew I was taking care of myself. We had shared more intimate parts of our lives than we ever had, despite Eric raising his irritated voice intermittently during our sharing.

I had stayed calm, and thought that I had expressed myself clearly and well. I was proud of myself. I concluded, "I'm glad we can be this honest and open because I love you and want to be close to you."

When Eric left me off at the airport, he hugged me quickly, and said "I love you," before I could, then did. Later, I wished that I had looked him in the eyes as I said those three special words that had gained more value during our trip of sharing beauteous nature, our true hearts.

While on the plane, I watched the movie "Life Once and Again," and cried when the boyfriend said to his girlfriend who had survived death, "I need to take this chance to say I love you." I was sad because I had not taken that chance with dad. Then, I was happy as I reflected on what Eric had said while in the midst of our hiking group on the last day, "Diane hardly got on my nerves."

"How did I?" I questioned.

"You really didn't," Eric replied with surprise in his basso voice.

When Johnny met me at the Buffalo airport, we greeted each other with loving eyes, a slow look: progression of attraction, intention, seeing the other, knowing that they love you. Cemented with a tender kiss. The intensity of feeling grows with the slow taking in, noticing, focusing a once black and white photo into vibrant colors. I had not felt sexual during the vacation, no need to masturbate, nor did I feel sexual anticipating seeing Johnny.

At midnight, I asked Johnny if I could undress him, slowly, stoking the flames of desire. Because I am not "in love" I am surprised how easily Johnny arouses me; it's like his positives spontaneously outweigh his negatives. A controlled burn until our matches strike – our bodies rub – our eyes meet. I noticed my eyes were open more often than Johnny's as we cooed, smiled, laughed softly in our bed of desire. Our kisses.

Johnny seemed more vocal, although his orgasm was more muted, fewer spasms, or aftershocks, as I liked to call them. It was new for him to orgasm before me, and I did not mind that when I moved on top, caressing his softer penis between my labia and over my clitoris, that I orgasmed more through my nipples, some near my vagina, leaving my clitoris to stew. Sweet waves of pleasure by which I slept dreamily.

Johnny awoke first, held me, then walked to the living room to do some work as I slept another hour. As I was aroused to the day, my clitoris and I brought Johnny back to bed to make love again. With my mouth on his Jack, I made him croon and spasm with pleasure, hearing three or four "Oh gods," which had been rare from Johnny's lips. I expressed many "Oh gods" and a couple "Oh Johnnys" as I rose toward orgasm with him inside and outside of me. I helped Johnny jump for joy! During 69, I had a long ride of pleasure and screamed until my mind went empty - dazed like a brilliant sun RISE.

I said, "I'm making love to you, and I love you," more than once, not hearing it back. It's really okay! Minutes later, in the calming afterglow, looking at each other with steadiness, Johnny said, "I love you." Somehow it felt more real being said outside the heat of passion; maybe it is absorbed more, instead of soft concrete, it is solidified into cement, less able to be taken lightly. I sense it is best to have both: passion with solidity.

The next day I spent with Johnny at his workplace, seeing his artistry in motion. At lunch, we talked about the importance of eye contact in feeling connected, Johnny stating that it affected his arousal, and without it he'd lose his erection. I shared how our greeting at the airport felt more loving than a sudden slobbering kiss. The slow progression of the dark brown eyes looking into the light blue eyes, our lips not touching, yet close, moving a few inches backwards, then forwards, looking, a small light kiss, looking, then another tender kiss, short, looking deeply into the eyes. Then, a longer kiss with an embrace, moving slowly into a passionate pressured kiss.

It's all about slowing down to notice instead of needing to be close so badly that one does not get to know or see the other without the fear of losing the closeness. Ultimately, the slowing intensifies the closeness, because one has taken the time to *look* and **know** the other, to see the love and then feel more. Love.

I am thinking that the ideal would be to have the passionate feeling before I meet "him" – in the anticipation, still be able to slowly look, be tender in kissing, then intensely kiss with passion. FEELING intensely and slowly is about KNOW-ING Love.

If I am very physically attracted and also emotionally heart-connected, then the PASSION does make a full circle of Love. "Passion is just the free flow of nat-ural emotional energy…emotional therapy is in order here." (pg. 266 *The Path to Love*)

"As nature created us it is normal to seek pleasure; a fearful person avoids pain instead…The spiritual answer to boredom is to open yourself to the very thing you have feared – the constant flow of desire that wants to express itself at every moment." (pgs. 268, 269, *The Path to Love,* by Deepak Chopra)

I will continue to heed my heart's lead because I know I can trust it! I know down deep that Love can be better, although it was wonderful that Johnny and I could talk about such thoughtful, deep, sometimes scary feelings. I love traveling to the unknown places inside of me where my spirit is trying to connect with my sexuality.

As well as with nature and creativity like music and poetry. Like while driving my car home, singing "Still" with Lionel Richie, crying many good tears as I thought of "still" loving Daddy, wanting to hold him, telling him "I love you, and always will." My tears continued to prove how profound Daddy's love was/is for me, therefore feeling more love for him as I recognize how deep my tears run.

When I read the poem I had written while hiking inside the Grand Canyon to Johnny, I was surprised as tears rose up when I read the line, "My hands reach out to touch, I look down to Bright Angel Creek, hearing it sing the same song." I had not felt sad when I wrote "Looking Up." The river of tears needing to be touched?

Looking Up

I see a baby mule deer trot down Grand Canyon's path,
Finding mother ripping green leaves from Bright Angel Creek bush.
Baby latches onto mama's udder with gusto,
Pulling and sucking in unison –
Mother standing two minutes worth.
Mother deer pulls away, stepping to another bush-
Now I have a view of her tush.
Her white charcoal tail raises like a can opener, and…
I see black easter eggs fall to the ground, one to ten I count.
A teenage buck raises eight inch antlers, stands parallel to mother,
His tush facing me.
I look surprised as he squeezes out seven black easter eggs – do I blush?
Never seen deer-poop falling; only solitary on the ground.
Everybody poops I know, but not before my eyes.
I look up. Straight up is crystal clear blue.
Not a fleck of any other color…
Deep blue; like it can only B blue.
I don't turn my head –
A red cardinal flashes its wings.
My body must turn –
Back and forth as I hike, over sand,
Sharp rocks, smooth stones…
Thirty pound pack on my back
Not to miss colors,
Playing major reds into minor pinks and lavenders.
An off key green rock accents quartz white,
Pin-striping my heart.
Looking up – not to miss pointed designs,
So high I feel the Grand Canyon walls holding me
With colors, shapes, beyond my deepest imaginations.
My hands reach out to touch…
I look down to Bright Angel Creek
Hearing it sing the same song.
Looking up – what about the stars?
The night black sky is gorged with twinkles -
The full moon giving guidance of wrinkles.
All I want is: to LOOK UP my father – the brightest star of all,

My love-light.
He is how I know my life is always **looking up**.

I was learning to "go with the flow," as Jerry had said; only I was going with the flow of tears, which he said he rarely accessed. I was disappointed yet understanding his fears. I notice the beautiful clouds; they flow and float with tears like I do, and then let them go as needed. Clouds of patience and trust to nourish me.

It is why I can be "so composed," as Johnny expressed when he realized that his harshness came from wanting me to be more vulnerable. In other words, my tears in front of him are good, but they are more about me than about him. I connected his pain under his harshness (anger) as wanting me to need him (therefore I would not be as independent or confident) and he would feel more loved by me. My strength was within mySelf, and not through him. It was very clear to me, and I believe to him as well.

This IS growing up, not <u>needing</u> someone, but <u>wanting</u> to be with. IN(ward) LOVE. A child <u>needs</u> to be with their parents, and mature adults <u>want</u> to BE with another. Passion makes it possible to find the courage to explore a deeper level of Love.

The kind of love I felt as I sang at the memorial service for my childhood friend Mary's mother in the Bethel Grove Bible church that I attended while growing up. Tears filled my voice with the words, "I am his own." I am god's (Daddy's) own daughter, meaning that I knew he (god) loved me. I had not known this divine love in the church, where guilt and fear predominated. I sang loud, strong, stood tall and proud, hearing rote words around me. I was grieving my own loss of birthright Love, while feeling compassion for others fear of vulnerability.

The vulnerability that has worn away my need to be as competitive, "Go out and play," popping out of my mouth as Denali stepped onto the soccer field. Her dad had just said, "Go out and win."

At that same soccer game, Erin had asked me to pipe down after hearing me yell and shout encouragements to Denali and her teammates. The woman on the blanket next to us said something like, "It's fine with me, they like it." I was surprised and dismayed that once again one's exuberance is questioned as not quite a good thing. The child being kicked like the soccer ball out of bounds.

As was my surprising full body orgasm, once again floating from a morning wakefulness feeling unaroused. There were no images, just a couple "Oh MY god's," coming easily. MY stood out as my god is me.

Our next lovemaking flowed from being in the shower together. Johnny wanted to make love standing up, with my legs wrapped around him, he lifting me up and down with intercourse. Then, he carried me to our bed, where I continued to feel distant because it became too much intercourse with not enough feeling. Even when I was on top. Then, he came in from behind, me on my stomach, coming hot and heavy with loud moans, no words.

Our relationship was a weather vane without direction as his tenderness afterwards held me as we fell asleep into the darkness of the night's rejuvenation. The morning dawned as Johnny's erection woke me even before we kissed. My nipples needed to be lightly turned with patience as I licked his penis for his pleasure. Then, I asked for flicks to my clitoris, which he needed to teach his tongue, as if with the lightness of an eagle's feather. I was riding a beautiful wave, not sure I'd surf to shore, or fly to the sky. But, I did as I said, "It's beautiful, it's delicious." I couldn't help but say those words. A moist silence from Johnny. After I had come back to earth, I said, "I love you, you know."

Johnny's lips could only smile. I knew he felt my distance. I knew I felt grateful and loving. I was ready for our imminent separation.

Not sure about my expansion that was reflected in my brassiere! I have not worn bras often in the past decade, as I feel more comfortable without them, freer to be me? I've worn 34B for years and had felt them to be more and more binding. Too tight like the religious box I had been put in. When I found an indigo blue lacey bra only in 36B, I tried it on and it fit just right.

It seems that my rib cage has become bigger, expanded, as I cry out my pain, I breathe more deeply, stand up straighter, and yoga may help too. I have not gained weight, nor lifted weights. Except, the weight of my past pain wept away.

When Johnny and I made love the next weekend, there were no "I love yous," less eye contact and only I orgasmed, while in the sixty-nine position. I didn't like his tongue in my mouth very much, as if something wasn't being said that needed to be. I wanted to be his friend, because larger pieces of the LOVE puzzle were missing for us to remaIN as LOVErs.

While we drove to the Wyalusing Arts Festival, where we would dance a tango demo, we discussed how he changes his thinking because of my influence and I don't except on less important aspects like what I wear. I do see the "bigger picture," which annoyed Johnny. He regretted his first marriage, believing it was a big mistake, because it caused too much pain, which he was still coping with because his ex-wife is the mother of his two daughters. I see these painful experiences as great teachers of Real Love. He admitted that he needed to work on acceptance and anxiety in his life, but didn't push that inward part of his life. And, I continue to grow in acceptance of the balance of dance, family, friends and writing in my life. Sometimes, I feel not generous enough with my time. Yes, grief over not receiving love from my mother, and then losing the love of my father circles like the moon with the tides and continues to show me Love in all its comforting vitality! Like dawn's early light. Then, noon's extra light. Finally, essential twilight.

I am happy to find that "twi" means doubly, or twice the amount of light in twilight. At a twilight dinner, a new friend told me after he saw my tears for the first time that he thinks women are beautiful when they cry. If only the world thought so. Or like I thought as I left my four-month-old granddaughter, Riley Shea, after a visit in October 2002. "I'm leaving this baby – myself!" Tears poured forth as I became conscious of how I had left mySelf behind as a baby, not able to endure the pain of feeling my mother not wanting or loving me. From the womb, and as a baby when mom tried to strangle me, a memory that came to me as I have been in touch with my grieving process.

I also noticed my stomach tighten up when Megan had me feed Riley from the bottle, although she nursed Riley most of the time. I was apprehensive because I did not want anything to get in the way of Riley and her mom's closeness. Clearly, I knew my hurt had been triggered by my mother and me not being close when I was a baby.

On the phone, tears rolled up yonder when I told my boyfriend of twenty years ago, Christian, about why I cried when leaving Megan and Riley Shea, as an example of how we need to come "home" and connect with our subconscious hurt, in order to leave our anger behind. Before I hung up I said, "I love you Christian." He replied, "That's good." And, it IS good that I didn't feel badly that I did not hear those three important words back.

After my visit, I emailed Megan tears as I wrote, "I love you so much my heart bursts." Tears are of Love is the best I can say and write. And, they result in "a hearty and exuberant laugh from her," which my dance friend Brian wrote in a poem after our trip to Italy, referring to me.

I am more rapidly courageous with each man in revealing my Self…this IS very good. Johnny and I laughed heartily when I told him that Jerry had said that he wished he had not told me that he was "very attracted to me." That fear thing - bursting out with honesty, then fearful of its consequences. I am noticing how laughter many times is a cover for our fear, not just for expression of joy, as I belly laughed in the mall with Johnny, climbing onto a funny piece of artwork that looked like a clown being sexy. Johnny told me that he really liked our conversation that day, and I asked why. He replied, "I am aware again of what a character you are." I took that as a compliment, knowing I would write that into my next children's book, *Everybody Laughs.*

Toward morning, I heard Johnny in the bathroom, washing? He carefully moves into our bed, where I feel his smooth shaven cheeks (he has a strip beard) on my knees. I knew we were in for sixty-nine, and I felt ambivalent, wanting to sleep, yet not wanting to reject Johnny. I knew from past experience I would be warmed up if he would be patient, which he generally was. I was mixed about not starting out kissing face to face because it felt impersonal, not about making love. Yet, I was feeling less close to Johnny. Still, we felt the pleasurable feelings, being high for fifteen or twenty minutes, my lips, tongue and hands making his penis grow, as he did for my clitoris, with one hand on my high voltage nipple. Many sucking moans before I come with a short scream of "Oh Johnny, oh god." Johnny is able to move into my birth canal with various positions for another twenty minutes. He doesn't orgasm before we are quiet in each other's arms.

Then, I ask, how he is feeling about us. "Not as close as this summer."

I concur. He tells me he is frustrated about how difficult it is for him to orgasm, even when he masturbates, although he had been freer with me until the past two or three weeks. I asked if he wanted my take on it. "Sure."

I told him that he needed to feel more grief of his past so that he could let go. He had been asexual for nearly a year after he left the mother of his two daughters, and had not had easy orgasms since then, even with his next wife. So it goes, the difficulty of being inward, facing and feeling one's pain.

We continued our conversation with great detail about our sexuality. How we need to be face to face. "It is your face that turns me on," Johnny smiled. Yes, that eye-to-eye soul-spirit connection is the lens that focuses Love in the other's eyes for each other. He told me that he was disappointed that he had not climaxed in my mouth because I did it very well, using my hand too, which other women had not done, as well as lick and tease him before sucking Jack.

I appreciated Johnny for his patience, tenderness and respectfulness, which made it easier to wake up, being willing to make love. We talked and talked; it was so easy. When I told him about my conversations with Erin and Niki and how Erin looked at me with "endearing eyes," I teared up at the moment that I could see love in her eyes. If only I could have looked back into my father's eyes as I am more able to now.

On Halloween, while in my office, I paused to look up at the 11x14 photograph of my father's face, into his kind eyes, missing him with tears. No wonder we take many photographs of one another, we so need to be SEEN. Another reason I wanted his photo in SUN magazine, to be Seen as the honored love IN my life. And as I continued to fall into my tears, I noticed the leaves falling "in love" with the earth, flying, letting go with blissful ease.

Green-bronze leaves fall "in love" with the beauty of color, oh what a tease.

Follow the leaves, fall "in love" with your heart, that says please, please, please.

Breaking away from fear, which is disease, and seize, seize, seize,

The love of my and your own life.

So too, do human BEings need to "fall in love" as a first-step in their process of letting go of past emotional pent-up pain; to find Real Love. "Falling in love" is the glue that helps the relationship stay together long enough to work through, grieve childhood pain, that causes disharmony in a committed partnership. "Only love can free us, because its truth is an antidote to fear,…of exposing our deepest fears and insecurities… The exhilaration of <u>falling in love</u> is an escape from the ego, (the defense we put up to protect our vulnerable feelings) its sense of threat and its selfishness. This escape is what we *really* want....Many other experiences that cannot be comprehended by ego apply to love – a lover is confused, spontaneous, vulnerable, exposed, detached, carefree, wondrous, and ever new....Love's journey would be terrifying if we didn't have passion to give us courage – the blind *wisdom of lovers*, because the ego's certainty is an illusion. Uncertainty is the basis of life." (pgs. 115-116, *The Path to Love*, by Deepak Chopra, parentheses mine)

As mentioned before "Oh god" or "Oh my god" is not said just at moments of loving bliss, but also when one is in extreme fear or pain. It is also the voice of a child, when I hear three-year-old Lucas' words to his Daddy, "I don't like you, I don't love you, go away, go back to work," shuts his door and says, "Don't come in." His mother, Tanya, reported that his father yelled back (he'd heard similar words from Lucas for some time), "I've made mistakes in my life, and the biggest one is you, Lukie!" I was so stunned that I could not cry, only say, "Oh my god" three or four times, until I heard Tanya repeat what I had said in another one of her sessions, "Luke is god's voice to you." Tanya fell into her tears as she said, that she was "enduring" life like her folks had, instead of loving and celebrating life. Her spirit was dying as her son was trying to wake her up to her dead-end marriage, and her fear to alienate her mother if she left the marriage. Lucas knew it was not loving, and Tanya knew enough not to silent her son's voice and feelings, to let him be spontaneous like my granddaughter Denali who when we part, presses her lips out for a mouth kiss and says "I love you" as easy as the blink of an eye. Isn't that the way Love should be? Spontaneously and easily given?

Why we love babies spontaneously, easily; why I dressed up as a baby for Halloween. Real cloth diapers, real bib, bottle (no pacifier☺), and teddy bear. I was innocent, beautiful and full of love, making others laugh. I am persistent in knowing that being a crybaby makes me happy. "Persevering" is what Tanya says is my best characteristic, and Connie said, "You are the most persistent person I know." Yes, I will be persistent with allowing my tears to heal my spirit into Love. Being a CRYBABE is a good thing. And it makes my sexuality sing a new hymn (him.☺)

I was surprised when Erin told me of what she remembered of her grandpa, my father, who had died when she was just six years old. When she said the big willow tree outside his picture window, a tear surprised me, running into the corner of my mouth. I made the smiling connection of why I love to look at the willow tree that now spreads out down the hill, its lacey tree top I can see from my picture window, standing out amidst a group of spruces. It was as if Daddy was present when we talk about him...it makes him important, be loved. When I told her that my client, Moe, had told me that I was his "guardian angel" and that Daddy was mine, Erin's eyes became misty.

Are the tears about me not having myself as my guardian angel, that I miss dad as my guardian angel, that I miss my own <u>angelic divine</u> being? Must be the last, especially as I spontaneously underlined "angelic divine" in my journal.

When I self-loved again, as usual those days, on awakening unaroused sexually, I began touching myself while thinking about a family I'd seen outside of Pizza Hut a few weeks earlier. A father was yelling at his three-or four-year-old son, as he rapped him on the head, with two brothers nearby. I wanted to intervene. I thought of how the father might respond that it was none of my business. I would have replied, "It's my business to protect children." As I said that to myself, I became highly aroused as I repeated, "It's my business to protect children!" And I felt the direct connection of sexuality with the divine spirit of the child, as one, as LOVE.

After that awesome moment, while on my back, open to the universe, I climaxed as I said, "Oh my god" about four times. Then, "Oh Jerry, let me in," thinking how I was to help him let his little boy in, as well as my little girl into me.

The little girl that cries so that she can help me feel more like a woman who can stand up for her own truth. When Johnny and I talked about the inequality of our relationship in the realm of influence, he brought up the example of me not giving into his opinion that it was "good art" that Georgia O'Keefe kept only 25-50 (the best quality) of her 150 paintings. I see it as his need to have me agree; we can't just have differing opinions. He was irritated that he is swayed by me most of the time, especially in the realm of relationship issues. He became mad when he felt I did not understand (the hurt underneath the anger) what he had said. Yet, when I repeated what he had said about O'Keefe's way of preserving quality art, he agreed that I had heard him. He left the table to walk outdoors, mostly mad that I "always" had to be right.

While sitting on the john, I had to agree that I am "right" much of the time, especially in relationship, awareness issues. Boy, was that last sentence had to write! When we came together, sitting in his Miata, I admitted that I am "right" a lot, and that it was hard to admit to without coming across as "superior" and that I don't think that I am any better than any other human being, yet superior, as an astrologer had said. "You know more about relationships than most people," so why can't I be "superior" in my field?

Later, Johnny apologized for leaving the table, and I understood and was easily accepting. It felt "good" to acknowledge my awareness emotionally and spiritually, as small bits of the ol' church message were still roamin' in the dark corners of my mind-heart. Nearly gone is the shame of saying "good" things about oneself, because of my tears tearing away false humility that squashes the true spirit within that is all "good."

As IS our relationship as it evolved into friendship, making love for the last time in early November. Not with the usual candles, and halfway through,

Johnny shut off the lamp as well. I caressed his penis with my tongue and mouth. Then, Johnny turned the lamp back on. His solid masculine body was on top of me as he lingered the words, "I love you." His "quirky and difficult" partner responded, "I haven't heard that in a while," letting a minute sound its voice, a whisper, "I love you too."

Two days later, Johnny writes in an email of November 6, 2002:

"I felt very close to you in a familiar kind of way, like old friends or family. I really do feel totally safe with you. Before I noticed Jennifer, I had been feeling out of place in this relationship with you, and trying to figure out how to explain it. But Sunday, when I was waiting for you in bed, I started to cry, feeling that we were drifting away from our relationship as lovers. I know it has been a good thing and you are a rare person and I want to say I really love you, <u>who you are, how you have loved me</u>..."

Tears made their usual appearance with those underlined words of love. It was very clear that I was connected to losing my dad grief, being intertwined with losing my Self. The love he gave me was the love for my Self. And, tears run as I type because it is the truth flowing from my eyes (I's), the windows to our soul-spirits.

Those tears were the same as the ones that came as I told one of my clients at the end of her session about the process of "getting myself back," by feeling all the feelings I had had to put away as a child.

"I felt last weekend that there was something much more durable than sex. I want it to go on," Johnny's email continued, and I knew it was an enduring love of friendship, like the love of a child renewed. Our lover-relationship had been a taste of a healthier open relationship's possibilities.

And I knew I must be IN LOVE, where you put the emphasis on IN, that's inside us – god IN us – being more aware of why we say offhandedly I need to feel "in love" with someone in order to grow and love more. Must be inwardly aw<u>are</u>, in order to know who we <u>are. All connected is our language, our spirits, our awareness! On page 69 of my journal</u>☺

The next weekend I attended a workshop about grief ritual, at Rowe Conference Center, led by Sobonfu Some, from West Africa. In talking with others about the layers of grief, I spoke of the helplessness and hopelessness underneath frustration and anger, ultimately helpless and hopeless to be good enough to *Be loved*. The **Beloved**. Unloved being the corest, deepest pain, like the shiniest diamond buried at the bottom of the *mine*.

In the group of twenty-five I introduced myself as Dianea (pronounced Diana), not the princess, which made many laugh. With Sobonfu open-mouthed, ready to protest, I added, "but I am the goddess," sparking more laughter. What was so funny? The fear of saying something so good about oneself raises its one eyebrow? Yet enjoying its possibility by saying "goddess" out loud?

I noticed that I still felt a bit apprehensive about speaking up, but didn't feel my heart pounding as it had in the past. We formed a circle at the end of the evening, where fifteen encircled ten who asked to be surrounded by special healing energy. My friend Becca cried with sobs, whereas I did not feel tearful. I hugged a couple women who were crying. I knew I was on the downside of the mountain of grief in my life.

My weekly crying sessions and writing in my journal was paying off even though I wrote one November day, "Sometimes I feel annoyed that I need to write *in you* journal☺ - "in you" – find out what is "in you" is what it is all about. So I am happy to, to know this is what I need to do! It's all intertwined. Journaling seems like such a time-consuming obligation and responsibility – but why not to my Self? The divine just wants to be recognized, right?" A divine obligation - or an obligation to the divine? Weeeeee.

During the grief ritual weekend we spent several hours building shrines, drumming, chanting African phrases that were very repetitious. I became tired of it, my voice as well, cried slow streams about wanting Daddy's presence and to tell him that I loved him. No sobbing or wailing as others were. I had let go of much of my grief, and could be there for others. One in particular, Sally, stands out. I was standing behind Sally, as she knelt before the shrine of nature's branches, colored leaves, stones, mushrooms, wildflowers collected by the participants. We had been instructed not to touch the person in front of us unless they laid in the fetal position. Sally had wanted to cry all weekend.

Sally was bent in yoga's child's pose, and I felt a strong sensitivity to lay my hand on her back. Within thirty to sixty seconds she was in tears, then sobbing. I had trusted my soul-spirit to touch. At Sunday lunch, Sally told me how my touch had brought up her tears, how surprised she was, and how *she had not even known to ask for touch.*

I thought of my Self as a child when I wrote those italized words in my journal. The parent needs to know when to touch and nurture their children like I had learned to do, through trusting my tears. A week later I received a note from Sally saying, "And thank you again for your sensitivity and that perfectly timed touch. It's making me cry again…"

When I was learning a West Coast swing choreography, I noticed that I was remembering the steps and sequences more quickly than in the past. As I remembered to grieve my childhood pain, I remembered more in the present! With less rain of tears, there was more space to shine in my dance!

When I self-loved again, still once or twice a week, I just wished to. I had awakened not aroused. After rolling over onto my stomach, the sensations became ten times more intense, suddenly bubbles were all over my body with fizzling pleasure, high intensity throughout my body for four to five minutes, then orgasm throughout my body. Only "Oh god, oh god," no images. I was connecting with god – no men involved.

Twleve days later, my experience of orgasm was similar. It felt like lightning shooting through my pelvis, my whole body feeling a soothing pleasure after the initial huge laser spark. The same "Oh god oh god" with no images of men. And, in the next bedroom was my loving friend, Ted, who wanted to be making love with me, but I did not. I needed to be "in love" and being "sexual" was obviously not a need of mine anymore, although I love being sexual when making love. I need a man who can turn me on – to Love! Love is the powerful key that turns on and over my heart.

It is why I was turned off when the audience of the *Vagina Monologues* was asked to repeat the word "cunt," to reclaim it in a new way. Susanne and I laughed at much of the performance, but I would not reclaim that degrading word, any more than I would reclaim "nigger" or slavery. I like to imagine my Self, writing my own version of the penis to clitoris dialogues!

I want to reclaim the words "Born Innocent," sung by Sarah McLachlan, which clearly connect me to the child, baby born innocent, for which my tears cry. I want to make the world hear *Born Innocent* over and over again, because when you look steadily into a baby's eyes, there is only pure innocent love called Real. The deepest pain is to lose that innocent spirit of Love we are all born with.

Also, more often synchronicity or connectedness seemed to make their entrance. I came across three pages of a ripped out journal writing of my mother's dated February 15, 1946, me being three months carried in her unwanting-womb. February 15th 2002 was the day my mother said, "I love you" to me, face to face for the very first time! I cried in telling of my find to Megan, who was supportive, not questioning my tears at 55 years old.

Tears that have led me to appreciate and love them more, to honor them with an article in the Ithaca Journal titled, "Thankful for Persistent Family Love." I was dismayed to see that the article did not identify my parents by name, although there was a small picture of me with my name. I sobbed in my session, saying, "I'm sorry mom and dad, and proud to be your daughter," and knew that I was crying about my own loss of identity for so many years.

I had learned to hold back my tears for years, like my client, Jen, who that same day had said that her parents had taken away her "right to cry." It is a *cryin' shame* how people walk around in a daze and do not talk about important things, like how Daddy and I never took the chance to talk about the distance between us created when I learned he was not my biological father. I did have that chance with my mother at the very end of her life. On the good side: not having that chance with Daddy is an essential chapter of my story that prompts me to search for the man who can be completely open and honest with me, and I with him. That's being "In Love." Therefore, to have a man in my life is important; I see, over and over again, that intimate relationships trigger feelings I need to feel, whether it is to let go of past emotional pain, or joy and love that is blissful.

I just noticed how Openness and Honesty are the two essentials in creating a deeply loving relationship with the Beloved. Those two words begin with "O" and "H," which when put together spell **Oh**, the beginning of "**oh** god." I love these synchronous connections!

When my brother, sister and I buried mom's ashes the day after Thanksgiving, the connection was not as clear when I cried as I said, "She loved flowers." Maybe, because she loved flowers more than me until our last two months together?

I had cried with Megan that day because I was disappointed that she needed to leave before going to the cemetery with me as she had planned. She was the one in the family I was closest to, who understands and loves me. (tears now) She held me close, and said, "I love you," more than once.

Earlier that morning, when I was playing with five-month old Riley Shea, I said to her, "You need my cheek near yours," as tears rolled: how much I had needed that from my mother, and more from dad. Megan was watching me cry as I rocked Riley Shea in my arms, saying how beautiful she is, so loving. Megan understood and that meant all the Love to me.

Megan was showing me the "grace" that was not said on Thanksgiving for the first time in our family's history! Mom was not there to insist, and I was surprised that my "born-again" sister did not either. There were fifteen of us at Connie's, and I missed saying out loud what we were most thankful for, which I had initiated when Thanksgiving was at my home. It was the same loss I felt with Daddy, not saying my feelings out loud to him. That is what **really** hurts us deeply, holding our feelings inside.

Ultimately, we desire to feel the union of Oneness with ourselves, to be wholly Love. Therefore, it makes sense to me why monogamy is important to our EVOLution. In monogamy, I am the only ONE you can Love physically and emotionally in combination. It is a metaphor (maybe an act out) of the Oneness that we wish to feel about ourselves –

One Love for all of me. It is why polyamory feels threatening, because we are not secure in the Love of Self, connected to the Oneness of the Universe.

With monogamy, we are forced to stay with one person, not flee to affairs, facing our feelings triggered by committed partners. It is truly an opportunity to heal our broken (inadequately loved) hearts. As John Welwood states, "Love's sadness is the *fullness of feeling* that arises out of our longing to open and connect. Thus at the core of devotion to another is a sweet, sad fullness of heart, which longs to overflow."

"Thus when we appreciate our aloneness, we can be ourselves and give ourselves most fully, and we no longer need others to save us or make us feel good about ourselves. Instead, we want to help them become themselves more fully as well. In this way, conscious love is born as a gift from our broken heart." (pgs. 205-206, *Journey of the Heart*)

I look forward to the day, and it feels closer, when I will not feel the rift inside me. That resistance to change we all feel as humans. Yet, I so desire change! The ultimate contradiction of life!

Coming out of the darkness of pain, into the light of love, which is reflected in me self-loving the majority of the time in the mo(u)rning.☺ One November morning, I touched myself for maybe twenty minutes, the <u>light</u> touch which sends me over the edge into an extraordinary full-body orgasm. I hardly touched my vagina these days; my labia and clitoris sing my song while lying on my back until I must roll over, using my stuffed polar bear's firm nose to electrify my nipples. I felt vibrations throughout my tensed body, powerful in the pit of my peach. No man, just "Oh god, oh god" times four.

A contrast to my orgasm a couple of days later, when I couldn't fall asleep, very unusual these days, as many different people crossed my thoughts. It was not a very satisfying orgasm, one "Ohhhhhhhh god," annoyed to be awake at 3am. I wondered what feelings were trying to make an appearance.

After I went dancing with Brad, a local man I met through Match.com, he wrote in an email, "As our bodies moved together I found myself reaching inside to feel every motion of your body…I did yearn to kiss you and to silently speak by peering into one another's eyes until we connected in a spiritual sense."

We danced on our third date, after enjoying dinner together and several heart-felt conversations. He told me that I was the first woman that understood him, and was able to converse deeply. He had been dancing to Texas country music for several years, a very energetic fifty-eight-year-old smooth dancer of 6'2." We seemed to be a good match, but what he said to me while dancing a swing number I could not match. "I love you dear," was swirling around my ears and eyes as he raised my arms in a twirl. I had never been told, for the first time, "I love you" while I was in motion. E-motion while in motion!

I have noticed throughout my growing EVOLution, that I have been told those three spiritual words, "I love you," more often outside of the bedroom when said for the first time. Usually, I've experienced that it has been easier to let go of those three words while experiencing sexual lovemaking passion. As I've grieved, I've picked partners who more readily say it before becoming sexual. There has been a growing progression of wanting to be physical in stages, like courses of a fancy meal. Dessert doesn't have to include intercourse on first lovemaking.

As it takes time for my heart-spirit to know someone, I want my body to be known in stages as well. Growing together like a well-anchored root that develops into an organic, whole ripe fruit full of the flavor of Love. I want to "*fall* in love" and be *caught* by Openness and Honesty of the heart. Not hunted down for my vagina. **Orgasm** and **being "IN LOVE,"** where the inward heart weaves into the outward skin, are the two greatest open doors to our spirit's vitality! Both are essential to find Real Love. Holy Love. As Chopra writes, "If you are honest in your search for your own feelings, you will hit upon love, even if it is the tiniest spark of attraction and desire…**You want the return of spirit within you, which is the return of God…It was your birthright to be that passion**…the source of enthusiasm…Spirit is waiting for you to rejoin her…whose only desire is to protect you and carry you in her arms **from fear to love**." (pgs. 270,271 *The Path to Love*, parenthesis and emphasis mine)

Carefree like I was at my friends Motown concert, where I filled the whole room with laughter, wondering why I was hearing my Self above everyone during a hilarious rendition of the song, "Walk Like a Man."

Wondrous like my Self-loving one December mid afternoon, lying on my red sofa, where my legs rose off the cushions and my head curved forward, instead of back, like the curve of a slivered moon. I screamed loudly, "Oh god," then "Oh my god" six or seven times into a huge full-body orgasm, bursting into tears. From ecstasy to tears, thinking to myself that god's existence in me had been hindered until now. How can I tell you, lovely reader, that I felt god was/is a part of me, and the sadness, that ushers divineness to join loving bliss?

On the phone, Brad told me, "You are extremely emotional and sensitive," which he liked. It was the first kissing, touching, drawn out with deep meaning that was (k)NEW to him; intrinsically its own thing – never been so consumed by kissing. Later, he emailed on December 9, 2002, "I sense we are connected together by something bigger than either of us can comprehend. We are being swept into a magical world of spirituality. The ears of our intuitions and the bodies of our spirits are forging ahead relishing in all that is happening to them right now."

No longer was I in the "box" of religion, or in the "box," slang for vaginal sex – the birthing place to get out of the box of what others expect of Me. I am honest in my search to source my feelings, and I continue to find Love. My deepest feelings, my wee voice within me, is returning my Spirit, which is the return of "god."

Passionate feelings have carried me out of fear into Love. The journey of IN LOVE to REAL LOVE. It is your birthright to be that Passion. That Compassion.

A rose has arisen from the grave

of our shut-down hearts.

Tears have offered its bloom.

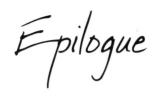

Oh god, I'm IN LOVE!

IF we truly follow our hearts, led by the IN LOVE feeling, traveling INward to the Great Spirit of REAL LOVE, there will be no prejudice, injustice, violence, anger, revenge. Only individual change can change the greater institutions of government, courts, education.

Therefore, my dream is that each of us will honor our god-given natural function of crying tears, that **tear** open our **heart**s so we can **hear** the hurt, grieving into healing compassion for all.

Just LOOK into the eyes of a baby, stay there, BE there, stay there. There, IS LOVE meant to Be. No fear, for perfectly possible love casts out **fear, dear** reader.

UNIVERSAL PRAYER

That which is called God by the Christians
Adonai by the Jews
Ultimate Reality by the Hindus
Buddhamind by the Buddhists
Allah by the Mohammedans
And which the Chinese call Tao,
That is the REAL SELF
And is all-pervading.
May we experience that!

This prayer has been displayed on a banner hanging in the Foundation of Light, Ithaca, New York, for more than twenty-five years. I'll add: The Great **Spirit**, by the Native Americans

"One's ability to grieve, is one's capacity to Love."
–*Dianea Kohl, Crybabe*

10 Steps to Access Healing Tears – your PEARLS of GOD

1   Notice your feelings! Focus on Feelings, not thoughts. I FEEL…sad, hurt, scared, alone, rejected, misunderstood, unheard, distrusted…

2   I feel like …I was hit by a Mac Truck is a thought, not a feeling.

3   When angry, ask what triggered it? (or triggered the sadness, hurt, or fear)

4   Write the feelings down, as well as the triggering event.

5   Close your eyes, ask yourself how this feeling feels familiar from your childhood – write down the memory (if you are crying, let yourself cry as much as needed first – same applies to anger/rage)

6   Give ROOM to FEEL…15 –45 minutes if you can. If angry: hit pillows, tear paper, go to your car and scream, throw pillows, stomp, etc.

7   Get support, such as re-evaluation counseling, or co-counseling or 12 step group

8   Let yourself feel tears: at movies, commercials, songs, looking at babies…☺

9   Find a picture of yourself as a small child, and put it up where you can't help but SEE it, LOOK into his or her eyes for at least a minute, then hold that picture close to your heart for at least a minute….daily!

10   Say out loud to that child's picture, "I love you," every day.

Notice what works best for you…and practice it as a spiritual practice of LOVE

Under Anxiety (**fear**) and Depression (**sadness, anger**) are these feelings!

Rage

Anger   Fear

Hurts:
unheard, misunderstood,
distrusted, shamed,
alone, helpless, hopeless

Rejection   Abandoned

Unloved

I feel confused is a step toward change. Uncertainty is good.
You are no longer in the box (of religion,)
but on your way to
retrieval of your "new born" Spirit,
where unconditional Love breathes.

Recommended Reading

1. Chopra, Deepak, *The Path to Love*. New York: Three Rivers Press, 1997.
2. Fox, Matthew, *Original Blessing*. Santa Fe: Bear and Publishing, 1983.
3. Freeman, Lucy, *Our Inner World of Rage*. New York: Continuum, 1990.
4. Hanh, Thich Nhat, *Peace Is Every Step*. New York: Bantam, 1991.
5. Hendrix, Harville, *Getting The Love You Want*. New York: Pocket Books, 1992.
6. Hesse, Hermann, *Siddhartha*. New York: Bantam, (1951), 1971.
7. Hillman, Anne, *The Dancing Animal Woman*. Connecticut: Bramble Books, 1994.
8. Janov, Arthur, *The New Primal Scream*. Wilmington,DE: Enterprise, 1991. *Why You Get Sick and How You Get Well*. Dove, 1996.
9. Klein, Marty, Emotional Cleansing. Bereley: Creative Arts Book Co., 2002.
10. Kornfield, Jack, *A Path With Heart*. New York: Bantam, 1993.
11. Lee, John, *The Flying Boy I, II, III*, and his other books.
12. Lerner, Harriet, *The Dance of Intimacy*. New York: Harper&Row, 1989. *The Dance of Anger*, 1988. *The Dance of Deception*, 1993.
13. Miller, Alice, *Drama of the Gifted Child*, revised edition, New York:Basic Books, 1994. *Thou Shalt Not Be Aware*, Meridian, 1990. *For Your Own Good*, 1984. (All her other books: an amazing evolution)
14. Montagu, Ashley, *The Natural Superiority of Women*. New York: Collier, 1992.
15. Moody, Raymond, *Reunions*. New York: Ivy Books, 1993.
16. Motz, Julie, *Hands of Life*. New York: Bantam, 1998.
17. Redfield, James, *The Celestine Prophesy*. New York: Warner, 1993.
18. Sheppard Alexander, Teresa, *Facing The Wolf*. New York: Dutton, 1996.
19. Solter, Aletha, *Tears and Tantrums*. California: Shining Star press, 1998.
20. Stettbacher, Konrad, *Making Sense of Suffering*. New York: Dutton, 1991.
21. Stone, Thomas A., *Cure By Crying*. Des Moines: Lightell Publishing, 1995.
22. Vissell, Barry & Joyce, *Risk To Be Healed*. Aptos, Ca.: Ramira Publishing, 1989.
23. Weiss, Brian, *Through Time Into Healing*. New York: Simon&Schuster, 1992. *Only Love Is Real*. New York: Warner, 1996.
24. Welwood, John, *Journey of the Heart*. New York: Harper, 1991.
25. Wisechild, Louise, *The Mother I Carry*. Seattle: Seal Press, 1993.
26. Woolger, Roger, *Other Lives, Other Selves*, New York: Bantam, 1988.

About the Author

Dianea has spent much of her life breaking down the myth, "Children are to be seen and not heard." After graduating from Cornell University's School of Nursing, she worked in various nursing arenas until she found her niche as a clinical nurse specialist on a psychiatric unit for five years. Since 1985, when she received her Master's Degree in Marriage and Family Therapy at Syracuse University, she has worked as a psychotherapist at Family and Children's Service and continues this work in private practice, in Ithaca, New York, where she was born and raised. For a year (96-97), she attended The Primal Center in Venice, California. Dianea's inspiration is greatly due to her deceased father, Michel's love, as well as from her two daughters, Erin and Megan. Her spirit is expressed most freely and joyously on the dance floor, and while hiking in the National Parks. She is a kid again.

Other books by Dianea:

TEARS ARE TRUTH…waiting to be spoken
Everybody Cries, children's picture book

Books in progress:
TEARS ARE TRUST…waiting to be felt
Everybody Laughs, children's picture book

Future book:
TEARS ARE TRUE LOVE…waiting be known

To order books:

Call 607-2776440, or write:

Chelan Publishing
4 Gray Road
Ithaca, New York 14850

Books can be ordered at any bookstore.

Dianea would like to hear from anyone willing to share their experience of crying at orgasm: what it means to you, what triggers the tears, and how you feel about the experience.

Email: dianeako@yahoo.com

www.lightlink.com/dianeal…
(expanded website soon)

If we do not allow:

Our skin to sweat......we overheat and die.

Our bladder or rectum to eliminate......we constipate, impact, and die.

Our genitals to orgasm......we become frigid, and smother joy.

Our muscles to exercise......we become immobile.

OUR TEARS to FLOW...we become anxious, depressed, unable to Really LOVE.

Oh God, please cry!

Oh God...
Please ask your Self:

Why is it that our bodies are made to cry?

TEARS are our body's NATURAL function for healing physical, emotional-spiritual pain.